61 N02851 AR

MFT Library Services
North Manchester

WITHDRAWN FROM STOCK
Servi...

D1433813

NORTH MANCHESTER
GENERAL HOSPITAL
JOINT EDUCATION LIBRARY
1 - FEB 2006

THE HIP
Second Edition

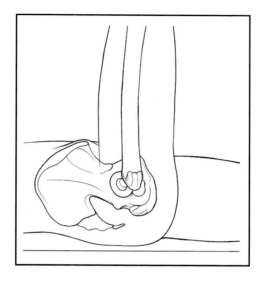

Editors

ROBERT L. BARRACK, M.D.
Charles and Joanne Knight Distinguished
Professor of Orthopaedic Surgery
Washington University School of Medicine
St. Louis, Missouri

AARON G. ROSENBERG, M.D.
Midwest Orthopaedics
Chicago, Illinois

Illustrators

Jennifer E. Fairman, CMI
Hugh Thomas

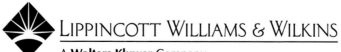

LIPPINCOTT WILLIAMS & WILKINS
A **Wolters Kluwer** Company

Philadelphia • Baltimore • New York • London
Buenos Aires • Hong Kong • Sydney • Tokyo

Acquisitions Editor: Robert Hurley
Developmental Editor: Grace R. Caputo, Dovetail Content Solutions
Managing Editor: Michelle M. LaPlante
Manufacturing Manager: Ben Rivera
Marketing Director: Sharon Zinner
Project Manager: Fran Gunning
Production Services: Maryland Composition
Printer: Quebecor World-Kingsport

© 2006 by Lippincott Williams & Wilkins
© 1998 by Lippincott-Raven Publishers

530 Walnut Street
Philadelphia, PA 19106

www.LWW.com

All rights reserved. This book is protected by copyright. No part of this book may be reproduced in any form or by any means, including photocopying, or utilizing by any information storage and retrieval system without written permission from the copyright owner.

The publisher is not responsible (as a matter of product liability, negligence or otherwise) for an injury resulting from any material contained herein. This publication contains information relating to general principles of medical care which should not be constructed as specific instruction for individual patients. Manufacturer's product information should be reviewed for current information, including contraindications, dosages, and precautions.

Printed in the United States

Library of Congress Cataloging-in-Publication Data
The hip / editor, Robert L. Barrack ; illustrators, Jennifer Fairman,
  Hugh Thomas — 2nd ed.
        p. ; cm. — (Master techniques in orthopaedic surgery)
     Includes bibliographical references and index.
     ISBN 0-7817-4634-5 (alk. paper)
     1. Hip—Surgery. I. Barrack, Robert L. II. Series: Master
techniques in orthopaedic surgery (2nd ed.)
        [DNLM: 1. Hip—surgery. 2. Hip Joint—surgery. 3. Hip Fractures—surgery.
4. Hip Prosthesis. 5. Orthopedic Procedures—methods. WE 855 H66715 2005]
RD549.H49 2005
617.5'81059—dc22

The publishers have made every effort to trace copyright holders for borrowed material. If they have inadvertently overlooked any, they will be pleased tomake the necessary arrangements at the first opportunity.

To purchase additional copies of this book, call our customer service department at (800) 638-3030 or fax orders to (301) 223-2320. For other book services, including chapter reprints and large quantity sales, ask for the Special Sales department.

For all other calls originating outside of the United States, please call (301) 223-2300.

Visit Lippincott Williams & Wilkins on the Internet: http://www.lww.com. Lippincott Williams & Wilkins customer srrvice representatives are available from 8:30 am to 6:30 pm, EST, Monday through Friday, for telephone access.

10 9 8 7 6 5 4 3 2 1

To my beautiful wife, Terri, and wonderful sons, Adam and Toby, for their love, support, and understanding, and to the memory of my brother, Michael.

RLB

■

TABLE OF CONTENTS

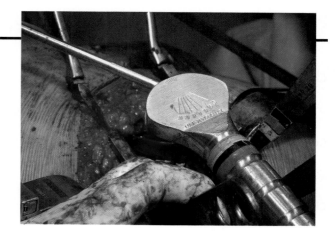

PART I   PREREQUISITE TO SURGERY

PART II   SURGICAL APPROACHES

PART III   NONARTHROPLASTY APPROACHES

PART IV   SURGERY FOR AVASCULAR NECROSIS

PART V   PRIMARY TOTAL HIP ARTHROPLASTY

SECTION A   THE STEM

SECTION B   ACETABULAR REVISION

PART VII   SPECIAL TECHNIQUES

CONTRIBUTORS

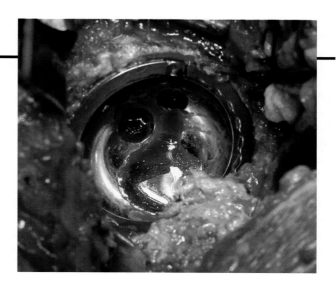

John Antonaides, M.D.
*Joint Replacement Institute,
Orthopaedic Hospital, Los Angeles,
California*

Michael J. Archibeck, M.D.
*New Mexico Center for Joint Replacement,
New Mexico Orthopaedics,
Albequerque, New Mexico*

Mark Barba
*Department of Orthopedics,
OSF Saint Anthony Medical Center, Rockford
Orthopedic Associates, Rockford, Illinois*

Robert L. Barrack, M.D.
*The Charles F. and Joanne Knight Distinguished Professor
of Orthopaedic Surgery, Department of Orthopaedic Surgery,
Washington University School of Medicine; Chief of Staff for
Orthopaedic Surgery, Director of Adult Reconstructive
Surgery, Barnes-Jewish Hospital, St. Louis, Missouri*

Christopher P. Beauchamp
*Orthopaedic Department, Mayo Clinic,
Scottsdale, Arizona*

Richard A. Berger, M.D.
*Assistant Professor of Orthopaedics,
Rush University Medical Center,
Chicago, Illinois*

Daniel J. Berry, M.D.
*Professor of Orthopaedics, Mayo Clinic College of Medicine;
Chair, Department of Orthopaedic Surgery, Mayo Clinic,
Rochester, Minnesota*

Hari P. Bezwada, M.D.
*Assitant Clinical Professor of Orthopaedic Surgery,
University of Pennsylvania School of Medicine, PENN
Orthopaedics, Pennsylvania Hospital, Philadelphia,
Pennsylvania*

Dennis W. Burke, M.D.
*Clinical Instructor, Harvard Medical School,
Boston, Massachusetts*

R. Stephen J. Burnett, M.D.
*Department of Orthopaedic Surgery, Washington University
in St. Louis, Barnes-Jewish Hospital, Barnes-Jewish West
County Hospital, St. Louis VA Medical Center,
St. Louis, Missouri*

John J. Callaghan, M.D.
*The Lawrence and Marilyn Dorr Chair and Professor,
University of Iowa Health Care, Iowa City, Iowa*

John Charity, M.D.
*Orthopaedic Fellow (Hip Unit), Princess Elizabeth
Orthopaedic Centre, Royal Devon and Exeter Hospital,
Exeter, UK*

John C. Clohisy, M.D.
*Associate Professor of Orthopaedic Surgery, Co-Chief, Adult
Reconstructive Surgery, Barnes-Jewish Hospital, Washington
University School of Medicine, St. Louis, Missouri*

Finnbar Condon, F.R.C.S., MCh
*Consultant Orthopaedic Surgeon,
Regional Othopaedic Hospital, Croom,
County Limerick, Ireland*

Alejandro González Della Valle, M.D.
*Assistant Professor of Orthopaedic Surgery, Weill Cornell
Medical College, Hospital for Special Surgery, New York,
New York*

Craig J. Della Valle, M.D.
*Assistant Professor, Department of Orthopaedic Surgery,
Rush University Medical Center, Chicago, Illinois*

Clive P. Duncan, M.B., F.A.C.S.
*Professor and Chairman, Department of Orthopaedic
Surgery; Head, Department of Orthopaedics, University of
British Columbia, Vancouver Hospital and Health Sciences
Center, Vancouver, British Columbia, Canada*

Donald S. Garbuz, M.D., M.H.s
*Assistant Professor, Division of Lower Limb Reconstruction
and Oncology, Department of Orthopaedics, University of
British Columbia, Vancouver, British Columbia, Canada*

Graham A. Gie, M.B.Ch.B., F.R.C.S.Ed
Hip Unit, Princess Elizabeth Orthopaedic Centre,
Royal Devon and Exeter Hospital, Exeter, United Kingdom

Andrew Glassman, M.D., M.S.
Associate Professor of Orthopaedic Surgery, Department of
Orthopaedic Surgery, Ohio State University College of
Medicine; Director, Total Joint Replacement Service, Ohio
State University Medical Center; Staff Surgeon, The
Halley-Glassman Orthopaedic Clinic, Columbus, Ohio

Allan E. Gross, M.D., F.R.C.S.C.
Orthopaedic Surgeon, Division of Orthopaedic Surgery,
Department of Surgery, Bernard I. Ghert Family Foundation;
Chair, Lower Extremity Reconstructive Surgery, Mount Sinai
Hospital, Professor of Surgery, Faculty of Medicine,
University of Toronto, Toronto, Ontario, Canada

Arlen D. Hanssen, M.D.
Professor, Department of Orthopedic Surgery, Mayo Medical
School; Consultant, Department of Orthopaedic Surgery,
Mayo Clinic, Rochester, Minnesota

Sanaz Hariri, M.D.
Resident, Harvard Combined Orthopedic Surgery Program,
Boston, Massachusetts

Donald W. Howie, M.B.B.S, Ph.D., F.R.A.C.S.
Professor and Head, Department of Orthopaedics and
Trauma, University of Adelaide; Clinical Director,
Orthopaedic and Trauma Service, Royal Adelaide Hospital,
Adelaide, South Australia, Australia

Waqqar Khan-Farooqi, M.D.
Chief Resident, Department of Orthopaedics and Sports
Medicine, University of Washington, Seattle, Washington

Anthony D. Lamberton, MBChB, F.R.A.C.S. (Orth)
Orthopaedic Surgeon, Tauranga Hospital, Tauranga,
New Zealand

Jo-ann Lee, MS
Nurse Practitioner, New England Baptist Hospital,
Boston, Massachusetts

Seth S. Leopold, M.D.
Associate Professor, Department of Orthopaedics and Sports
Medicine, University of Washington School of Medicine,
Seattle, Washington

David G. Lewallen, M.D.
Professor, Department of Orthopedic Surgery, Mayo Medical
School; Consultant, Department of Orthopaedic Surgery,
Mayo Clinic, Rochester, Minnesota

Steve S. Liu, M.D.
University of Iowa Health Care, Iowa City, Iowa

Andrew D. MacDowell, M.D.
Arthroplasty Fellow, Department of Orthopaedics and
Trauma, Royal Adelaide Hospital and University of
Adelaide, Adelaide, South Australia, Australia

David W. Manning, M.D.
Assistant Professor, Division of Orthopaedic Surgery,
Department of Surgery, University of Chicago,
Chicago, Illinois

Bassam A. Masri, M.D.
Associate Professor and Head, Division of Lower Limb
Reconstruction and Oncology, Department of Orthopaedics,
University of British Columbia, Vancouver,
British Columbia, Canada

David Mattingly, M.D.
Associate Clinical Professor of Orthopaedic Surgery,
Tufts University School of Medicine; Department of
Orthopaedic Surgery, New England Baptist Hospital,
Boston, Massachusetts

Joseph C. McCarthy, M.D.
Clinical Professor of Orthopaedic Surgery, Tufts University,
New England Baptist Hospital, Boston, Massachusetts

Robert W. McGraw, M.D.
Vancouver Hospital HSC,
Vancouver, British Columbia, Canada

R. Michael Meneghini, M.D.
St. Vincent Center for Joint Replacement, St. Vincent
Hospital, Indianapolis, Indiana

Michael A. Mont, M.D.
Sinai Hospital of Baltimore,
Baltimore, Maryland

Maurice E. Müeller
Lindenhof Hospital
Bern, Switzerland

Shawn J. Nakamura, M.D.
Orthopaedic Surgeon, Austin Medical Center,
Mayo Health System, Austin, Minnesota

Michael R. O'Rourke, M.D.
Assistant Professor, Department of Orthopaedics and
Rehabilitation, University of Iowa Hospitals and Clinics,
Iowa City, Iowa

Douglas E. Padgett, M.D.
Associate Professor of Orthopaedic Surgery, Weill
Cornell Medical College, Hospital for Special Surgery,
New York, New York

Wayne G. Paprosky, M.D.
Associate Professor, Rush Medical College,
Rush-Presbyterian-St. Luke's Medical Center,
Chicago, Illinois; Staff Orthopaedic Surgeon
Department of Adult Reconstructive Surgery
Central DuPage Hospital, Winfield, Illinois

Javad Parvizi, M.D., F.R.C.S
Associate Professor, Department of Orthopaedic Surgery,
Rothman Institute, Thomas Jefferson University,
Philadelphia, Pennsylvania

Paul J. P. Pongor, M.D.
Instructor in Surgery, Director of Orthopaedic Registry,
Department of Surgery, Beth Israel Deaconess Hospital,
New England Baptist Hospital, Boston, Massachusetts

Phillip S. Ragland, M.D.
Center for Joint Preservation and Reconstruction,
Rubin Institute for Advanced Orthopaedics,
Sinai Hospital of Baltimore, Baltimore, Maryland

Amar S. Ranawat, M.D.
Attending Orthopaedic Surgeon, Department of Orthopaedic
Surgery, Lenox Hill Hospital, New York, New York

Chitranjan S. Ranawat, M.D.
The James A. Nicholas Chairman, Department of
Orthopaedic Surgery, Lenox Hill Hospital,
New York, New York

Aaron G. Rosenberg, M.D.
Midwest Orthopaedics
Chicago, Illinois

Harry E. Rubash, M.D.
Chief of Orthopaedic Surgery, Massachusetts General
Hospital; Edith M. Ashley Professor, Harvard Medical
School, Boston, Massachusetts

Richard F. Santore, M.D.
Clinical Professor of Orthopaedic Surgery, University of
California, San Diego; Senior Orthopaedic Surgeon, Sharp
Memorial Hospital, San Diego, California

Thomas P. Schmalzried, M.D.
Associate Medical Director, Joint Replacement Institute,
Los Angeles, California; Chief of Joint Replacement,
Harbor-UCLA Medical Center, Torrance, California

Peter F. Sharkey, M.D.
Professor, Department of Orthopaedic Surgery,
Rothman Institute, Thomas Jefferson University Hospital,
Philadelphia, Pennsylvania

Craig D. Silverton, D.O., Lt Col, U.S.A.F. Reserves
Chief, Adult Reconstruction, Department of Orthopaedics
Henry Ford Hospital, Detroit, Michigan; Wilford Hall
Medical Center (USAF), Lackland AFB, Texas

Franklin H. Sim, M.D.
Department of Orthopedic Surgery, Mayo Clinic College of
Medicine, Rochester, Minnesota

Scott Sporer, M.D.
Rush University, Chicago, Illinois;
Central DuPage Hospital, Winfield, Illinois

Craig M. Thomas, M.D.
Center for Joint Preservation and Reconstruction,
Rubin Institute for Advanced Orthopaedics,
Sinai Hospital of Baltimore, Baltimore, Maryland

Andrew John Timperley, M.B., ChB, F.R.C.S. Ed
Hip Unit, Princess Elizabeth Orthopaedic Centre, Royal
Devon and Exeter Hospital, Exeter, United Kingdom

Robert T. Trousdale, M.D.
Professor of Orthopaedics, Mayo Graduate School of
Medicine, Rochester, Minnesota

Thomas R. Turgeon, M.D.
Assistant Professor, Department of Surgery, University of
Manitoba, Concordia Hospital, Winnipeg, Manitoba, Canada

David A. Vittetoe, M.D.
Des Moines Orthopaedic Surgeons, West Des Moines, Iowa

Frazer E. Wade, F.R.C.S.(Ed), F.R.C.S.(Tr&Orth)
Consultant Orthopaedic Surgeon, Royal Infirmary of
Edinburgh, Edinburgh, United Kingdom

Lucian C. Warth, M.D.
University of Iowa Health Care, Iowa City, Iowa

Richard E. White, Jr., M.D.
Medical Director, New Mexico Center for Joint
Replacement Surgery, New Mexico Orthopaedics,
Albuquerque, New Mexico

SERIES PREFACE

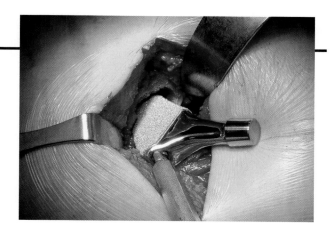

Since its inception in 1994, the *Master Techniques in Orthopaedic Surgery* Series has become a well-accepted "must" for surgeons in training and in practice. The user-friendly style of providing and illustrating authoritative information on a broad spectrum of orthopaedic techniques has filled a void in orthopaedic education materials. The exceptional success of the series may be traced to the leadership of the original series editor, Roby Thompson, whose clarity of thought and focused vision sought "to provide direct, detailed access to techniques preferred by orthopaedic surgeons who are recognized by their colleagues as 'masters' in their specialty" (Series preface, Volume I). The essential elements of success are clear. In addition to the careful selection of the *Master* volume editor, the format of the presented material has almost become classic. I am personally rewarded by numerous comments by both residents and practicing orthopaedic surgeons regarding the value of these volumes to their training or in their practice. The format has become a standard against which others are to be compared, "A standardized presentation of information replete with tips and pearls through years of experience with abundant color photographs and drawings to guide you step by step through the procedures" (Series preface, Volume II).

Eight second edition volumes are currently in print, and two more are in preparation. Building on the success of the current ten-volume series, we are in the process of expanding the texts to include an even broader range of relevant orthopaedic topics. New volumes will appear on surgical exposures as well as peripheral nerve surgery. Other topics are being actively explored with an expectation that the series will expand to 15 titles over the next several years.

I am honored to be assuming the responsibility of the series editor. The true worth of this endeavor will be measured by the ongoing and ever-increasing success and critical acceptance of the series. I am indebted to Dr. Thompson for his inaugural vision and leadership, as well as to the *Master* volume editors and to the numerous contributors who have been true to the style and to the vision. Ultimately, as is stated by the Mayo brothers, "The best interest of the patient is the only interest to be considered." It is hoped that the information in the *Master* Series equips the surgeon to realize this patient-centric view of our surgical practice.

Bernard F. Morrey, M.D.
Series Editor

PREFACE

The first edition of *The Hip* was published in 1998. Since that time, the number of total joint procedures performed annually has approximately doubled, and all data indicate that this rapid rate of growth will continue for the foreseeable future. There has been a dramatic increase in technology and surgical techniques in hip surgery that has occurred at the same time. This is reflected in the substantial expansion in length and breath of the second edition of this volume. This now includes 33 chapters compared with 17 in the original edition, with contributions from 54 new authors. Some new chapters focus heavily on new techniques, such as minimal incision surgery, hip arthroscopy, and surgical approaches for avascular necrosis, including hip resurfacing. Other chapters focus on applications of specific implants, such as the megaprosthesis, total femoral placement, acetabular cages, and the PROSTALAC technique for infection. The use of cementless femoral stems has increased in popularity, particularly in North America, and this is reflected in the four chapters devoted to the nuances of surgical technique of different types of cementless stems compared with the single chapter in the earlier edition. Another recent trend in medicine, which has equal relevance to hip surgery, is the use of more analytical systematic techniques of interpreting medical data. For this reason a chapter has been added on evidence-based surgery as well as a section on surgical decision making. Because of the proliferation in the number of

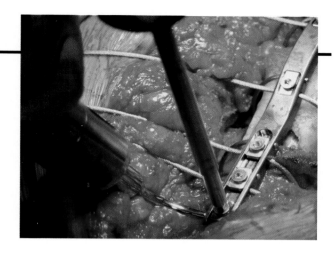

implants and techniques available, planning prior to entering the operating room assumes more importance. Therefore, two extensive chapters on preoperative planning—both for the primary and the revision hip arthroplasty—have also been added. Even with the growth of the new edition, the original theme of the volume remains the same, which is to provide a well-illustrated, step-by-step guide to reflect the current state of the art in hip surgery. It is hoped *The Hip* will serve as a guide to assist orthopaedic surgeons in understanding and adapting new techniques with greater efficiency and safety.

Robert L. Barrack, M.D.

Prerequisite to Surgery

PART I

Prerequisite to Surgery

1

Evidence-based Orthopaedics

Waqqar Khan-Farooqi and Seth S. Leopold

"The failure of most surgeons to stick to one type of operation, or to one surgical exposure. . . implies underlying discontent."
—Sir John Charnley, *Low Friction Arthroplasty of the Hip: Theory and Practice,* 1979

Despite extraordinary knowledge increases since Charnley's landmark work, areas of controversy in adult hip surgery—including indications, surgical approaches, and implant selection—populate the intellectual landscape as fully as topics on which consensus has been reached. Whether in fact this is a function of "underlying discontent," a lack of high-quality evidence on which to base clinical decisions, or divergent interpretation of available data, is not so important. Finding the best available evidence with which to perform clinical decision-making and interpreting that evidence thoughtfully, on the other hand, is critical. The related enterprise of deciding whether published results apply to one's own practice—and if not, why not—is as essential. Taken together, the steps of finding, interpreting, and applying the highest-quality research to the care of patients form the core of the evidence-based medicine (EBM) paradigm; EBM has been popular in general internal medicine for decades (1,2), but one would have a difficult time identifying an orthopaedic reference on the topic before the late 1990s.

Orthopaedists frequently dismiss EBM as not relevant to the "art" or practice of surgery. There is a perceived absence of unbiased evidence in orthopaedics to guide patient evaluation and treatment decision-making; industry influences and psychological factors undoubtedly impact surgeon-developers, and there may be systematic bias against the publication of "negative" results (3). Problems with study quality are also brought up as "evidence" against evidence-based orthopaedics. Randomization is uncommon, and some have gone so far as to say unethical; in any case only about 3% of orthopaedic trials randomized patients or study subjects (3). Practical surgeons say that we simply do not have the liberty to wait, paralyzed by indecision, for first-order evidence to answer every important clinical question—there are patients in the waiting room *now.* As a result of these factors and others, surgeons rely on their own or experts' anecdotal experiences to guide practice; experienced practitioners often take an empirical ("it works for me") approach, which indeed can be hard to dispute. However, several insidious influences, including recall, transfer, and selection bias, potentially diminish the validity of this experiential "evidence" and falsely elevate practitioners' confidence in long- and dearly held approaches. Patients who fail to follow up with their surgeons, on average, score worse on standardized outcomes instruments and are more likely to have failed treatment than patients who follow up regularly (4,5); since the surgeon only sees those people who report for follow-up, this impact, called transfer bias, is only one influence that may inappropriately reassure well-intentioned providers who depend excessively on their own observations to assess their own outcomes.

When considering indications to perform adult hip surgery—indeed any surgery—the key question becomes not "which approach is better," but "how can I use a reasonable balance of evidence-based orthopaedics and my own clinical experience to care for my patients most effectively?" So rather than summarizing the senior author's approach to surgical indications in the adult hip, this chapter reviews available means to identifying the best-quality evidence and resources that help busy providers identify the "pearls" from those sources and apply them in practice.

EVIDENCE-BASED ORTHOPAEDICS: THE KEY STEPS

With the goal of minimizing the effects of bias and lower-quality studies on the practice of orthopaedic surgery, surgeons have begun to discover the EBM paradigm and begun the evolution of evidence-based orthopaedics. The principles of EBM have been articulated (in both print and online formats) by a variety of sources including a group at McMaster University in Canada (6,7) and the Cochrane Collaboration (8), among others; more recently, *The Journal of Bone and Joint Surgery* (*JBJS*) has made preliminary offerings in the area of evidence-based orthopaedics (9,10). While those sources differ in numerous details, they all follow a similar general approach to clinical decision-making, and that approach involves four key steps:

1. Ask an answerable question.
2. Perform searches that yield relevant sources.
3. Evaluate the evidence.
4. Apply the results to an individual patient.

Asking a good question is deceptively difficult. We often seek to ask the "big" question and are discouraged when it is not answerable as phrased. But frequently, nested within the key "unanswerable" question there often are several important (and eminently answerable) subqueries, which, when addressed in sequence, will result in the desired moment of clarity. Once the surgeon articulates the key question, (s)he needs to search the source or sources most likely to yield relevant results; once, this might have been simply the index of a multivolume textbook of orthopaedic surgery. Perhaps sometime later, this might have been the CD-ROM containing the last 10 years' worth of a review journal. However, today, this step can be so daunting as to halt the process itself; depending on the question, this process might include Medline, the Cochrane Collaboration, Clinical Evidence, Orthopaedics Web Links, journal Web sites, textbooks, and/or an Internet search engine. Search results then are culled to return a list of the most relevant sources to the question at hand.

With relevant sources in hand, surgeons should consider employing now-standardized techniques (4,7,10–18) to analyze the quality of the recommendations, identify any particularly strong sources of bias in the articles reviewed, and estimate what impact those biases may have on the result. Once study quality has been assayed, the surgeon should view the evidence in light of his/her own practice and clinical experience; discrepancies between individuals' observations and published findings occur frequently, but those discrepancies should provoke further inquiry. Some studies that are extremely well conducted (studies with good "internal validity") may have no impact on our own practices because of obvious surgeon-dependent factors, lack of access to necessary equipment, or irreconcilable differences between the patient population studied and our own. Those studies have little "external validity" with respect to our search and need to be viewed cautiously. Finally, the thoughtful surgeon will consider his/her findings in light of individual patient factors, including values, functional goals, and fears or concerns; often, the patient's own personal outlook contributes heavily to the decision-making.

ASK AN ANSWERABLE QUESTION

When a patient presents to a surgeon, (s)he generally arrives seeking advice in managing a problem. In clinical medicine, difficult or ambiguous cases will provoke questions of diagnosis, prognosis, treatment, and/or efficient use of medical resources (costs of care); in adult hip surgery, the most common questions arise over treatment decisions—whether surgical indications or choosing from an array of surgical options once it is clear that surgery is desired—but other types of questions also arise. The key skill at this phase of the EBM process is posing an "answerable" question, which will drive the search process.

With respect to the adult hip, surgery is most commonly indicated to alleviate pain; in most cases, functional improvements follow pain relief but are secondary drivers of the decision process. Accordingly, the choice to proceed with surgery usually is a "quality of life" decision that the patient needs to make, using appropriate educational input from the surgeon to help weigh risk and benefit and to be sure that all reasonable nonsurgical options have been considered. However, there are several common conditions in the adult hip where surgery is a reasonable—and sometimes the optimal—choice even in the absence of activity-limiting pain. Tumors, early presentations of osteonecrosis of the femoral head, developmental dysplasia of the hip in its prearthritic stages, periprosthetic osteolysis following total hip arthroplasty, and other conditions all may mandate surgery in certain scenarios even if the patient is asymptomatic or relatively so. However, the choice of when to operate on patients with those diagnoses or others, which procedures to consider, and how best to perform them should not be the topic of a book chapter that may be outdated by the time it is printed. Rather, using the principles of EBM, surgeons will be able to make good choices about those problems with the best-quality and most current data available at the time the patient presents to the office.

The first and most important step in EBM is to pose a succinct clinical question. This question should be pertinent to the care of a particular patient and should be formulated so as to guide a search of specific, relevant literature. When devised to answer a question about a given therapy, it should seek to compare the results of the proposed treatment with the known alternatives for the presenting problem of that particular patient. It is useful to consider four elements in the preparation of the clinical question: patient or problem, intervention, comparison intervention, and outcomes (6,7). Use of this basic format to generate a clinical query helps guide the seeker through a precise search of the literature.

SEARCH AND LOCATE RELEVANT EVIDENCE

Once a clinical question has been formulated, the surgeon then should seek current evidence from the peer-reviewed literature to guide action. There are several ways to access the relevant literature. With the large and ever-expanding roster of biomedical journals and databases, a description of every resource to the literature is beyond the scope of this chapter. Rather, we have provided examples of the most commonly used resources for searching the available literature.

PubMed is currently the most popular engine for the primary search of journal articles. It provides access to Medline, a bibliographic database including over 12 million citations from 4,600 international biomedical journals, over 100 of which are of orthopaedic focus. PubMed provides links to full-text articles from selected journals, and many biomedical libraries provide such access to even more publications. Tutorials on how to use the PubMed database are provided at the Web site. Through PubMed, the surgeon can perform an exhaustive literature search dating back to the 1960s.

The large number of orthopaedic journals makes staying current through subscriptions essentially impossible for the busy clinician, and even a specific PubMed search can yield an unwieldy number of journal articles, only a fraction of which are truly relevant, and even fewer of which are of sufficient quality to guide clinical practice. Fortunately, several resources exist that systematically evaluate and summarize the available evidence for a given topic. Familiarity with how to access and use these sites can be very helpful in the search process.

Perhaps the most popular resource for systematic analysis of the literature is the Cochrane Library. Updated quarterly, this library is available in full-text form via subscription; extremely informative abstracts of Cochrane reviews are available for free online. The Cochrane Collaboration offers access to these resources in a convenient, searchable manner. This group of investigators systematically reviews the available evidence of various medical and surgical treatments. The list of reviews is not exhaustive, but it is surprisingly rich; although musculoskeletal issues are currently somewhat heavy in rheumatologic focus, "bread-and-butter" orthopaedic surgical topics are well covered. In addition, several relevant reviews are underway or proposed, and each quarter this resource becomes more helpful to the practicing surgeon.

Clinical Evidence provides another useful resource for systematic evaluation of available literature. Updated monthly by the *British Medical Journal*, Clinical Evidence is designed along the format of EBM, providing an assessment of the literature relevant to specific clinical questions. By starting with a question, publishers of Clinical Evidence also inform the investigator when sufficiently good evidence does not exist to address common clinical problems.

The American College of Physicians (ACP) Journal Club, a journal of evidence-based medicine, is designed, in the words of the journal club founders, "to select from the biomedical literature those articles reporting original studies and systematic reviews that warrant immediate attention by physicians attempting to keep pace with important advances in internal medicine" (19). While it focuses on internal medicine, a search of the term *arthroplasty* in September 2003 resulted in 44 reviews returned, and "hip" yielded 143 orthopaedic reviews and summaries on common and important topics. Like Clinical Evidence, the ACP journal club performs a critical review of the literature, saving the investigator time and assisting in assessment of the quality of the search results.

The National Institutes of Health provides a registry of unpublished, ongoing clinical trials. This registry provides information on the goals and conductors of the trial. Creators of these trials are often thought leaders within the field and can provide another source of review of the relevant literature. The existence of a prospective registry of ongoing clinical trials is considered an essential element in controlling the problem of positive-outcome (publication) bias in the published literature, which, when not corrected for, risks causing overestimation of treatment effects in systematic reviews (meta-analyses) of published reports (3).

EVALUATE THE EVIDENCE

After the search is performed, the surgeon needs to cut through the volumes of anecdotal reports and case series in order to identify the highest-quality information on which care should be based. "Information" and "evidence" are not the same; *The Journal of the American Medical Association* (*JAMA*) has published guidelines to help the surgeon separate the two (14–16,18,20,21). Known as the *JAMA* Users' Guides, they help the reader to assess the quality and applicability of a given research study. These can be found in their original form in *JAMA*. The Users' Guides have also been summarized by several groups, including by the Centre for Health Evidence (CHE) in Canada. In similar fashion, Bhandari, Swiontkowski, Guyatt, and others have published articles in *JBJS* guiding the use and evaluation of orthopaedic literature (11–13,17,22), which are reminiscent of the *JAMA* Users' Guides but may be more directly applicable to orthopaedic searches.

While a central tenet of EBM is that the highest-quality evidence should be used to address the clinical question at hand, it is a practical exercise that helps surgeons to analyze the adequacy of available information—whether in the form of randomized, controlled trials (RCTs) or lower levels of evidence. Many surgical topics are not (and will not ever be) addressed by adequately powered RCTs. EBM is a paradigm that guides surgeons not only to utilize the best available evidence but also to be cognizant that the strength of the available literature should affect our level of confidence in our recommendations. It coaches us to be sensitive to the possibility that lower-quality studies may be tainted by bias so severe that the conclusions may in fact be the opposite of what was previously perceived and that this may not be discovered until adequately designed studies address topics that were earlier thought to be beyond the reach of research of that quality and scope—as has happened recently with arthroscopy for the degenerative knee and hormone-replacement therapy in postmenopausal women (23,24). The central goal is the thoughtful analysis and application of current evidence in terms of its relevance to care of the individual patient; the CHE states, as part of its mission, to "know what to do, do what is known, and understand what is done" by having providers "assess problems, ask questions, and acquire, appraise, and apply knowledge" (6).

JAMA's series of Users' Guides, now expanded and summarized by the CHE online, classifies 25 common types of journal articles. However, the vast majority of orthopaedic literature falls into only four of those types: articles about therapy, articles about diagnostic tests, articles about prognosis (natural history), and systematic reviews (meta-analyses). According to the guidelines, the reader should seek to answer three basic questions regardless of the article type:

1. Internal validity: Will the study methods yield believable results?
2. Results: What are the results of the study?
3. Applicability (sometimes called external validity): Will the results help me in caring for my patients?

However, the study's design—therapy, diagnostic test, prognosis, or meta-analysis—mandates the use of specific criteria in order to answer those three important questions. Tables 1–4 outline the Users' Guides' recommended approaches for each of those study types.

Critical Appraisal of Published Literature

The Users' Guides' articles are worth reviewing for each of the four common types of orthopaedic clinical research; it is possible to obtain them in their original form in *JAMA* (14–16,18,20,21). They also have been posted online by CHE (22) and presented with orthopaedic examples in *JBJS* (11–13,17,22). To gain efficiency in one's own reading, it is reasonable to employ the following two-step approach (7):

1. Read the title and (if necessary) the abstract section, and ask, "If the results offered were true, would they be interesting to me?" Do not try to determine at this stage if they are true—often that can be difficult after reading the entire article—just try to decide if everything the authors suggest is correct, whether it would have an impact on your practice. If the answer is "no," skip the article; if "yes," read on.
2. Scan the methods section briefly, use the EBM criteria for the particular article type (Tables 1–4), and ascertain whether the major criteria for that type of article are met. If the basic methodological elements for that type of article—for example, adequate follow-up and outcomes assessment for an article about therapy—are not met, the likelihood of that study concluding with results that are reasonably free from bias is so low that it is reasonable to skip the article.

Simply applying those two questions to each potentially interesting article will dramatically reduce the size of the pile of journals on the nightstand, and use of the EBM criteria in greater detail will increase the yield from those articles that are worth reading. The most important criteria for each of the common types of orthopaedic articles are summarized here.

The key elements of an article about therapy are the method of allocation to treatment groups (and use of control groups), the length and completeness of follow-up, and the methods used to assess the outcomes of treatment, including blinding, independent assessment, and validated outcomes instruments (see Table 1). In essence, the analysis of an article about therapy should determine whether the methods used have a reasonable likelihood of identifying true effects of treatment, the magnitude of any treatment effect and how potential biases might have impacted that treatment effect, and the applicability of the study's results to the reader's patients. Unlike studies in internal medicine, where treatment endpoints are more often readily quantifiable (mortality, blood pressure, rate of deep vein thrombosis),

Table 1. *How to Assess an Article about Therapy*

Question

Internal Validity
1. Were the patients similar at the start of the trial, and was their assignment to study groups randomized?
2. Is there an appropriate control group?
3. How long and complete is the follow-up?
4. Are the study personnel blinded to patient allocation?

Results
1. What were the results?
2. Is the outcome measure valid?
3. What is the statistical probability that the results are real?

Generalizability
1. Are the study patients similar to mine?
2. Is the technology employed in the study available to my practice today?
3. What is the cost of performing the studied treatment in my practice?
4. Are the results worth the costs?

From Centre for Health Evidence Web site; available at: http://www.cche.net/; accessed July 15, 2005; Guyatt GH, Sackett DL, Cook DJ. Users' guides to the medical literature. II. how to use an article about therapy or prevention. B. what were the results and will they help me in caring for my patients? Evidence-Based Medicine Working Group. *JAMA* 271:59–63, 1994; Sackett DL, Straus SE, Richardson WS, et al. *Evidence-based Medicine: How to Practice and Teach EBM*. New York: Churchill Livingstone; 2003.

outcome measures in orthopaedic surgery can be difficult to standardize and somewhat subjective. There is a general movement toward using validated outcomes tools, such as functional scoring systems and quality of life assessment tools. However, the fact that, for example, all articles comparing hip prosthesis designs do not use the same (or even similar) outcomes instruments renders comparisons among studies challenging (25). The reader must therefore pay close attention to the treatment results within each study evaluated and assess whether these results would be important to the reader's own patients and whether the costs or risks of the treatment would be worth the potential benefits.

An internally valid article about a diagnostic test (see Table 2) will apply the test in question to a cohort of patients that is likely to include a representative spectrum of disease incidence and/or severity, will compare the test to an accepted gold standard, and will not let the results of the test in question affect the decision to perform the gold standard on all study subjects. Again, the validity of the study design rests in the ability to eliminate or minimize

Table 2. *How to Assess an Article about a Diagnostic Test*

Question

Internal Validity
1. Is there an appropriate comparison to a "gold standard?"
2. Is the study population a representative cohort of the spectrum of disease severity and incidence?
3. Did the results of the studied test influence the choice to perform the "gold standard" test?

Results
1. What are the sensitivity, specificity, positive predictive, and negative predictive values of the test?
2. How do these compare with the values of the reference standard?

Generalizability
1. Are the study patients similar to mine?
2. Is the technology employed in the studied test available to my practice?
3. Will the test results change the management of my patients?

From Bhandari M, Montori VM, Swiontkowski MF, Guyatt GH. User's guide to the surgical literature: how to use an article about a diagnostic test. *J Bone Joint Surg Am* 85-A:1133–1140, 2003; Centre for Health Evidence Web site; available at: http://www.cche.net/; accessed July 15, 2005; Jaeschke R, Guyatt G, Sackett DL. Users' guides to the medical literature. III. how to use an article about a diagnostic test. A. are the results of the study valid? Evidence-Based Medicine Working Group. *JAMA* 271:389–391, 1994.

Table 3. *How to Assess an Article about Prognosis*

Question

Internal Validity
1. Are the patients at a similar course in the disease at the beginning of the study?
2. Is the follow-up of sufficient length to identify all possible outcomes or complications?
3. Is there adjustment for known important prognostic factors?

Results
1. Is the outcome of interest clearly defined?
2. What is the stated likelihood of occurrence of the outcome?
3. What is the precision of this estimated likelihood?

Generalizability
1. Are the studied patients similar to mine?
2. Do the results help guide treatment or counseling of my patients?

From Bhandari M, Guyatt GH, Swiontkowski MF. User's guide to the orthopaedic literature: how to use an article about prognosis. *J Bone Joint Surg Am* 83-A:1555–1564, 2001; Centre for Health Evidence Web site; available at: http://www.cche.net/; accessed July 15, 2005; Laupacis A, Wells G, Richardson WS, Tugwell P. Users' guides to the medical literature. V. how to use an article about prognosis. Evidence-Based Medicine Working Group. *JAMA* 272:234–237, 1994.

systemic sources of systematic bias. Just as in articles about therapy, the magnitude of the difference made by the new test—measured by the test's sensitivity, specificity, and positive and negative predictive values—should be an important consideration to the reader. Because the positive and negative predictive values depend on disease incidence, the characteristics of the reader's own patient population play a large role in determining the applicability of the new diagnostic test. In addition, not all technology is universally available, further making the applicability of an article about a diagnostic test specific to the individual reader.

Useful articles about prognosis or natural history (see Table 3) begin by assembling an inception cohort that has a representative and well-defined sample of patients at a similar course in the disease and then carries out follow-up over a time period that is long enough to identify either the complications of interest or disease resolution, while keeping loss to follow-up to a minimum. These studies optimally also will use validated outcomes tools and will adjust for important prognostic factors. There is usually a well-defined outcome that is being studied, and the reader should know what this is and what the stated likelihood of the occurrence of the outcome. The precision of the study's estimate is also important, and this again is usually expressed in confidence intervals. Narrow confidence intervals usually represent a higher-quality study. Once again, the patient cohort being studied should adequately represent the reader's patient. Finally, a useful study about prognosis should either guide treatment or give the reader data by which to counsel the patient and his family.

A well-constructed study about risk or harm (see Table 4) should identify baseline comparison groups that are similar with respect to the outcome of interest, except for

Table 4. *How to Assess an Article about Harm*

Question

Internal Validity
1. Are the study groups similar in every respect except the exposure being studied?
2. Was follow-up of sufficient length to identify all possible outcomes?

Results
1. What is the association between exposure and harm (relative risk)?
2. Is there a dose–response relationship?
3. How precise is the estimate of risk?

Generalizability
1. Are the studied patients similar to mine?
2. Do the results help guide treatment of my patients?

From Centre for Health Evidence Web site; available at: http://www.cche.net/; accessed July 15, 2005; Levine M, Walter S, Lee H, et al. Users' guides to the medical literature. IV. how to use an article about harm. Evidence-Based Medicine Working Group. *JAMA* 271:1615–1619, 1994.

Table 5. *Common Types of Bias*

Bias	Description
Forms of Bias That Are Potentially Detectable by the Critical Reader	
Susceptibility bias	Comparing results between prognostically dissimilar groups (improved by randomization; stratified randomization even better)
Performance bias	Dissimilar levels of surgeon skill or confounding by "coprocedures" (single-surgeon or expert surgeon series and studies with historical controls are very vulnerable)
Detection bias	Using nonstandardized or inconsistent study endpoints (improved by blinding, independent examiners, and validated outcomes instruments)
Transfer bias	Differential loss to follow-up or excessive loss to follow-up
Some Types of Bias Cannot Be Detected by the Reader (Even a Good Reader); One Such Example	
Publication bias	Disproportionate publication of work based on nonscientific factors (outcome bias and investigator/study site preference are two well-studied examples); this can be hard to eliminate; may only be detectable when large numbers of papers are read or when the process itself is audited

differences in the exposure in question; the outcomes and exposure also should be similarly measured, and follow-up needs to be adequate. These studies also need to present a biologically plausible temporal relationship and, depending on the type of exposure, a dose–response gradient. As with other types of studies, the questions about validity of study design, magnitude and precision of results, and generalizability (external validity) to the reader's practice are all important (6,16).

In summary, the *JAMA* Users' Guides provide one approach to evaluating the importance of a particular study to the practice of an individual physician as regards the patient. Use of these guides should make the reader more efficient, increase the return on the time spent reading, and over time, even improve experimental design as investigators use these criteria to design higher-quality studies. Considering the elements covered in these Users' Guides helps the reader identify potential sources of bias (see Table 5), although not every type of bias is evident on even a careful reading of a particular article. Some more systematic biases, such as publication bias, require analyses of an entire body of literature for them to be uncovered (3).

Levels of Evidence

Another tool that readers can use is the Levels of Evidence ratings. These were described initially in nonsurgical journals (26) but recently have been introduced into *JBJS* to provide another measurement of study quality (10,26). The editors divide research articles into four types: therapeutic studies, prognostic studies, diagnostic studies, and economic and decision analyses. These articles are then assigned a hierarchical number, designated by Roman numerals, based on the study design employed. For example, Level I articles on therapy are randomized clinical trials, Level II studies typically are controlled cohort studies that are not randomized, Level III studies employ a case-control design, Level IV studies are case series, and Level V articles represent expert opinion only. Similar distinctions are drawn, based on study design, for studies about prognosis and natural history, diagnosis, and medical economics.

With this system, the editors hope to provide the reader with an idea of the relative influence a study or article should have on the resolution of clinical questions. Furthermore, by knowing ahead of time what features of an article will make it more powerful to the readers, the creator of a study will be motivated to embark on a higher-quality research effort.

Whatever the conclusion regarding a study's strength of design, it is important to remember that prospective, randomized, double-blinded, placebo-controlled studies are not always possible in orthopaedic surgery. Therefore, within the Levels of Evidence schema, the only evidence available to answer a given clinical question may not be "Level I." In such situations, the surgeon should not simply abandon the clinical question as unanswerable because of lack of objective research. Rather, the surgeon should keep in mind that the available evidence has a low or indeterminate certainty of representing the truth and proceed accordingly. Conversely, sometimes a single high-quality study exists among a myriad of lesser reports; in these cases, the answer to the clinical question should be based on a critical review of all the available literature, but the weight placed on each report considered will vary according to quality. No single study, regardless of its quality, is likely to contain all that is needed to answer an important clinical question.

APPLY THE RESULTS TO THE INDIVIDUAL PATIENT

The entire exercise of EBM begins with a single patient provoking a clinical question, leading the surgeon to embark on a quest for evidence to answer the question. The journey should result in an idea of what the magnitude of the effect of a surgical treatment is, the associated risks and their likelihoods, the costs of the treatment, and the relative strength of the evidence supporting the treatment. However, the art of EBM comes in educating the individual patient, who then should put this knowledge in the context of his/her own values and ultimately guide the treatment decision. Unfortunately, no systematic or objective assessment of patient values exists, making the final practice of EBM a subjective one based on individual surgeon and patient values.

However, applying the results of research to one's own practice deals with the question of external validity, or generalizability, of the studies themselves. There are no lists of criteria for external validity as there are for internal validity, which are covered earlier in this chapter. However, several key questions are worth considering with respect to generalizability of surgical research; these focus on the providers, the patients, and the technologies employed:

1. Who performed the study and where was it done? Surgical trials by a single (or small number) of subspecialty-trained, high-volume providers at one center are often less generalizable than studies that recruit from practices of multiple surgeons at diverse sites of practice. One type of trial is not "better" than the other; it is just important to decide whether one's own practice and skill set mirror the subspecialty practice or the general practice and interpret published results in light of this decision.
2. Were the patients included similar to the ones I see in my own practice? Typical confounding variables here include the proportion of compensation claims pending, the medical and surgical complexity of the patients included in the study (which may be greater or less than the reader's), and sometimes discrete patient factors such as smoking, diabetes, or other specific predictors of outcome.
3. Is the technology employed in the study available to me today? This most commonly comes into play in studies about new diagnostic tests, but can apply to studies on therapy—for example, hypotensive epidural anesthesia has been shown to favorably affect rates of thromboembolic disease after joint replacement surgery (27,28); however, not every hospital has anesthesia providers who are skilled in this technique and who can perform it safely. Determining whether the technology in question is available locally is important; if it is not, and the study is sufficiently convincing, the work may serve as an impetus to gain access to newer equipment (if the study deals with a diagnostic test) or additional training (if it is about a surgical technique).

What is evident from reviewing the issue of external validity is that it usually comes at a cost to internal validity, and vice versa. That is, the more homogeneous the study population and the fewer variables permitted in the performance of techniques under study (such as the number of surgeons involved), the tighter the study appears methodologically—but the less generalizable the study becomes to other providers and their practices. The more "real world" variability permitted in the study design—in terms of patient qualities like age and comorbidities, or the number of participating surgeons—the more confounding variables usually find their way into the methods. The right balance of internal and external validity depends on the clinical question at hand and on the specific needs of the reader, his/her practice patterns, and the demographics of the patients (s)he sees in the office.

THE ROLE OF TEXTBOOKS

So where does a textbook like this one fit in an EBM schema? This chapter has focused on finding the most current, least biased, and most appropriate evidence that speaks to a specific clinical question and then interpreting that evidence in light of local factors (external validity). Given that high-quality objective evidence is not available to answer all questions, and given that this evidence does not exist independent of real-world surgeons' experiences, expert opinion continues to have a role. Textbooks not only provide a forum for this opinion but also often represent a published documentation of experts' quests through the current evidence—as well as experience—that have led those individuals to perform procedures a certain way or for certain indications. In addition, textbooks provide fast, easy, convenient, and graphic references for complex surgical techniques. The quality and number of descriptive illustrations and photographs presented in high-quality textbooks usually are not found in journal articles. Therefore a good textbook provides an invaluable supplement to the peer-reviewed literature and should remain a part of every surgeon's guide to the practice of EBM.

ACKNOWLEDGMENT

The authors gratefully acknowledge the assistance of Debbie Ames, whose help was invaluable during manuscript preparation.

REFERENCES

1. Evidence-Based Medicine Working Group. Evidence-based medicine. A new approach to teaching the practice of medicine. *JAMA* 268:2420–2425, 1992.
2. Gibson P. Asthma guidelines and evidence-based medicine. *Lancet* 342:1305, 1993.
3. Leopold SS, Warme WJ, Braunlich EF, Shott S. Association between funding source and study outcome in orthopaedic research. *Clin Orthop Relat Res* 415:293–301, 2003.
4. Guyatt GH, Sackett DL, Cook DJ. Users' guides to the medical literature. II. How to use an article about therapy or prevention. A. are the results of the study valid? Evidence-Based Medicine Working Group. *JAMA* 270:2598–2601, 1993.
5. Wright CC, Sim J. Intention-to-treat approach to data from randomized controlled trials: a sensitivity analysis. *J Clin Epidemiol* 56:833–842, 2003.
6. Centre for Health Evidence Web site. Available at: http://www.cche.net/.
7. Sackett DL, Straus SE, Richardson WS, et al. *Evidence-based Medicine: How to Practice and Teach EBM.* New York: Churchill Livingstone; 2003.
8. Cochrane Collaboration Web site. Available at: http://www.cochrane.org/.
9. Wright JG, Swiontkowski MF, Heckman JD. Editorial. Introducing a new journal section: evidence-based orthopaedics. *J Bone Joint Surg Am* 82:759–760, 2000.
10. Wright JG, Swiontkowski MF, Heckman JD. Introducing levels of evidence to the journal. *J Bone Joint Surg Am* 85-A:1–3, 2003.
11. Bhandari M, Guyatt GH, Montori V, et al. User's guide to the orthopaedic literature: how to use a systematic literature review. *J Bone Joint Surg Am* 84-A:1672–1682, 2002.
12. Bhandari M, Guyatt GH, Swiontkowski MF. User's guide to the orthopaedic literature: how to use an article about a surgical therapy. *J Bone Joint Surg Am* 83-A:916–926, 2001.
13. Bhandari M, Guyatt GH, Swiontkowski MF. User's guide to the orthopaedic literature: how to use an article about prognosis. *J Bone Joint Surg Am* 83-A:1555–1564, 2001.
14. Guyatt GH, Rennie D. Users' guides to the medical literature. *JAMA* 270:2096–2097, 1993.
15. Jaeschke R, Guyatt G, Sackett DL. Users' guides to the medical literature. III. How to use an article about a diagnostic test. A. are the results of the study valid? Evidence-Based Medicine Working Group. *JAMA* 271:389–391, 1994.
16. Jaeschke R, Guyatt GH, Sackett DL. Users' guides to the medical literature. III. How to use an article about a diagnostic test. B. What are the results and will they help me in caring for my patients? The Evidence-Based Medicine Working Group. *JAMA* 271:703–707, 1994.
17. Laupacis A, Wells G, Richardson WS, Tugwell P. Users' guides to the medical literature. V. How to use an article about prognosis. Evidence-Based Medicine Working Group. *JAMA* 272:234–237, 1994.
18. Levine M, Walter S, Lee H, et al. Users' guides to the medical literature. IV. How to use an article about harm. Evidence-Based Medicine Working Group. *JAMA* 271:1615–1619, 1994.
19. ACP Journal Club Web site. Available at: http://www.acpjc.org/ACP.
20. Guyatt GH, Sackett DL, Cook DJ. Users' guides to the medical literature. II. How to use an article about therapy or prevention. B. What were the results and will they help me in caring for my patients? Evidence-Based Medicine Working Group. *JAMA* 271:59–63, 1994.

21. Oxman AD, Sackett DL, Guyatt GH. Users' guides to the medical literature. I. How to get started. The Evidence-Based Medicine Working Group. *JAMA* 270:2093–2095, 1993.

22. Bhandari M, Montori VM, Swiontkowski MF, Guyatt GH. User's guide to the surgical literature: how to use an article about a diagnostic test. *J Bone Joint Surg Am* 85-A:1133–1140, 2003.

23. Hulley S, Grady D, Bush T, et al. Randomized trial of estrogen plus progestin for secondary prevention of coronary heart disease in postmenopausal women. Heart and Estrogen/Progestin Replacement Study (HERS) Research Group. *JAMA* 280:605–613, 1998.

24. Moseley JB, O'Malley K, Petersen NJ, et al. A controlled trial of arthroscopic surgery for osteoarthritis of the knee. *N Engl J Med* 347:81–88, 2002.

25. Beaton DE, Schemitsch E. Measures of health-related quality of life and physical function. *Clin Orthop Relat Res* 413:90–105, 2003.

26. Siwek J, Gourlay ML, Slawson DC, Shaughnessy AF. How to write an evidence-based clinical review article. *Am Fam Physician* 65:251–258, 2002.

27. Haas SB. Effects of epidural anesthesia on incidence of venous thromboembolism following joint replacement. *Orthopedics* 17(Suppl):18–20, 1994.

28. Sharrock NE, Salvati EA. Hypotensive epidural anesthesia for total hip arthroplasty: a review. *Acta Orthop Scand* 67:91–107, 1996.

SECTION I BASIC CARDIOLOGY

[references list, largely illegible]

PART II

Surgical Approaches

2

Anterolateral Approach

Paul J. P. Pongor and Maurice E. Müeller

Originally described by Watson-Jones (1), the anterolateral approach allows for excellent exposure of the femoral neck and acetabulum without the need for a trochanteric osteotomy. By largely passing in front of the gluteus medius, the anterolateral approach limits damage to this important hip abductor. However, to obtain an adequate exposure, the more anterior fibers of the gluteus medius require division.

The anterolateral approach may be indicated for patients with scarring or otherwise inappropriate soft tissues for either direct, lateral, or posterior approach. It is particularly useful for patients in whom the risk of posterior dislocation is great or who have neurological conditions such as Parkinson's disease, spasticity, or severe flexion deformity. The anterolateral approach is particularly useful in patients undergoing bilateral simultaneous total hip arthroplasty in that the patient is operated on in a supine position, making it unnecessary to reposition, reprepare, and redrape the patient. An assessment of leg length is facilitated by having the patient in the supine position with both lower extremities available for visual inspection.

Having the patient in the supine position improves airway access and control, as well as pulmonary mechanics. This is a particular advantage in elderly patients and in patients with respiratory difficulties, particularly patients with ankylosing spondylitis, in whom limited chest expansion may be further compromised by the lateral decubitus position. The position of the acetabular component is easier to judge from the anterolateral approach than from lateral or posterior approaches, and the dislocation rate is very low, probably due to a combination of visualization of the acetabular component from this approach and the ability to judge its position more accurately. The incidence of heterotopic ossification is also very low. A particular advantage of the anterolateral approach is that the incidence of injury to the abductor muscles is extremely low, particularly when compared to the direct lateral approach.

The anterolateral approach is contraindicated in obese and/or heavily muscled patients, and the incision is not easily extended if wider exposure is needed—for example, if there are unexpected defects in the posterior rim of the acetabulum that need to be addressed.

PREOPERATIVE PLANNING

Careful preoperative planning is essential to ensure the expected operative outcome. Preoperative planning provides information about the appropriate prosthesis, the depth of acetabular reaming, and the level of the femoral neck resection, as well as correct positioning and orientation of the components. The plan ensures that the surgeon has anticipated potential intraoperative difficulties, such as the resection of osteophytes, acetabular bone grafting, or need for a trochanteric osteotomy. Significant leg length discrepancies are also addressed within the preoperative plan. A carefully prepared preoperative plan requires an anteroposterior (AP) radiograph of the pelvis including the proximal third of both femurs, component templates, tracing paper, a black pencil to silhouette the bones, and a red pencil to silhouette the implant.

After selecting the appropriate implant, three tracings are made of the preoperative AP radiograph. The first tracing (tracing A) follows the bony contours of the healthy hemipelvis, the greater and lesser trochanters, and the inner borders of the medullary canal. The second tracing (tracing B) follows the bony contours of the diseased hemipelvis. The last tracing (tracing C) is of the diseased femoral head and neck, greater trochanter, lesser trochanter, and medullary canal contours. The actual planning is a four-step process.

Step 1: Tracing A, the healthy hemipelvis, is superimposed on the template of the chosen implant. When the outer diameter of the acetabular component corresponds with the weight-bearing segment of the acetabular contour, the socket is outlined on the drawing. At the same time, the medial edge of the femoral stem has to touch the inner border of the medial femoral cortex. With offset reproduced, the trochanteric reference line (T), the femoral resection line (F), and the outlines of both trochanters and the femoral prosthesis are added to the tracing.

Step 2: Tracing B, the diseased hemipelvis, is now superimposed on an inverted tracing A. The pelvic silhouettes roughly coincide. The acetabular component is now copied at its anatomic locations. This helps determine the depth of acetabular reaming.

Step 3: Tracing C, the diseased femoral silhouette, is superimposed on the inverted tracing A in such a way that the trochanters are at the same level. The trochanteric reference line (T) and the resection line (R)—as well as the silhouette of the chosen femoral prosthesis—are carefully drawn onto tracing C. If the medullary canals do not match, the stem size may be adjusted with the aid of an appropriate femoral component template.

Step 4: Finally, tracing B, the diseased hemiplevis, is superimposed on tracing C, the diseased proximal femur, and the nonresected femoral portion and the chosen prosthesis are drawn in. The composite corresponds to the anticipated postoperative result.

Although the procedure at first may seem confusing, the four steps allow the surgeon to base the reconstruction on the healthy hip, helping to ensure the correction of the leg length discrepancies and reproducing appropriate biomechanical offset.

OPERATIVE TECHNIQUE

Patient Positioning

The procedure can be performed with the patient supine or in the lateral decubitus position using a modified Kocher approach. The supine position may be preferred with its advantage in facilitating correct positioning of the prosthetic components during the procedure. In addition to the standard instruments used for the insertion of a total replacement, special instruments, such as narrow-tipped retractors, greatly facilitate exposure and help avoid damage to surrounding neurovascular structures.

Initial Incision and Superficial Dissection

Originally, the incision was described as curved, 12 to 15 cm in length, and starting from the midpoint of a line joining the anterosuperior iliac spine to the tip of the greater trochanter. The distal part of the incision was to parallel the femoral shaft with the angle between these two arms of the incision approximately 130 degrees, the apex of the incision positioned just behind the greater trochanter (2). Correct position of the apex was felt to be important for allowing adequate access to the exposed femoral neck later in the procedure (see Fig. 1). More recently, however, a straighter, less curved incision has been advocated (see Fig. 2). A similar incision is used to incise the underlying iliotibial band. In obese patients, the incision should be straight and longer in length.

Deep Dissection

The hip joint is approached in the interval between the tensor fascia lata and glutei, sparing the nerve to the tensor fascia lata (see Fig. 3). The branch of the superior gluteal nerve to the tensor fasciae lies in this interval and should be carefully protected during this approach.

A transverse incision is used to release the anterior third of the distal attachment of the gluteus medius from the lateral aspect of the trochanter. Development of the interval between the gluteus medius and minimus may be aided by placing a bone hook around the gluteus medius, applying proximal tension, and then sharply dividing the anterior fibers of the medius until the bursa between the gluteus minimus and the greater trochanter is opened (see Fig. 4). This will expose the gluteus minimus tendon underneath. The tendon of the gluteus minimus is cut approximately 1 cm from its attachment to the ventral aspect of the greater trochanter and tagged for later repair (see Fig. 5B). If necessary, more of the gluteus medius may be released to avoid damaging the muscle during the procedure.

Joint Capsule Exposure

Three long, narrow-pointed lever-retractors are carefully positioned within the wound: Two are placed on the capsule on each side of the neck, and the third is placed behind the

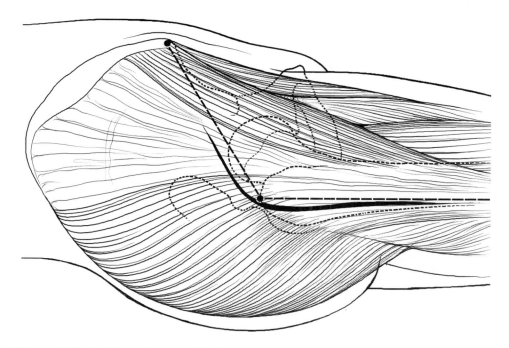

Figure 1. The incision as it was originally described is curved, 12 to 15 cm in length, beginning at the midpoint of a line from the anterosuperior iliac spine to the tip of the greater trochanter. The distal portion is parallel to the femoral shaft with an angle of approximately 130 degrees between the two arms of the incision. The apex of the incision is positioned just behind the greater trochanter to allow adequate access to the femoral neck.

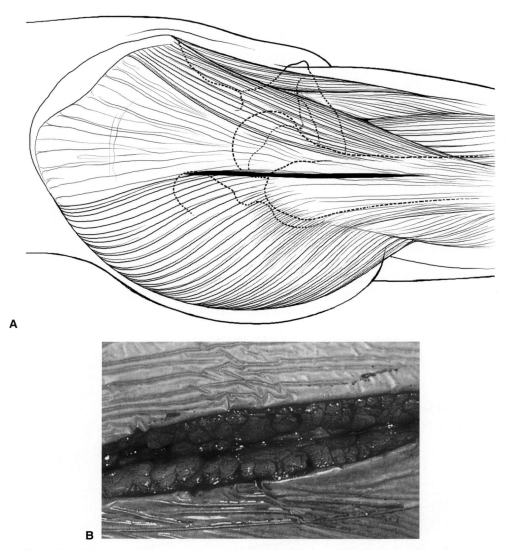

A

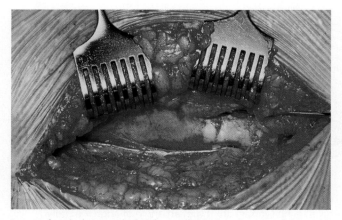

B

Figure 2. A less curved incision than described in Figure 1 has also been described and should be used in obese patients.

Figure 3. The tensor fascia lata and glutei are divided, being careful to spare the nerve to the tensor fascia lata.

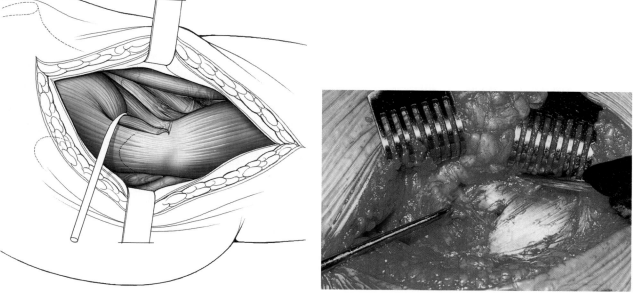

Figure 4. A: The anterior third of the distal attachment of the gluteus maximus is released from the lateral aspect of the trochanter by means of a transverse incision. The interval between the gluteus medius and minimus is aided by placing a bone hook around the gluteus medius, applying proximal tension, and sharply dividing the anterior fibers of the medius to open the bursa between the gluteus minimus and the greater trochanter. **B:** Intraoperative photograph showing the division of the gluteus medius and minimus.

anterior rim of the acetabulum (see Fig. 6). Great care must be taken to ensure that this last retractor is in contact with bone rather than slipping into the soft tissues anterior to the acetabular rim and damaging the femoral nerve (Fig. 4A). A large, T-shaped capsular incision is then made. On either side of the exposed femoral neck, two blunt-tipped retractors are placed between the neck and the joint capsule. These three retractors encircle the neck and protect the structures behind the joint (see Fig. 7). Excision of the capsule should be as complete as possible in order to permit an easy dislocation of the stump of the neck. Often, especially with an external rotation contraction, the short external rotators require division during capsular excision (3).

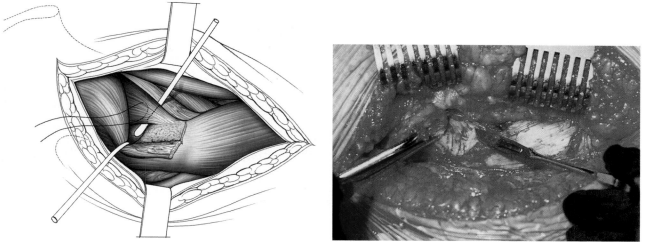

Figure 5. A,B: The tendon of the gluteus minimus is cut and tagged for later repair.

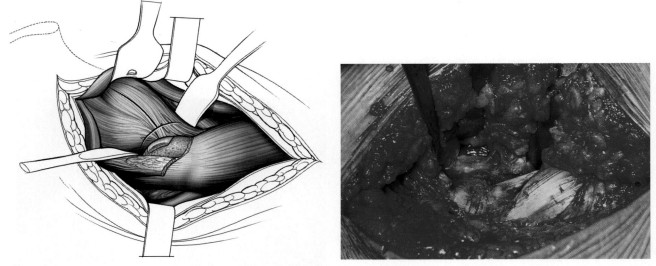

Figure 6. Two long, narrow-pointed retractors are placed on the capsule on each side of the neck, and a third long, narrow-pointed retractor is placed behind the rim of the acetabulum.

Femoral Neck Division and Femoral Head Removal

The femoral neck is now adequately exposed to allow for a safe, controlled division with the aid of an oscillating saw. A flat chisel is then introduced between the bony surfaces and is used to spread the osteotomy (see Fig. 8). This helps ensure that the division of the femoral neck is complete. A corkscrew is deeply inserted into the femoral head with a lever introduced between the two articular surfaces to aid in dislocation of the resected femoral head (see Fig. 9). If dislocation is not possible because of a severely deformed joint, fragmentation of the head with a chisel may be necessary (4).

Completion of the Femoral Neck Division

The leg is now gently externally rotated. With the oscillating saw, the femoral neck is definitively trimmed 1 or 2 cm above the lesser trochanter as previously calculated on the

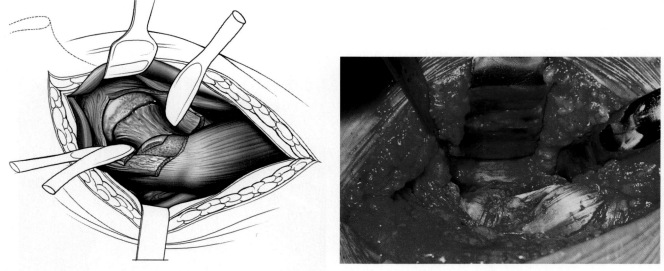

Figure 7. The three retractors are used to encircle the femoral neck and protect the structures behind the joint.

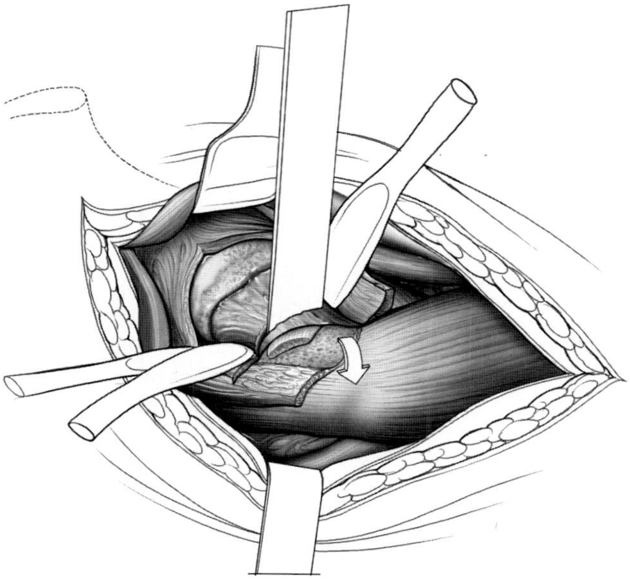

Figure 8. Use of a flat chisel to spread the osteotomy.

graphic preoperative plan (see Fig. 10). The line of resection should be almost perpendicular to the bicondylar axis of the knee and should also form an angle of 45 degrees with the femoral diaphysis. With the knee orientation used as the point of reference, the goal of 10 degrees of femoral anteversion is also carefully considered during the trimming of the femoral neck.

Capsular Excision

The remainder of the anterior aspect of the capsule is excised along with the incision of the posterior aspect of the capsule to permit easy delivery of the femoral neck stump into the wound (see Fig. 11). To protect the iliopsoas tendon, it is necessary to identify its course prior to incision of the capsule. One must also remain attentive to the course of the femoral nerve, the femoral artery, and the femoral veins running along the anteroinferior aspect of the capsule. A

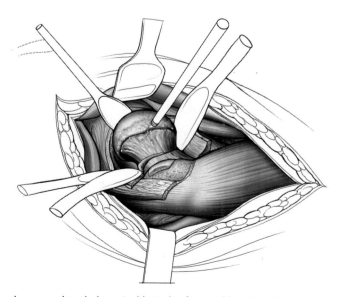

Figure 9. A corkscrew, deeply inserted into the femoral head, with a lever introduced between the articular surfaces, aids in dislocation of the femoral head.

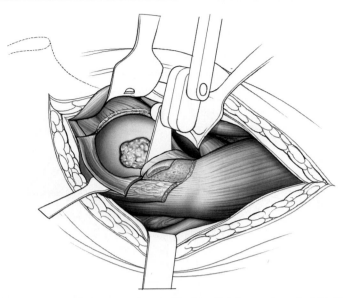

Figure 10. An oscillating saw is used to trim the femoral neck definitively.

separate incision is occasionally necessary to repair these structures if they are inadvertently injured while the remainder of the capsule is addressed. With excessively thick capsules, it is occasionally difficult to incise the posterior capsule or excise the remainder of the anterior capsule. The use of a bone hook helps facilitate this step. Care should be taken to identify and coagulate all bleeding vessels exposed during capsular excision.

Positioning of Acetabular Retractors

In order to gain adequate exposure of the acetabulum, correct positioning of the acetabular retractors is essential. A long-handled curved retractor is inserted over the anterior lip of the acetabulum. The teeth of a second retractor are positioned around the posterior

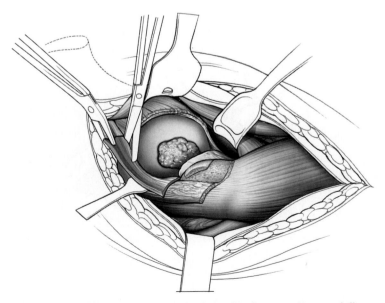

Figure 11. The anterior aspect of the capsule is excised to permit easy delivery of the femoral neck stump into the wound.

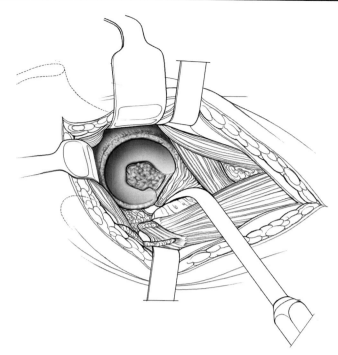

Figure 12. Three retractors are placed around the acetabulum: a long-handled curved retractor over the anterior lip of the acetabulum, a tooth retractor around the posterior inferior acetabular rim, and a short-pointed retractor into the superior rim of the acetabulum.

inferior acetabular rim and used to depress the proximal femur. In placing this femoral retractor, it is necessary slightly to abduct and flex the thigh. This will allow the teeth of the retractor to be placed underneath the posterior inferior acetabular rim. The femoral retractor may then be fixed in place by hammering the points into the bone. Hooking a weight to the retractor and clamping it to the patient's thigh drape eliminates the necessity of manual retraction. Finally, a third, short-pointed retractor is placed into the superior rim of the acetabulum (see Fig. 12). This should allow for full 360-degree exposure of the acetabulum. Again, care should be taken to ensure that the retractors are kept close to bone to avoid serious neurovascular complications.

Preparation of the Acetabular Bed/Insertion of Component

The acetabulum is now optimally exposed to allow preparation of the bed for insertion of the component. Classically, the acetabulum is fashioned with flat and swan neck chisels to first remove the osteophytes. Deepening of the acetabulum is performed with hand or power reaming. Care must be taken to avoid excessive weakening of the floor, which could eventually lead to fatigue fractures of the pelvis. The component may be inserted after adequate preparation of the bed. Proper orientation of the socket is essential. The aim is to achieve 42 to 45 degrees of inclination (see Fig. 13A) and 5 to 15 degrees of anteversion (Fig. 13B) in order to obtain a range of flexion of 110 degrees or more.

Periacetabular Soft Tissue Examination

After completion of the insertion of the acetabular component, an examination of the soft tissue tension is in order. With preoperative external rotation deformities, division of the piriformis muscle may be required. This can be examined by placing the limb in internal rotation. If excessive tension is noted, the piriformis may be pulled forward with a bone hook and carefully divided near its insertion to the tip of the greater trochanter (see Fig. 14).

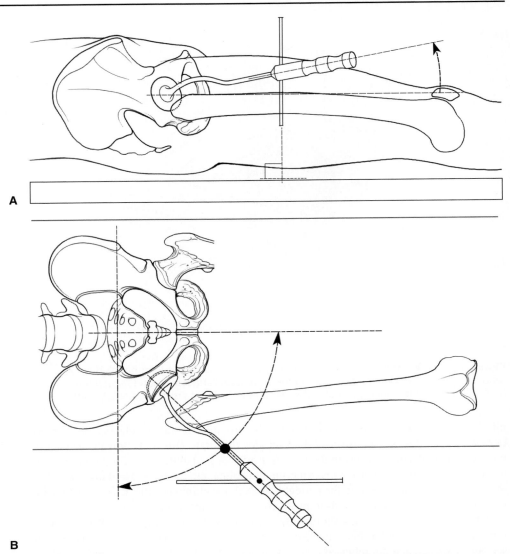

Figure 13. After preparation of the acetabular bed and insertion of the component, the socket is oriented with **(A)** an inclination of 42 to 45 degrees and **(B)** 5 to 15 degrees of anteversion in order to obtain a range of flexion of 110 degrees or more.

With very stiff hips, all external rotators may require division; however, the quadratus femoris should not be divided. Transection of the quadratus femoris with inadvertent division of its accompanying artery could lead to a serious postoperative hematoma. All sources of bleeding should be visualized and coagulated at this point.

Femoral Neck Exposure and Preparation

A wide self-retaining retractor is placed under the greater trochanter to aid in lifting the femur anteriorly. The leg is then pulled in external rotation and maximal flexion and adduction until the heel touches the contralateral shoulder (see Fig. 15A). The glutei are protected by a second small retractor. A third small retractor is placed under the psoas (Fig. 15B). The distance between the division of the neck and the lesser trochanter is first palpated and then measured. This measurement is compared to the distance previously estimated on the preoperative plan, and the neck cut is adjusted as required. The base of the femoral neck is first prepared using a chisel to gouge out cancellous bone from the center of the neck (Fig. 15C).

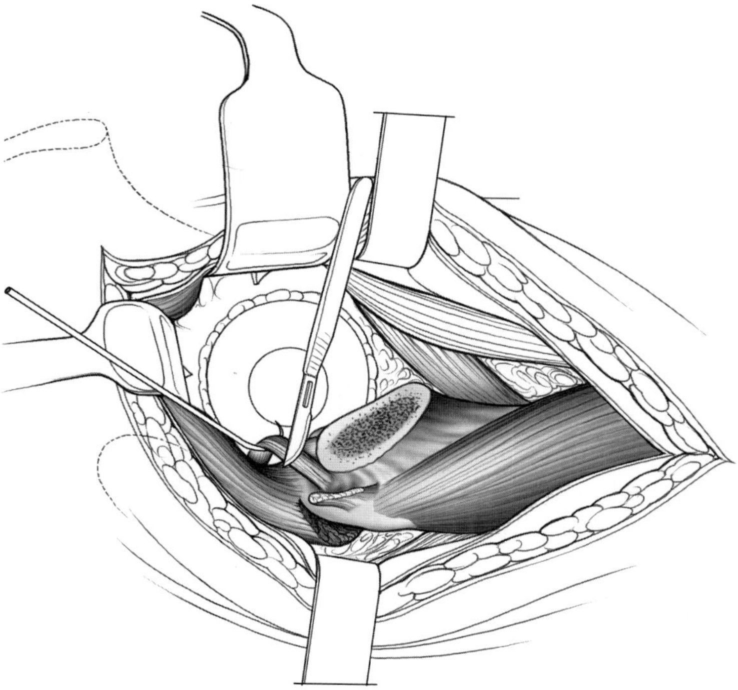

Figure 14. Division of the piriformis near its insertion to the tip of the greater trochanter can be used to release excess tension.

Femoral Medullary Canal Preparation

The femoral canal is explored using a long curette (see Fig. 16). This exploration is essential; without a proper exploration, it is difficult to establish the exact direction of the canal and determine whether the cut surface of the neck is sufficiently clear for reaming. This step also helps avoid perforation of the cortex with the rasp. The neck must be perfectly visualized, and if it is not, adjust the position of the leg. The remainder of the medullary canal is prepared guided by the hip system chosen and its instrumentation (see Fig. 17). Regardless of the system, care should be taken to ensure that the anteversion of the new canal is no more than 10 degrees. During preparation of the femur, the broaches must be inserted as laterally as possible to avoid damage or perforation of the femoral shaft.

Trial Prosthesis Insertion

The trial prosthesis is inserted after adequate canal preparation. The glutei are easily pushed aside with two fingers (see Fig. 18). If a collared prosthesis is chosen and if the seat of the collar on the femoral cortex is not satisfactory (or if the distance between the lesser trochanter and the collar is not as previously calculated), the necessary corrections may be made with the oscillating saw. The hip is then gently reduced.

Assessing Component Orientation and Position

Once reduced, the orientation between the head and the cup can be carefully examined. Note the angle formed between the acetabular component and the base of the femoral head (see Fig. 19); it is equal to the sum of the anteversion of the neck and the cup. This sum should measure approximately 20 to 30 degrees to allow for flexion of more than a right angle. Retracting the glutei with a right-angle retractor, a Kirschner wire is passed along the tip of the greater trochanter at right angles to the shaft, aiming toward the midline (Fig. 19). The

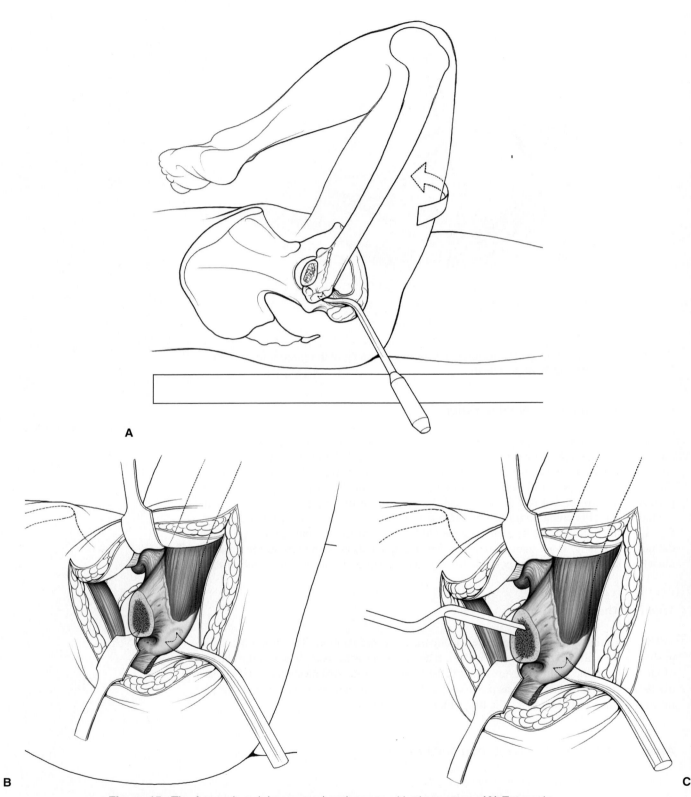

Figure 15. The femoral neck is exposed and prepared in three steps: **(A)** External rotation is used to achieve maximal flexion and adduction until the heel touches the contralateral shoulder, **(B)** the glutei and psoas muscles are retracted, and **(C)** a chisel is used to gouge out cancellous bone from the neck.

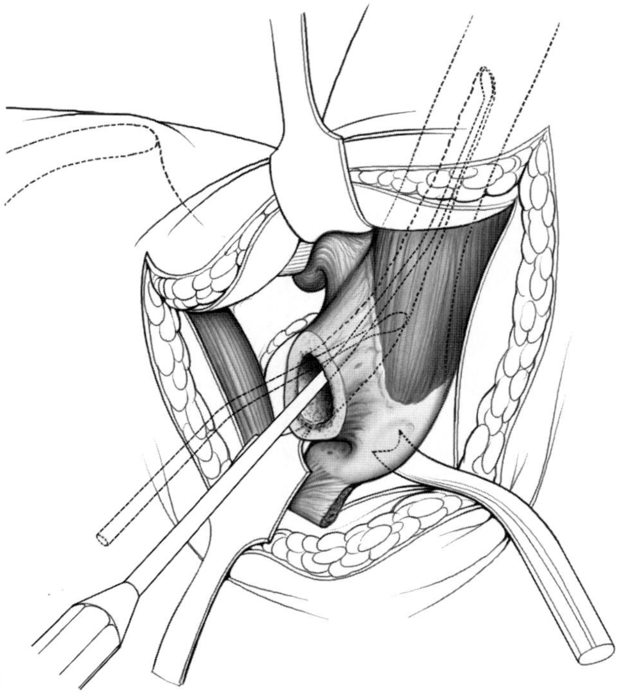

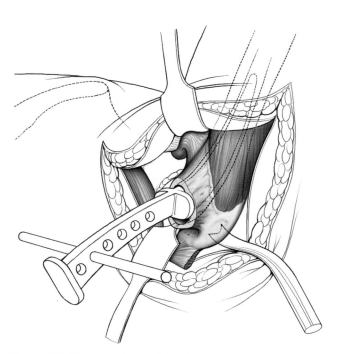

Figure 16. A long curette is used to explore the femoral canal.

Figure 17. The remainder of the femoral canal is prepared using the hip system instrumentation.

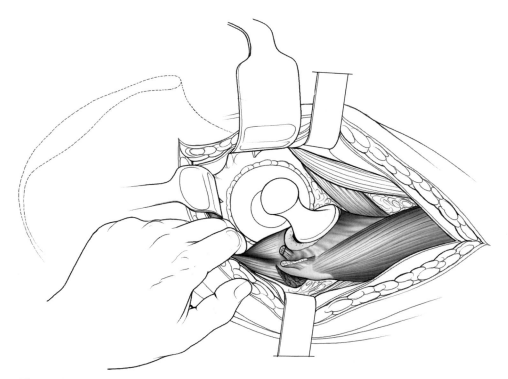

Figure 18. Two fingers are used to push the glutei aside and allow for prosthesis insertion.

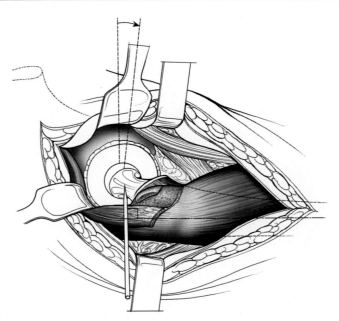

Figure 19. The angle between the acetabular component and the base of the femoral head is 20 to 30 degrees to allow for flexion of greater than 90 degrees.

distance between this Kirschner wire and the middle of the prosthetic femoral head can be measured and compared to the preoperative graphic plan. Again, adjustments in depth of insertion or orientation of the femoral component may be necessary. With the hip in extension, the leg is rotated to bring patellar orientation in the sagittal plane to neutral. Anteversion of the femoral component in this position should measure approximately 10 to 15 degrees.

Assessing Component Stability

The hip is next flexed to 90 degrees (see Fig. 20). If internal rotation is restricted, further division of the posterior capsule and/or short external rotators may be necessary. Any tendency to dislocate should be assessed along with potential causes such as posterior impingement of the trochanter on residual posterior acetabular osteophytes. The prosthesis is then dislocated. The dislocation is aided by passing a hook around the neck of the prosthesis and applying traction to the leg in abduction and external rotation (see Fig. 21).

Final Medullary Canal Preparation/Component Insertion

A sharp curette is used to remove all debris left during rasping of the canal (see Fig. 22). If a cemented component is used, a medullary canal plug is placed, and its depth is carefully checked. A small suction tube is inserted into the medullary canal to the level of the canal plug to allow air and blood to escape during the pressurization and placement of the femoral component (see Fig. 23).

After aggressive irrigation and antegrade insertion of cement using a cement gun fitted with a pressurization collar, the femoral prosthesis is inserted. Orientation of the prosthesis during insertion is important. Care must be taken to ensure that the prosthesis is introduced in a slightly valgus or neutral position.

During the last 2 cm of cement insertion, the suction tube is removed, and the prosthesis is driven to its final position (Fig. 23B). Measurements are taken between the prosthesis and the lesser trochanter during insertion to ensure that the device has been precisely placed at its predetermined level. All excess cement and debris are removed while waiting for the cement to harden.

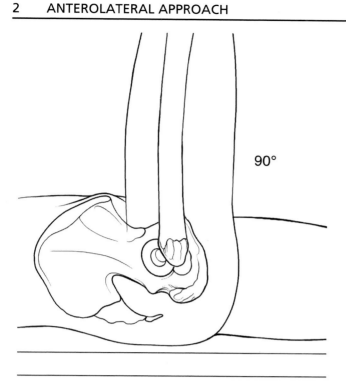

Figure 20. To assess component stability, the hip is flexed to 90 degrees.

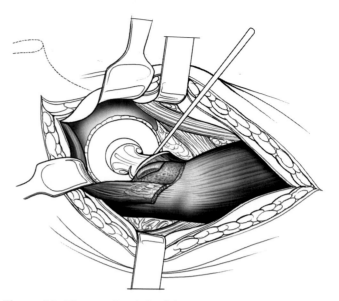

Figure 21. The prosthesis is dislocated by passing a hook around the neck of the prosthesis and applying traction to the abducted and externally rotated leg.

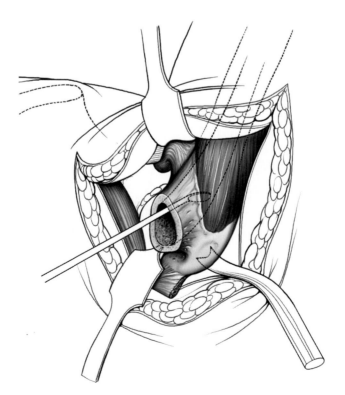

Figure 22. With a sharp curette, the femoral canal is cleaned of all debris left from rasping.

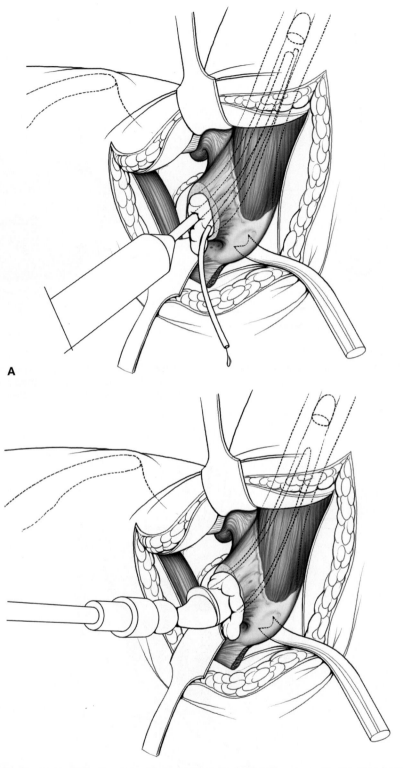

Figure 23. A: A small suction tube, inserted into the medullary canal to the level of the cement plug, allows air and blood to escape during pressurization and insertion of the femoral prosthesis. **B:** The tube is removed, and the prosthesis is driven to its final position during the last 2 cm of cement insertion.

Closure

The prosthesis is reduced. The distance between the lesser trochanter and femoral head, as well as the distance between the perpendicular from the tip of the greater trochanter and the femoral head, is remeasured and compared to the preoperative plan. Any evidence of posterior impingement may be addressed at this time. A careful check for bleeding, interposition of cement, bone debris, or soft tissue is carried out. With traction applied to the leg, the wound is copiously irrigated (see Fig. 24).

The gluteus minimus tendon is sutured to its attachment. Also, the released anterior aspect of the gluteus medius is now sutured to the vastus lateralis. The soft tissue is carefully inspected for injured or crushed glutei and bony debris. If left behind, these may serve as a source of ectopic bone formation. Suction drains are placed, one at the level of the prosthesis and the second subcutaneously.

POSTOPERATIVE MANAGEMENT

Excessive soft tissue retraction, particularly when exposing the anterior aspect of the acetabulum, can predispose to heterotrophic ossification. An excessive medius release with a poor repair may lead to a postoperative limp, another known complication of the antero-lateral approach. Because of the concern with the abductor repair, ambulation is initiated with the aid of a cane on the contralateral extremity for the first 6 weeks. Once abductor strength is regained, full weight bearing may be allowed. Even with initiation of full weight bearing, abductor strengthening continues to be a focus of concentration.

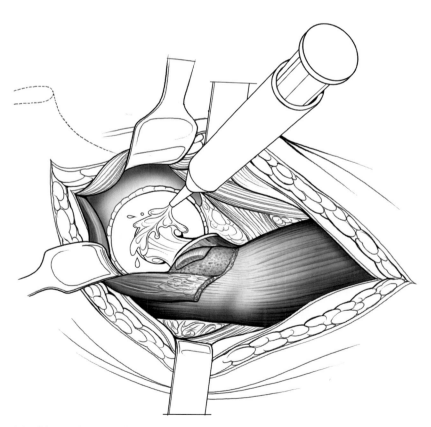

Figure 24. After reduction of the prosthesis, traction is applied to the leg, and the wound is copiously irrigated before closure.

COMPLICATIONS

As mentioned, major complications are less frequent with the anterolateral approach than with other approaches. Femoral nerve damage may occur either from improper placement of the anterior acetabular retractor with the tip not being kept on bone during insertion or by injury during coagulation of nearby vessels. The femoral nerve may also be damaged either directly during the process of drilling for acetabular fixation holes in the case of cemented component use or by screw fixation in an uncemented acetabular component. In addition, if perforation occurs in the anterior acetabular shell and a cemented component is being used, cement extrusion may occur and damage the femoral nerve. Most injuries to the femoral nerve are transient and resolve spontaneously within 4 to 8 months.

Damage to the femoral artery and vein is also possible because of their proximity in this exposure. However, the portion of the operation during which these vascular structures are most vulnerable is during excision of the anterior capsule. With the anterolateral approach, the anterior capsule can be directly visualized, thus lessening the likelihood of injury to the anterior neurovascular structures.

RECOMMENDED READING

1. Watson-Jones R. Fracture of the neck of the femur. *Br J Surg* 23:787, 1935.
2. Müeller ME. Total hip replacement: planning, technique, and complications. In: Cruess RL, Mitchell NS, eds. *Surgical Management of Degenerative Arthritis of the Lower Limb*. Philadelphia: Lea & Febiger; 1975: 91–113.
3. Müeller ME. Total hip prostheses. *Clin Orthop Relat Res* 72:46–68, 1970.
4. Müeller ME. Osteotomy of the greater trochanter. Part I: total hip replacement without trochanteric osteotomy. In: Harris WH, ed. *The Hip: Proceedings of the Second Open Scientific Meeting of the Hip Society*. St Louis: Mosby; 1974.

3

Posterolateral Approach

Richard E. White, Jr., and Michael J. Archibeck

INDICATIONS/CONTRAINDICATIONS

The posterior approach remains the most popular approach in primary and revision total hip replacement. Advantages of the posterior approach include its simplicity and ease of dissection in internervous planes, its preservation of the abductor musculature, its potential to be an extensile approach, and its ability to be used with a variety of trochanteric osteotomies (standard osteotomy, trochanteric slide, extended trochanteric osteotomy) (1).

While several approaches exist for routine hip surgery, indications for the posterior approach can include primary and revision total hip replacement, hemiarthroplasty for fracture, open reduction and internal fixation of posterior column or wall fractures of the acetabulum, and drainage of the septic hip. While the choice of approach in primary and revision hip replacement depends on surgeon comfort and experience, there are situations in which the posterior approach is preferable. Primary hip replacement cases that may necessitate a posterior approach include developmental dysplasia of the hip with a high riding dislocation that may require femoral shortening osteotomy. In addition, a posterior approach is preferable in primary hip replacement cases that may require a trochanteric osteotomy (ankylosis, protrusio, extensive heterotopic ossification), as the standard posterior approach can be easily converted to a transtrochanteric exposure. Revision hip replacement that may require a more extensile exposure generally is best performed via a posterior approach. These include cases of acetabular reconstruction that may require allograft, posterior column plating, or cage reconstruction. Femoral revision that will require osteotomy (trochanteric slide or, more commonly, extended trochanteric osteotomy) also should generally be approached posteriorly. While it is possible to perform these osteotomies through a modified direct lateral approach, the closure is complicated by the need for anterior abductor repair in addition to osteotomy fragment reattachment.

Contraindications to the use of the posterior approach to the hip are limited. Anterior approaches are generally preferred in nonarthroplasty cases requiring arthrotomy (open reduction and internal fixation of anterior femoral head fractures, loose body removal, drainage of septic arthritis), as the posterior blood supply (branches of the medial femoral circumflex artery) provides the majority of femoral head vascularity and is often disrupted by a posterior approach and arthrotomy. In primary total hip replacement, a modified direct lateral approach may be preferable in patients at high risk for dislocation such as neuromuscular disorders, Parkinson disease, substance abuse, or cognitive impairment. In revision total hip replacement, an anterior approach may be preferable in cases that are known to have a high rate of postoperative instability such as polyethylene and femoral head exchange. The anterior approach provides adequate exposure for such cases and potentially reduces the risk of posterior dislocation. However, these are relative contraindications, and many surgeons successfully use a posterior approach for all reconstructive hip procedures.

Controversy remains regarding the superiority of the posterior or modified direct lateral approach in total hip replacement. One issue is the incidence of dislocation. Generally, the rate of dislocation has been reported to be lower following the direct lateral approach ranging from 0.3% to 2% (2–5). Reported rates of dislocation following total hip replacement using the posterior approach range from 2% to 7%. (3,5–7). While the etiology of dislocation is multifactorial, it has been postulated that disruption or attenuation of the posterior soft tissues (capsule and short external rotators) as well as the potential for inadequate acetabular anteversion on implantation may have led to these findings. As most surgeons currently using the posterior approach routinely perform posterior soft tissue repair, the rate of dislocation has been shown to be reduced. At our institution, we found a reduction in the rate of dislocation from 4.8% to 0.7% as a result of routine posterior capsular repair in primary total hip replacement (8). Another controversy is that of a reduced incidence of limp following posterior approach compared to approaches that disrupt the abductor musculature, such as the modified direct lateral approach (9). While literature on this topic is limited, the incidence of limp in the early postoperative period does appear to be higher in patients who undergo a direct lateral approach (3). While the limp resolves in most patients, it may persist. This may be secondary to avulsion or attenuation of the repaired anterior abductors, a concern not generally found with the posterior approach.

PREOPERATIVE PLANNING

We obtain an anteroposterior view of the pelvis, an anteroposterior view of the affected hip, and a frog lateral of the affected hip. The two views of the hip are taken with magnification markers. Standard templates generally allow for 20% magnification, which may or may not be accurate depending on x-ray magnification.

The goals of preoperative templating are to guide proper sizing of components and to guide intraoperative restoration of soft tissue balance of the hip (leg length and hip offset). Templating begins with the anteroposterior view of the pelvis. Drawing a line along the bottom of the ischium or obturator foramen provides a pelvic reference for determining leg length discrepancy (LLD). A common point on the lesser trochanter is then marked on both sides. Generally, its most prominent point as this point is less affected by rotational asymmetry. The distance between the previously drawn line and the marks on the lesser trochanters is then used to determine LLD. Clinical measures of LLD should also be performed to include discrepancies arising from differences below the hip or fixed pelvic obliquities. The anteroposterior view of the hip is then used to template the acetabular size and position. The center of rotation of the proposed acetabular component is marked. A line is then drawn above the acetabular center of rotation at a distance of the desired leg lengthening (i.e., if 4 mm of lengthening is desired, the line is drawn 4 mm above the acetabular center of rotation). The femoral component is then templated. The appropriately sized component is placed such that the zero neck length (zero modular femoral head) intersects this line. The need for an extended offset femoral and/or acetabular component(s) is anticipated if the proposed reconstruction results in reduced offset. In this scenario, we generally prefer to add offset to the femoral component as this provides improved abductor mechanics and thus a reduced joint reactive force. The desired length of neck cut is then measured and marked for guidance of intraoperative femoral neck osteotomy.

SURGERY

Positioning

The patient is placed in the lateral decubitus position on a standard operating room table. A Foley catheter is routinely inserted, and preoperative antibiotic prophylaxis is administered. While a variety of hip patient positioning devices are available, we use a posterior pad applied at the level of the sacrum (just proximal to the gluteal fold), an anterior pad applied at the level of the pubis, and an anterior chest bolster applied at the level of the nipples or just below the breasts to prevent the chest and pelvis from rotating anteriorly, which can result in placement of the acetabular component in reduced anteversion or retroversion if unrecognized. An axillary roll is inserted distal to the axilla under the chest wall. We then check to confirm that the pelvis is level and secure. The dependent arm is placed on a well-padded arm board in an extended position. Two to three pillows are placed between the arms and taped in place. We use a vertical laminar flow room with battery-powered body exhaust suits routinely.

Draping

After a nonsterile adhesive U-drape is applied to the hip region, a standard Betadine soap and paint scrub is performed. The anticipated field is cleaned with alcohol to allow, once dried, improved adherence of the iodine-impregnated adhesive skin barrier. A sterile down drape is applied below the leg as an assistant holds the leg. An impervious plastic U-drape is placed to drape out the perineum. A large stockinette is placed to just above the knee and wrapped in a 6-inch ace bandage. Towels are applied around the hip and clipped to skin using two towel clips. The hip drape is applied. Ioband is then placed covering all exposed skin.

Approach

With the current trend in less invasive hip replacement or smaller incisions, it is important to be sure visualization is "adequate." The length of the incision needed for adequate visualization depends on many variables including surgeon factors (level of comfort, experience, etc.) and patient factors (patient size, muscularity, etc.). The posterior approach, while traditionally performed through an 8- to 10-inch (20- to 25-cm) incision, can be done through a smaller incision without loss of significant visualization. As the incision is made to be smaller (8 to 12 cm), the technique becomes more difficult, requiring modified retractors, broach handles, and offset acetabular insertion devices. For purposes of illustration, we will demonstrate the approach with approximately a 15-cm incision. The senior author's routine posterior approach is done through an 11- to 14-cm incision.

The position of the incision is dictated by the location of the tip of the greater trochanter and the anatomy of the proximal femur. While the incision in generally centered 1 to 2 cm distal to the tip of the greater trochanter, excessive coxa valga or hip dysplasia may require adjustment of the incision location. The standard incision extends at a 30- to 40-degree angle posterior and proximal to the tip of the greater trochanter for approximately 5 cm. It gently curves proximally to approach the anterior boarder of the femur and extends about 5 to 8 cm distal to the tip of the trochanter (see Fig. 1). As the incision becomes smaller, its location becomes more critical.

Dissection is carried down to the fascia lata sharply (see Fig. 2). The fat is elevated off the fascia with a dry laparotomy sponge along the length of the incision for a width of about 2 cm. The fascia is sharply incised along the length of the incision. Proximally, the fibers of the gluteus maximus are divided deep to the superficial fascia. A Charnley retractor is then placed.

Proximally, the plane between the capsule and the gluteus minimus is identified and developed proximal to the piriformis tendon. The plane is dissected with a Cobb or Key eleva-

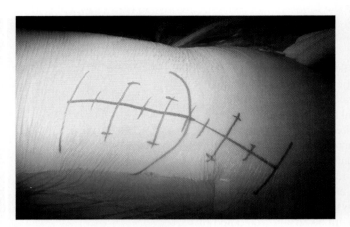

Figure 1. This figure illustrates the standard incision for a posterior approach to the hip performed for total hip arthroplasty. While the incision in generally centered 1 to 2 cm distal to the tip of the greater trochanter, excessive coxa valga or hip dysplasia may require adjustment of the incision location. The standard incision extends at a 30- to 40-degree angle posterior and proximal to the tip of the greater trochanter for approximately 5 cm. It gently curves proximally to approach the anterior boarder of the femur and extends about 5 to 8 cm distal to the tip of the trochanter.

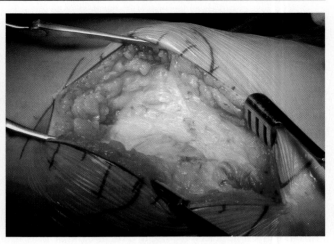

Figure 2. Dissection is carried down to the fascia lata sharply. The fat is elevated off the fascia with a dry laparotomy sponge along the length of the incision for a width of about 2 cm.

tor, and a sharp Hohmann retractor is inserted (see Fig. 3). Fat can be gently elevated off the short external rotators and quadratus femoris posteriorly. The sciatic nerve should be palpated. The sciatic nerve exits the pelvis via the greater sciatic foramen distal to the piriformis. It then travels distally superficial to the short external rotators in a sleeve of fatty tissue and deep to the gluteal sling into the thigh. Palpation is adequate to localize and protect the sciatic nerve. Dissection of the nerve risks devascularization and increases the risk of nerve palsy.

The posterior capsule and short external rotators are detached from the trochanteric crest in a single layer in anticipation of repair at the time of closure (see Fig. 4). The capsular incision is initiated at the acetabulum proximal to the piriformis and extends distally to the capsular insertion on the proximal femur. It then extends along the trochanteric crest, including the external rotators and capsule in a single layer directly off bone (see Fig. 5). The capsular flap should include 30% to 50% of the circumference of the acetabulum. The quadratus femoris is released in a subperiosteal fashion distally to visualize the lesser trochanter. If a more extensile exposure is needed, as in many revision cases, the gluteal sling can be released from the proximal femur, allowing for greater anterior excursion of the proximal femur.

Posterior labrum and/or osteophytes can be removed to facilitate hip dislocation. The hip is then dislocated with flexion, adduction, and internal rotation. Once dislocated, the lesser trochanter should be well exposed so as to guide the level of neck osteotomy as templated preoperatively. Using a femoral neck-cutting guide, the femoral neck osteotomy is made (see Fig. 6).

Exposure of the acetabulum begins with placement of an anterior retractor. A tonsil or long hemostat is used to open a small rent in the anterior capsule just peripheral to the labrum and adjacent to the acetabulum in the anterior-superior region of the acetabulum (10 or 2 o'clock for left or right hip, respectively). A large, sharp-tipped acetabular retractor is placed through this small rent onto the anterior wall of the acetabulum and used to retract the proximal femur anteriorly. This should be placed directly adjacent to the bone, as deeper placement risks injury to the adjacent neurovascular structures. Inferior placement of this retractor should be avoided for similar reasons. A sharp Hohmann retractor is inserted posteriorly, adjacent to bone, just superior to the ischium. Care is taken, when placing posterior retractors, to avoid injury or excessive retraction on the sciatic nerve. An inferior broad Hohmann retractor is placed caudad to the transverse acetabular ligament into the obturator foramen for circum-

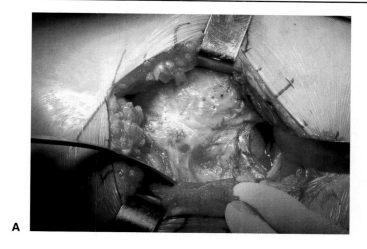

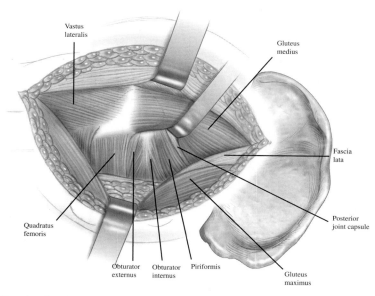

Figure 3. Proximally, the plane between the capsule and the gluteus medius is identified and developed proximal to the piriformis tendon. The plane is dissected with a Cobb or Key elevator, and a sharp Hohmann retractor is inserted.

ferential exposure (see Fig. 7). The pulvinar is removed from the cotyloid notch using a large curette to allow visualization of the acetabular floor as a guide medial reaming depth. If osteophytes have overgrown the notch, they should be removed using an osteotome.

After implantation of the acetabular component, the proximal femur is exposed. The leg is held perpendicular to the floor, allowing a reference point for femoral component anteversion. A femoral elevator is placed under the anterior neck to bring the proximal femur out of the wound. A sharp Hohmann is placed proximally under the gluteus medius insertion to expose the lateral femoral neck (see Fig. 8). The femur is then prepared, and final components are implanted.

Closure begins with a posterior capsular repair. The position of the leg during the capsular repair should be in approximately 20 degrees of internal rotation and neutral abduction (see Fig. 9). Placement of the leg on two Mayo stands (one under the knee and one under the foot) maintains this position. A no. 5 Ethibond suture is passed into the cut surface of the piriformis and passed into the capsule as one layer. It is then passed from

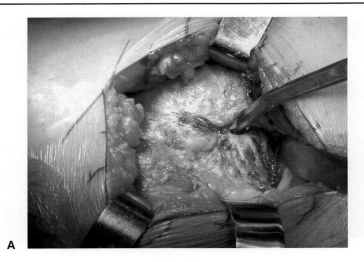

A

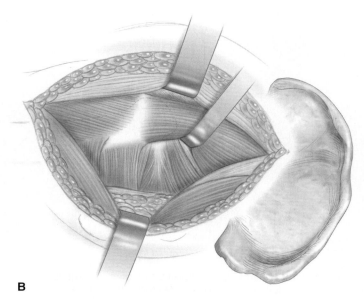

B

Figure 4. The posterior capsule and short external rotators are detached from the trochanteric crest in a single layer in anticipation of repair at the time of closure.

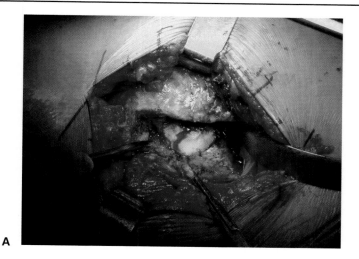

A

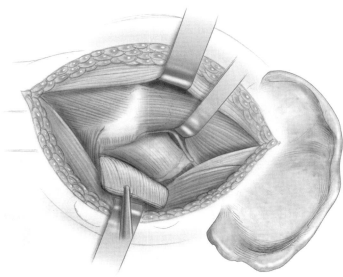

B

Figure 5. The capsular incision is initiated proximally at the acetabulum proximal to the piriformis and extends distally to the capsular insertion on the proximal femur. It then extends along the trochanteric crest, including the external rotators and capsule in a single layer directly off bone.

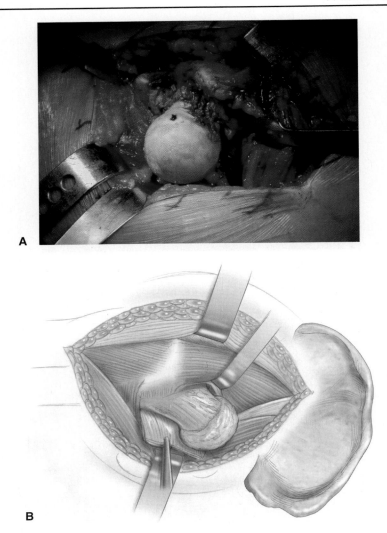

Figure 6. Posterior labrum and/or osteophytes can be removed to facilitate hip disloca-tion. The hip is then dislocated with flexion, adduction, and internal rotation. Once dislo-cated, the lesser trochanter should be well exposed so as to guide the level of neck os-teotomy as templated preoperatively. Using a femoral neck-cutting guide, the femoral neck osteotomy is made.

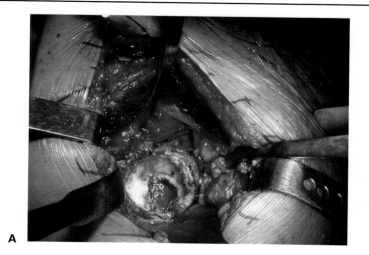

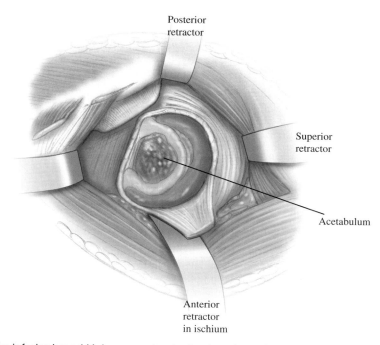

Figure 7. An inferior broad Hohmann retractor is placed caudad to the transverse acetabular ligament into the obturator foramen for circumferential exposure. The pulvinar is removed from the cotyloid notch using a large curette to allow visualization of the acetabular floor as a guide to depth of medial reaming. If osteophytes have overgrown the notch, they should be removed using an osteotome.

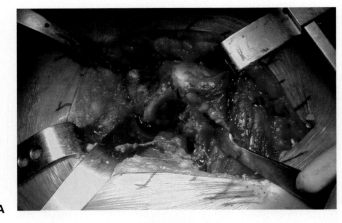

A

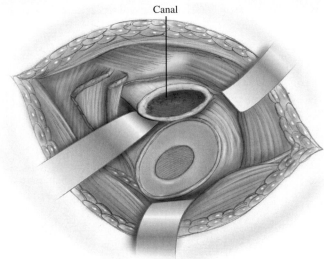

B

Figure 8. After implantation of the acetabular component, the proximal femur is exposed. The leg is held perpendicular to the floor allowing a reference point for femoral component anteversion. A femoral elevator is placed under the anterior neck to bring the proximal femur out of the wound. A sharp Hohmann is placed proximally under the gluteus medius insertion to expose the lateral femoral neck. The femur is then prepared, and final components are implanted.

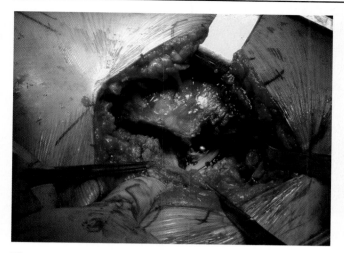

Figure 9. Closure begins with a posterior capsular repair. The position of the leg during the capsular repair should be in approximately 20 degrees of internal rotation and neutral abduction. Placement of the leg on two Mayo stands (one under the knee and one under the foot) maintains this position.

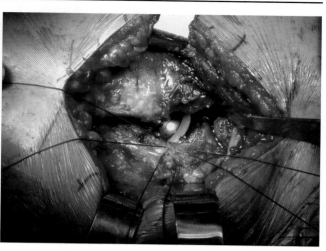

Figure 10. A no. 5 Ethibond suture is passed into the cut surface of the piriformis and passing into the capsule as one layer. It is then passed from within the capsule as a cross stitch, then from in to out of the capsule and piriformis. A second and third capsular suture is passed proximal and distal to this piriformis suture.

within the capsule as a cross stitch, then from in to out of the capsule and piriformis (see Fig. 10). A second and third capsular suture is passed proximal and distal to this piriformis suture. Four holes are drilled with a 2.7-mm drill bit in the posterior aspect of the trochanter. The most proximal hole is near the junction of the posterior aspect of the gluteus medius and the trochanter. Each subsequent hole is 5 to 8 mm distal, depending on the size of the femur (see Fig. 11). The sutures are passed through the drill holes (see Fig. 12) using a Huson suture passer. If difficulty is encountered in advancing the musculocapsular flap to the trochanter, a proximal and distal release of the capsule from the acetabulum can be performed to facilitate apposition. The sutures are then tied (see Fig. 13).

The posterior approach can be an extensile exposure and, in revision hip replacement, is often used in conjunction with an extended trochanteric osteotomy. In such cases, the posterior extent of the deep dissection is continued from the quadratus femoris into the posterior aspect of the vastus lateralis. The vastus lateralis is split, leaving a 1- to 2-cm cuff posteriorly. Care must be taken to ligate or electrocauterize arterial perforators when dissecting in the muscle. This split in the vastus lateralis can extend as far distally as needed. At the time of closure, the fascia of the vastus lateralis is closed using a running 0 Vicryl absorbable suture. The posterior approach also allows exposure of the posterior column and ischium in revision cases requiring plating (pelvic discontinuity) or cage reconstruction. The soft tissues can be elevated in a subperiosteal fashion off the posterior wall and column with care being taken to avoid violation of the greater sciatic notch and its neurovascular structures. Distally, the origin of the hamstrings can be elevated off the ischium in a subperiosteal fashion. This gives exposure of the entire posterior column. Proximally, the abductors can be elevated off the outer table of the ilium for placement of flanges of cage constructs as well. Care must be taken to avoid avulsion of the superior gluteal artery as it exits the sciatic notch.

POSTOPERATIVE MANAGEMENT

Patients are left at bed rest the day of surgery. Physical therapy, twice daily, begins on the first postoperative day and continues daily until discharge. Drains are removed, and dressings are changed on the second postoperative day. Patients use a walker and generally can bear weight as tolerated for both hybrid and cementless modes of fixation. Active abduction is allowed immediately except if an extended trochanteric osteotomy is performed.

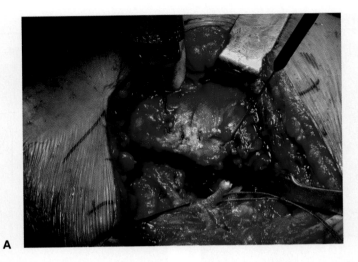

A

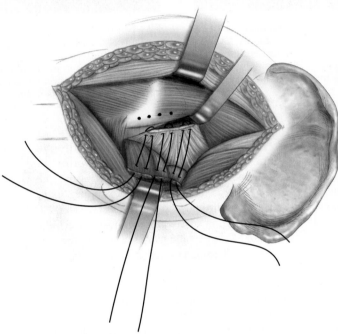

B

Figure 11. Four holes are drilled with a 2.7-mm drill bit in the posterior aspect of the trochanter. The most proximal hole is near the junction of the posterior aspect of the gluteus medius and the trochanter. Each subsequent hole is 5 to 8 mm distal, depending on the size of the femur.

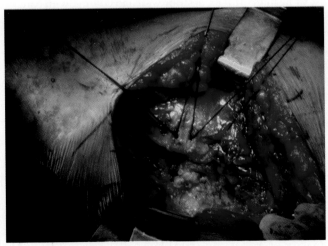

Figure 12. The sutures are passed through the drill holes using a Huson suture passer.

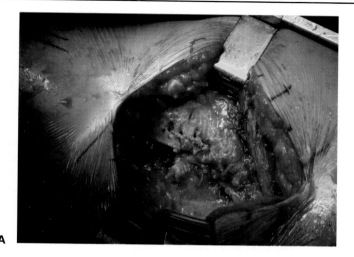

A

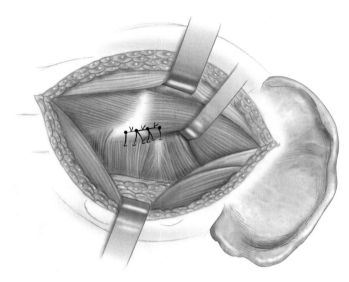

B

Figure 13. If difficulty is encountered in advancing the musculocapsular flap to the trochanter, a proximal and distal release of the capsule from the acetabulum can be performed to facilitate apposition. The sutures are then tied.

COMPLICATIONS

The most common complication of the posterior approach is that of postoperative dislocation. While this is discussed in more detail early in the chapter, the rate of dislocation is generally reported to range from 2% to 7% (3,5–7). It has been shown to be reduced when a posterior capsular repair is performed during closure (8).

Neurovascular injury is an uncommon complication of hip surgery. Vascular injuries associated with total hip replacement range from 0.1% to 0.2%. Vascular injury can be minimized by careful placement of anterior retractors and minimizing the time that the leg is held in extreme positions. This can help reduce the incidence of deep venous thrombosis as well. Sciatic nerve injury can occur and has been reported to occur in 0% to 3% of total hip replacements. The risk is higher in revision hip surgery. Care should be taken to gently palpate the nerve and avoid undue traction on it.

RECOMMENDED READING

1. Archibeck MJ, Rosenberg AG, Berger RA, Silverton CD. Trochanteric osteotomy and fixation during total hip arthroplasty. *J Am Acad Orthop Surg* 11:163–173, 2003.
2. Demos HA, Rorabeck CH, Bourne RB, et al. Instability in primary total hip arthroplasty with the direct lateral approach. *Clin Orthop Relat Res* 393:168–180, 2001.
3. Masonis JL, Bourne RB. Surgical approach, abductor function, and total hip arthroplasty dislocation. *Clin Orthop Relat Res* 405:46–53, 2002.
4. Mulliken BD, Rorabeck CH, Bourne RB, Nayak N. A modified direct lateral approach in total hip arthroplasty: a comprehensive review. *J Arthroplasty* 13:737–747, 1998.
5. Woo RY, Morrey BF. Dislocations after total hip arthroplasty. *J Bone Joint Surg Am* 64:1295–1306, 1982.
6. Callaghan JJ, Heithoff BE, Goetz DD, et al. Prevention of dislocation after hip arthroplasty: lessons from long-term followup. *Clin Orthop Relat Res* 393:157–162, 2001.
7. von Knoch M, Berry DJ, Harmsen WS, Morrey BF. Late dislocation after total hip arthroplasty. *J Bone Joint Surg Am* 84-A:1949–1953, 2002.
8. White RE Jr, Forness TJ, Allman JK, Junick DW. Effect of posterior capsular repair on early dislocation in primary total hip replacement. *Clin Orthop Relat Res* 393:163–167, 2001.
9. Hardinge K. The direct lateral approach to the hip. *J Bone Joint Surg Br* 64:17–19, 1982.

4

Trochanteric Osteotomy

Craig D. Silverton

Most surgeons today find that trochanteric osteotomy has limited value in primary hip arthroplasty. Most total hip replacements are performed utilizing either a direct lateral (Hardinge) or posterior approach. The comfort afforded by utilizing the same operative approach in each case prevents us from deviating to another, less secure approach. Attempting a first-time trochanteric osteotomy on a difficult primary hip arthroplasty can be uncomfortable. B. M. Wroblewski, a true disciple of Sir John Charnley, performs a trochanteric osteotomy on all primary hip replacements. He feels that the experience gained at Wrightington Hospital in performing thousands of trochanteric osteotomies has resulted in their very low nonunion rate. The most difficult primary and revision cases are then approached with ease, resulting in a higher likelihood of success. Nonunion rates are typically two to three times higher for those surgeons who are not experienced in trochanteric osteotomy.

So, is there really a need for trochanteric osteotomy in primary hip arthroplasty? The patient with protrusio acetabuli, developmental dysplasia of the hip (DDH), or severe ankylosis may require an osteotomy to gain adequate exposure. Charnley felt that restricted exposure of the hip led to more complications than the actual detachment of the trochanter. He believed that trochanteric osteotomy was an essential part of the operation, not only for exposure but also to restore more normal biomechanics to the hip joint by advancing the trochanter.

The purpose of this chapter is to acquaint the arthroplasty surgeon with several techniques of trochanteric osteotomy that have a relatively shallow learning curve and can aid in the exposure of the difficult primary or revision hip arthroplasty. The classic chevron trochanteric osteotomy will be described, followed by several different exposure options that you may find useful in your practice. The decision as to when to use these techniques is based on the surgeon's comfort level and the anticipated difficulty in exposure. I would recommend that you begin with a less demanding case and progress to the more difficult cases as your comfort level permits.

INDICATIONS/CONTRAINDICATIONS

The decision to perform a trochanteric osteotomy is based on the surgeon's ability to gain adequate access to the hip joint. Cases of DDH, protrusion acetabuli, prior hip fusion, or stiff or ankylosed hip all may benefit from the exposure afforded by removal of a portion of the trochanter or all of the trochanter. Patients with prior hip surgery or deformities of the proximal femur or trochanter either posttraumatic or secondary to primary bone diseases such as Paget or fibrous dysplasia all may necessitate a more extensile exposure. The occasional patient with ipsilateral knee stiffness or a prior knee fusion can make the standard exposures challenging. Malunion or nonunion of a previous trochanteric osteotomy may require further advancement and fixation. Selected cases of hip instability where leg lengthening becomes excessive and tension on the abductors must be restored may benefit from advancement of the trochanter.

Trochanteric advancement can improve hip mechanics and was originally a popular reason for trochanteric osteotomy in hip arthroplasty. With the multiple offsets in femoral components, modular necks, and offset cup liners available today, that rationale for removal of the trochanter has less validity. In cases where the trochanter is removed for the purpose of femoral lengthening (congenital dislocated hip) or advancement (addressing abductor tensioning as in femoral shortening), nothing short of complete removal of the trochanter will suffice. A soft tissue approach is not adequate in these unique cases.

In the case of revision arthroplasty, a well-fixed femoral component, either cementless or cemented, is difficult to remove leaving the trochanter intact. The use of the extended trochanteric osteotomy affords the surgeon safe access to the femoral component and lessens the risk of iatrogenic fracture of the femur. Attempting to perform revision surgery without adequate exposure risks injury to the sciatic nerve, iatrogenic fractures of the femur, trochanter, and acetabulum, as well as malposition of both femoral and acetabulum components. Certain types of femoral components with a large shoulder or antirotation wing can fracture the trochanter upon removal through standard soft tissue approaches. In most of these cases, the extent and level of osteotomy required can be determined preoperatively.

Contraindications to trochanteric osteotomy include those patients with a deficient trochanter bed in which to reattach the bone fragment. The patient with an eggshell trochanter secondary to severe osteolysis or osteopenia would be best served keeping the trochanter intact and using an alternate soft tissue approach. Patients that are at high risk for heterotopic bone formation and may require radiation postoperatively are not ideal candidates for any type of trochanteric osteotomy. Patients who have had high-dose radiation around the hip are not candidates for a trochanteric osteotomy because of the high risk of nonunion. Nonunion of the trochanter remains the most common complication, and poor bone stock preoperatively is a relative contraindication.

PREOPERATIVE PLANNING

The decision to use a more extensile approach should be made preoperatively. The danger lies in beginning a less extensile approach or minimally invasive approach and then realizing a more extensile approach is needed. Trying to convert a minimally invasive Hardinge approach to a trochanteric osteotomy or trochanteric slide is fraught with complications. If, however, one begins with the posterior approach, conversion to a more extensile exposure is usually more readily accomplished. In determining the type of osteotomy needed, adequate exposure remains the key in performing any difficult primary or revision arthroplasty.

Preoperative standard full-length radiographs will usually give the surgeon enough information about the trochanteric or femoral deformity present and implants in place. The trochanter should be carefully evaluated for bone quality, areas of lysis, and impingement on the insertion or removal of the femoral implant. Preoperative templating will give the surgeon an idea as to how much trochanter needs to be removed for straight insertion of the prosthesis, preventing a varus attitude. In cases of a malunion of the trochanter or deformity of the proximal femur, nothing short of a standard trochanteric osteotomy may suffice. Gaining access to the femoral canal is the priority; however, reattaching the trochanter is the "Achilles' heel" of the trochanteric osteotomy. A sufficient bone bed has to be present, or a nonunion may result.

Planning the extent of a proposed trochanteric osteotomy in the revision setting requires the surgeon to understand several additional key factors.

1. The total length of the femoral implant.
2. The amount and extent of porous coating (cementless).
3. The extent of the cement mantle (cemented).
4. The total length of the required osteotomy measured from the tip of the trochanter to the transverse cut of the osteotomy.
5. Remaining host bone diaphysis.
6. Reconstructive options following repair of the osteotomy.
7. Area of lysis around the trochanter.

In the revision setting, a more extensive osteotomy seems to be common practice. If femoral implant removal is required, a more limited osteotomy (trochanteric slide) may not give the surgeon adequate exposure to the full extent of the implant surfaces. Generally, trochanteric osteotomies cannot be converted to a more extensile osteotomy without complications.

Proper prior planning is a key to success and may prevent a disaster in surgery. For surgeons who rarely use the trochanteric approach, the availability of another surgeon with experience may provide additional assurance during these challenging cases.

SURGERY

The standard trochanteric osteotomy has been the "gold standard" for exposure since it was first introduced by Sir John Charnley. Few would argue that this exposure still provides the best access to the difficult primary or revision hip. According to Charnley, who was taught the method of trochanteric osteotomy by Sir Harry Platt, "If it could be guaranteed that the greater trochanter would unite within three weeks when reattached, and without imposing restrictions which would impede rehabilitation, few surgeons would fail to avail themselves to the easy and beautiful access to the hip joint provided by the transtrochanteric approach." Nonunion still remains the most common complication following standard trochanteric osteotomy. Despite the use of multiple-wiring techniques, cables, claws, bolts, and other devices, trochanteric healing is the "Achilles' heel" of this approach. This chapter will describe the classic chevron trochanteric approach, followed by several trochanteric osteotomy techniques that keep the abductor-vastus muscle sleeve mechanism intact. Maintaining the continuity of the gluteus medius and vastus lateralis has several advantages: (a) a compressive force is placed across the osteotomy site aiding in healing (see Fig. 1); (b) superior migration of the trochanteric fragment is limited by the tethering of the vastus lateralis; (c) blood supply to the trochanter is maintained; and (d) fixation techniques are simple and reproducible.

Chevron Trochanteric Osteotomy

The classic trochanteric osteotomy as described by Charnley was a flat cut that was then transferred distally and secured in place. Recognizing the inherent stability problems with a flat cut, the French and Swiss popularized the chevron or "dihedral self-stabilizing" trochanteric osteotomy. The advantages were obvious: The rotation is more rotationally stable, and the bone contact area is increased. Distal transfer can be carried out as well to tension the abductors. The use of a biplane osteotomy has decreased the rate of nonunion as compared to the flat cut trochanteric osteotomy.

Although the access provided by this trochanteric osteotomy is superb, nonunion still is a common problem, with rates reported from 1% to 15%. Clearly, the more practice one has in reattaching the trochanter, the better union rates will follow. For the occasional case, this

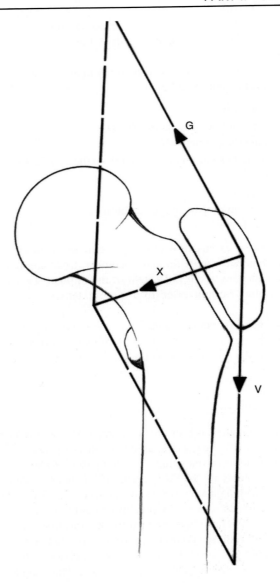

Figure 1. Leaving the gluteal *(G)* and vastus *(V)* muscles attached produces a medial component *(X)* that exerts a compressive force on the plane of osteotomy.

classic trochanteric osteotomy may not be the best choice available. Detaching the vastus lateralis creates a bone fragment that is inherently unstable and wants to migrate anteriorly and superiorly. With the difficulty in reattachment techniques, one may be better served using a technique that keeps the vastus lateralis attached to the fragment (i.e., trochanteric slide).

Technique. The standard incision is made, and the fascia is split in the midportion. The osteotomy is planned 4 to 5 cm distal to the tip of the trochanter. The vastus lateralis insertion is divided 1 cm distal to its insertion so that a cuff of tissue remains for repair. The external rotators can be tagged and retracted, protecting the sciatic nerve from harm. The bone fragment should be at least 3 to 5 cm in length and should include the attachments of the gluteus medius and minimus tendons. The osteotomy can be done intracapsularly or extracapsularly. The idea is to create a biplane surface much like the roof of a Swiss chalet. The anterior and posterior segments should be cut at an angle of about 30 degrees from the parasagittal plane. This cut can be made with a Gigli saw, with an oscillating saw, or with chevron-shaped osteotomes (see Figs. 2–4). If the decision is to use an oscillating saw, it is important to cool the blade with cold water during the cutting process to minimize thermal necrosis of the delicate

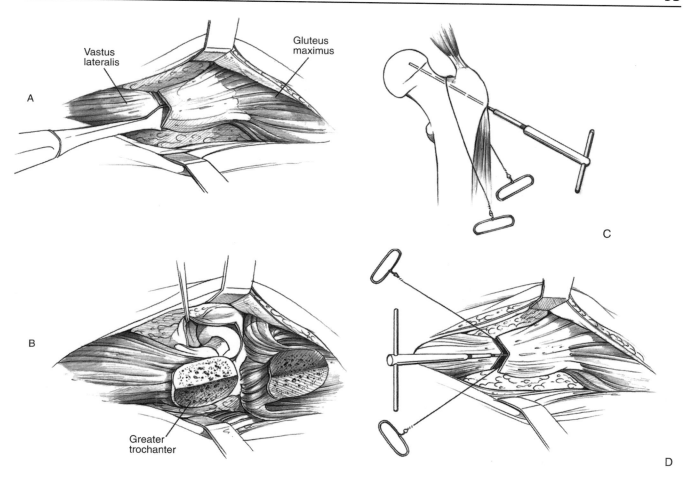

Figure 2. **A:** The chevron osteotomy performed with an osteotome. **B:** The dihedral cut provides for stable approximation of the cut surfaces. **C:** The chevron osteotomy performed with a Gigli saw over a smooth Steinmann pin. **D:** The Gigli saw is directed distally, cutting anteriorly and posteriorly and creating a dihedral osteotomy.

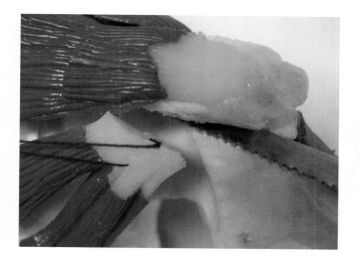

Figure 3. Charnley osteotomy. The external rotators are retracted, and an oscillating saw is used from posterior to anterior. This method creates a relatively flat osteotomy that is inherently unstable. A biplane or chevron osteotomy is more stable and is the method of choice.

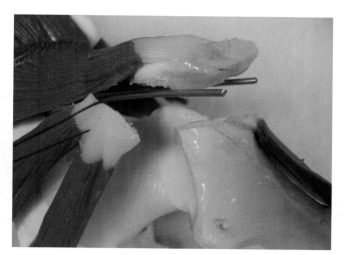

Figure 4. Once the osteotomy is cut, it should be retracted in a superior direction and held with 1/8-inch Steinmann pins.

underlying cancellous bed. If a Gigli saw is chosen, two methods seem to be reliable and reproducible. Wroblewski's technique requires that a 4-mm pin be directed just below the vastus ridge at about a 45-degree angle toward the femoral head. The Gigli saw is then passed between the superior aspect of the femoral neck and the trochanter. The saw lies proximal to the Steinmann pin and is directed distally, cutting anteriorly and posteriorly, creating a two-plane osteotomy (see Figs. 2C and 2D). The other technique involves passing a large Kelly clamp either intracapsularly or extracapsularly from posterior to anterior and attaching the Gigli saw. Internally rotating the leg 20 degrees will place the plane of the osteotomy parallel to the floor. This technique, however, will not produce a biplane osteotomy, only a relatively flat cut. The osteotomy should end just distal to the vastus ridge. The fragment can now be retracted cephalad and held with retractors or 1/8-inch Steinmann pins. The arthroplasty is carried out in the normal fashion, making sure leg lengths are checked. Without the trochanter in place for tensioning of the abductions, excessive lengthening can occur.

Reattachment of the trochanteric fragment can be carried out with wires or cables. Most recommend vertical and horizontal wires (see Figs. 5 and 6). The idea is to resist the forces acting on the trochanteric fragment while providing compression across the osteotomy site. Rotational forces across the osteotomy site in an anteroposterior plane are stronger than the vertical forces. This shearing effect challenges the most intricate reattachment system. Even in the most experienced hands, nonunion remains a problem despite the use of multiple wires, cable, cable grips, and a cable plate system. The four-wire technique seems to be simple and reproducible; however, there is a significant learning curve using monofilament wires. The ability to tension the wires, provide compression across the osteotomy site, and then secure them is an art few surgeons will master. For this reason, cables seem to be

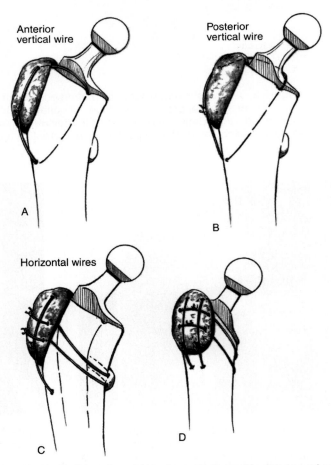

Figure 5. The four-wire technique of trochanteric reattachment is simple and reproducible, and it yields a 97% union rate.

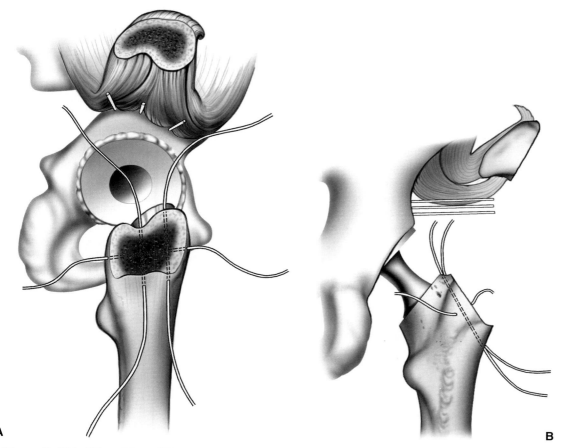

Figure 6. Side **(A)** and front **(B)** views of the hip showing wires passing deep to the trochanteric bed for a three-wire technique.

easier to work with and are easier for the novice to master. However, the use of cables around the hip joint has been fraught with complications as well. There is no evidence that any of these devices changes the rates of nonunion. Some of the newer cable grip plates may have a role in the difficult case when standard techniques have failed (see Fig. 44).

Anterior Trochanteric Osteotomy

Taking advantage of the continuity of the gluteus medius and the vastus lateralis, a slice of the anterior trochanter is removed, leaving the majority of the gluteus medius attached to the remaining trochanter. This is a modification of the Hardinge approach. The exposure is similar; however, the advantage of this modification is the bone-to-bone apposition afforded by the osteotomy. Popularized by Dr. Des Dall (Dall-Miles) and also known as the Liverpool approach (Liverpool, UK), this easily accomplished partial trochanteric osteotomy is an entry-level osteotomy that provides excellent exposure in primary total hip arthroplasty. Dall claims the following advantages:

1. Continuity of the anterior half of the gluteus medius and vastus lateralis prevents superior migration of the fragment.
2. Reattachment is easier than fixation of the entire trochanter.
3. Strength of tendinous attachments is maintained.
4. An intracapsular exposure is optional for additional hip stability.
5. Denervation of muscles is avoided.
6. Power of abductors is preserved.

In the revision setting, this osteotomy may not be adequate; however, it can be converted to a more extensile exposure. Head et al. have published their experience with a similar approach taking a 5-mm slice of the anterior trochanter and extending the incision further distally. The exposure afforded by this anterior trochanteric osteotomy in the simple revision setting may be adequate; however, one must remember that this approach cannot be converted to either a trochanteric slide, conventional trochanteric osteotomy, or extended trochanteric osteotomy. It can, however, be converted to the more extensile Stracathro approach, which will be discussed later.

Another indication for this approach is the patient with a previous Hardinge approach that may have a thin and atrophic anterior attachment of the gluteus medius tendon. Reattachment of a bone fragment is more secure and may prevent compromising this tenuous junction.

A modification of this technique involves leaving the gluteus medius insertion intact and only taking the insertion of the gluteus minimus and vastus lateralis. The advocates of this modification (R. Ganz) claim a more rapid recovery of abductor power and gait. They also claim that by not splitting the gluteus medius tendon, the risk of damaging the superior gluteal nerve is decreased. Exposure may be more difficult with this modification; however, occasionally the gluteus minimus tendon is scarred and contracted. In these cases, the minimus is released to prevent a tethering effect on the fragment. The additional support of the gluteus medius insertion would be important in these cases.

Technique. The incision is made directly over the trochanter with a length from 3 to 7 inches. The use of this osteotomy can be combined with a "minimally invasive approach."

The cutting diathermy is used to divide the gluteus medius and vastus lateralis, leaving one half to three fourths on the posterior portion of the trochanter. The anterior one fourth to one half of the gluteus and vastus extends 2 cm above the trochanter and 3 cm distally. A large curved forceps is passed deep to the gluteus minimus and medius over the capsule exiting proximally in the interval previously developed (see Fig. 7A). A Gigli saw is passed and with the hip adducted, slightly flexed, and internal rotated (Fig. 7B). The fragment should be at least 1 cm thick and should include the insertion of the gluteus medius and minimus as well as the vastus lateralis (Fig. 7). An alternative to the use of the Gigli saw is a standard oscillating saw with a thin kerf blade (see Figs. 8 and 9). One has to be careful not to angle the saw into the femoral neck. The saw blade should follow the contour and anteverted direction of the femoral neck. A modification by Dall recommends including the insertion of the capsule for those cases where instability may be a problem. We have not found it necessary to include the capsule. The fragment with the attached soft tissue is retracted anteriorly and placed under the anterior Charnley retractor carefully to prevent its fracture (see Figs. 10 and 11; see Fig. 7C). The anterior capsule is removed or opened in a T-type fashion. The hip is dislocated in an anterior direction. Arthroplasty is carried out in the normal fashion.

Following reduction of the hip, the fragment will lay in its bed without difficulty. It is attached with no. 5 sutures, cables, or monofilament wires (see Fig. 12). This stable osteotomy can be approximated in many different ways (see Figs. 13–15). Excessive hardware or trochanteric grip devices are not necessary. The use of two cables, wires, or sutures is sufficient. Drill holes in the fragment and through the lateral cortex are sufficient (see Fig. 16). The hardware should not be placed around the neck of the prosthesis. After fixation of the fragment, a repeat of the extremes of motion should be done to ensure adequate stability of the hip and make sure no impingement of the anterior trochanter occurs. Closure and postoperative rehabilitation is routine.

Trochanteric Slide

McFarland and Osborne and Debeyre and Duliveux originally described the advantages of keeping the tendinous portions of the gluteus medius and vastus lateralis intact during exposure of the hip. Unhappy with this soft tissue approach recommended by McFarland and Osborne, English modified this technique to include a portion of the trochanter. Leav-

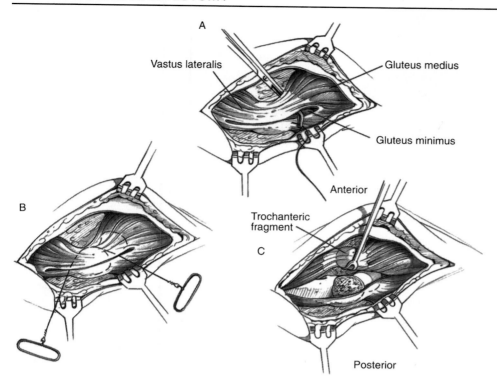

Figure 7. **A:** The Gigli saw is passed deep to the gluteus medius and vastus lateralis insertions. **B:** The hip is adducted, flexed, and internally rotated prior to cutting the fragment. **C:** The trochanteric fragment is retracted anteriorly prior to dislocation.

ing the gluteal and vastus muscle attachments and external rotators intact, English felt that this musculotendinous sleeve would create a compressive force on the osteotomy site, preventing migration and encouraging rapid union. Further modification by Fulkerson et al. was done so that this slide could be performed through an anterior approach. The Keggi slide modification left the posterior cortex intact, and as the femur is brought anterior an "open-book" hinge is created posteriorly. This stable modification requires minimal fixation after reduction since the posterior hinge is kept intact (see Fig. 17).

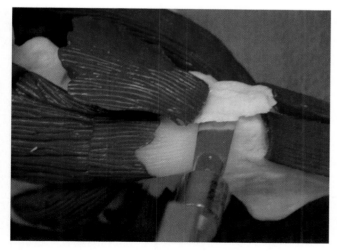

Figure 8. An oscillating saw is used to create a sliver of bone and keep the continuity of the anterior gluteus medius and anterior vastus lateralis.

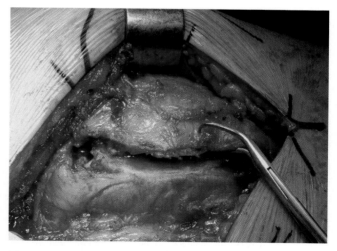

Figure 9. The anterior fragment is controlled with a towel clip and elevated with or without the attachment of the gluteus minimus.

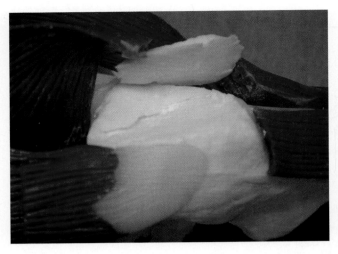

Figure 10. The fragment is now retracted anteriorly, exposing the hip capsule. The fragment can be carefully placed under the Charnley retractor anteriorly.

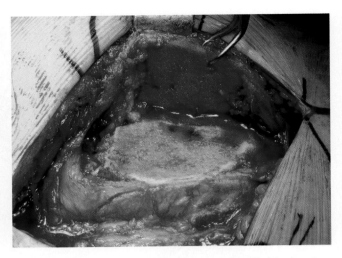

Figure 11. Once the fragment is elevated, a Cobb elevator is used to define the margins of the hip capsule, and the capsule is incised or excised.

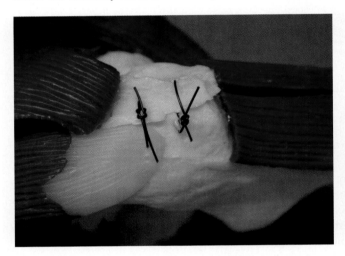

Figure 12. Following completion of the arthroplasty, the osteotomy fragment is secured with no. 5 Ethibond sutures, monofilament wires, or cables.

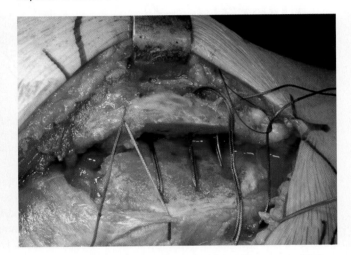

Figure 13. Fixation in this case was done with no. 5 Ethibond sutures. Choice of fixation is up to the surgeon. One may want to consider the cost of a monofilament wire or suture compared to the cost of a cable and crimp.

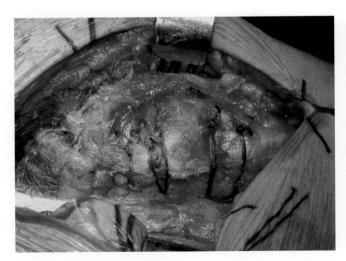

Figure 14. Secure fixation of the trochanteric fragment. Note the sutures placed in the gluteus medius tendon for additional support. Postoperatively, there is no change in the standard protocol of weight bearing as tolerated from day 1.

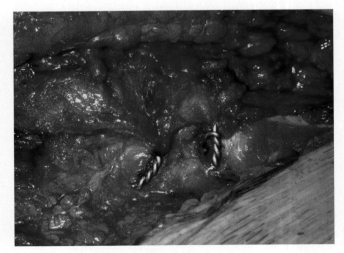

Figure 15. Once the monofilament wires are twisted, they should be turned back on themselves and carefully tapped into the soft tissues.

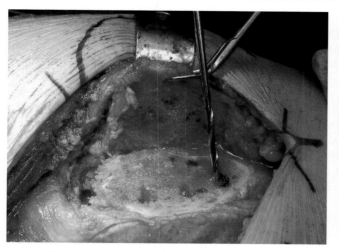
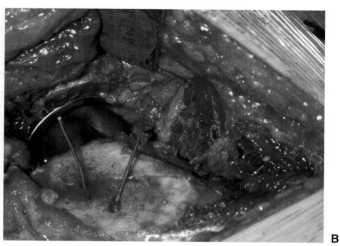

A   B

Figure 16. A: Drill holes made through the cortical margins for repair. Only the lateral cortex needs to be secured with fixation. **B:** Excellent exposure is afforded by this osteotomy. Fixation in this case was done with monofilament wires.

As revision surgery emerged in the 1980s, the need for greater exposure became evident. A. Glassman modified the English technique, taking the external rotators down prior to the osteotomy and reattaching them following reapproximation of the fragment. The trochanteric slide is an excellent technique in difficult primary hip arthroplasty and can be used for exposure during most revision surgery. In the unlikely case that additional exposure is required, the trochanteric slide can be converted to a conventional osteotomy by simply removed the insertion of the vastus lateralis and repairing it at the completion of the case. The striking advantage of this technique over the classic Charnley trochanteric osteotomy is the continuity of the vastus with the gluteus medius and the prevention of the migration of the trochanteric fragment.

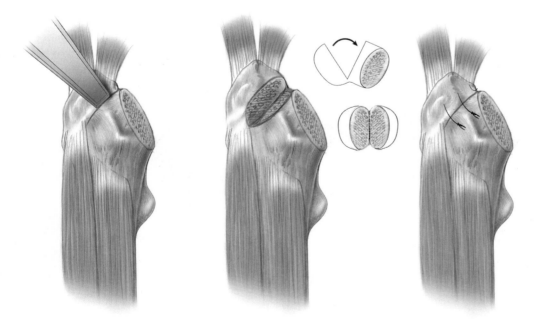

Figure 17. Fulkerson and Keggi described a trochanteric slide modification in 1977 through an anterior approach. The gluteus medius and vastus lateralis remain attached to the trochanteric fragment; however, the trochanter is folded back like an "open book," delivering the proximal femur into the wound.

The indications for a trochanteric slide are the same as for the standard conventional trochanteric osteotomy. Proponents of the classic Charnley trochanteric osteotomy claim that advancement of the trochanter is not possible with the trochanteric slide. Distal advancement is possible up to approximately 1 cm. If additional advancement is required, then the slide can be converted to a traditional osteotomy and advanced further. Trochanteric advancement over 1 cm is noted to have a significant increased rate of nonunion. Another advantage is in the revision setting; should a proximal femoral allograft be required, the trochanteric slide provides the ideal situation for reattachment with its compressive forces acting on the allograft bed. The learning curve with the trochanteric slide is relatively easy as compared to a conventional osteotomy, and fixation is not as crucial since the tethering of the vastus lateralis helps prevent superior migration of the fragment. This may be the "gold standard" for difficult primary and routine revision cases.

Technique. A standard posterior approach is used centered over the trochanter. A bent Hohman retractor is placed just superior to the piriformis tendon. The external rotators are identified, tagged with no. 2 sutures, and cut at their insertion (see Fig. 18). The vastus lateralis is elevated off the femur about 1 cm anterior to the lateral intermuscular septum for a distance of about 5 to 10 cm. A single cobra retractor holds the vastus lateralis anterior (see Fig. 19). An oscillating saw with a thin kerf blade is used beginning posterolateral to the insertion of the gluteus medius (see Figs. 20 and 21). The trochanteric fragment should be at least 1 cm thick proximally tapering to 0.5 cm distally at the level of the vastus ridge (see Figs. 22 and 23). The gluteus minimus may stay attached to the trochanteric fragment. The attachment of the minimus to the osteotomized fragment may tether the fragment anteriorly and can affect external rotation following reattachment. For this reason, leaving the minimus attached to the femur may aid in the exposure. The trochanteric fragment, in continuity with the gluteus medius and vastus lateralis, can now be retracted anteriorly, exposing the hip capsule (see Figs. 24 and 25). The hip pseudocapsule is now excised, and the hip is dislocated either anteriorly or posteriorly on the basis of the pathology, the anatomy, and the surgeon's preference.

An alternative method involves leaving the external rotators and piriformis intact on the posterior trochanter and beginning the osteotomy just lateral to their insertion. This has the advantage of leaving an intact posterior capsule and muscle sling that theoretically may prevent any posterior instability.

Repair is done with wires or cables passed around the femur through separate drill holes and around or through drill holes in the fragment (see Figs. 26 and 27). One of the cables or wires should pass through a separate hole in the lesser trochanter or proximal femur to pre-

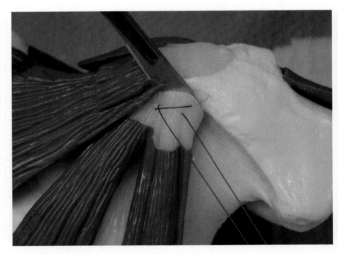

Figure 18. The posterior approach is utilized, and the external rotators are isolated, tagged, and released from their insertion on the trochanter.

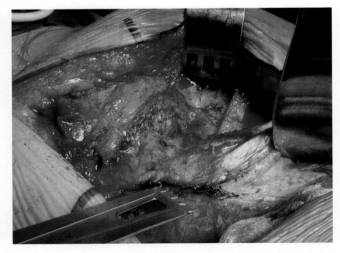

Figure 19. The vastus lateralis is elevated off the lateral femur prior to the osteotomy. A cobra retractor keeps tension on the soft tissues.

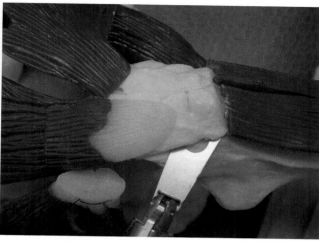

A

B

Figure 20. A thin kerf blade is directed anteriorly, keeping the insertions of the vastus lateralis and gluteus medius and minimus attached to the fragment.

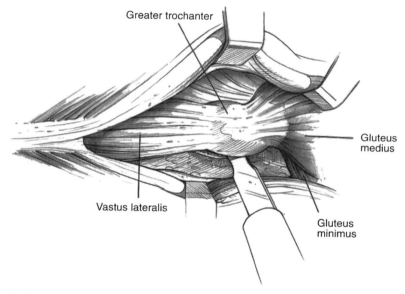

Greater trochanter

Gluteus medius

Vastus lateralis

Gluteus minimus

Figure 21. The sliding trochanteric osteotomy performed with an oscillating saw, keeping the insertions of the vastus lateralis and gluteus medius in continuity.

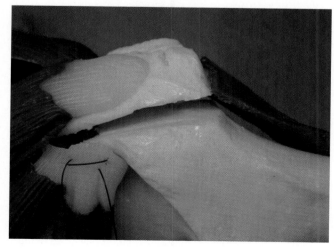

Figure 22. The fragment is now displaced anteriorly with the soft tissue attachments intact.

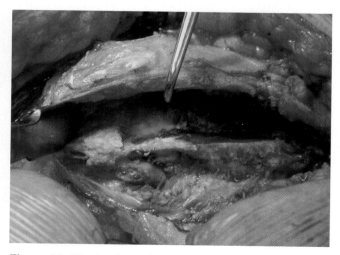

Figure 23. The trochanteric fragment is now elevated with a bone hook, exposing the back of the femoral prosthesis.

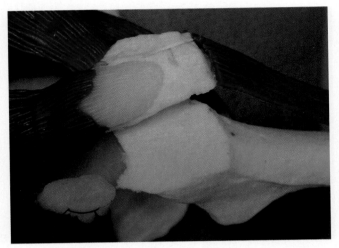

Figure 24. Dislocation can now occur anteriorly or posteriorly on the basis of the exposure required and the surgeon's preference.

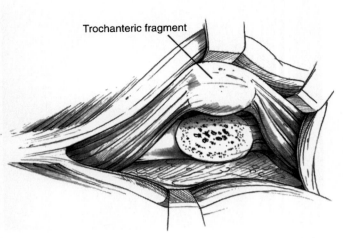

Figure 25. The trochanteric fragment can now be retracted anteriorly, exposing the hip joint.

vent migration. A trochanteric grip device is not generally required unless significant lengthening occurs and reapproximation to the original bed is not possible (see Figs. 28 and 29).

No special precautions are necessary postoperatively; weight bearing as tolerated is allowed on the basis of the stability of the construct and method of fixation.

Extended Trochanteric Osteotomy

Removal of well-fixed implants from the femur can be extremely difficult, time-consuming, and is occasionally a disastrous undertaking. Standard osteotomies (including the trochanteric slide) do not give adequate exposure of the more distal cementless interfaces or to the cement mantle distally. Although the trochanteric slide gives some access proximally, its usefulness is limited for the cemented or cementless implant that is well fixed distal to the trochanteric ridge. When access to the femoral canal is required in a precise, controlled fashion, the extended proximal femoral osteotomy combines the advantages of an extremely wide exposure of component interfaces with the preservation of soft

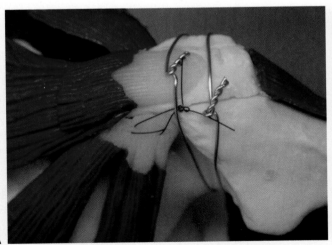

A

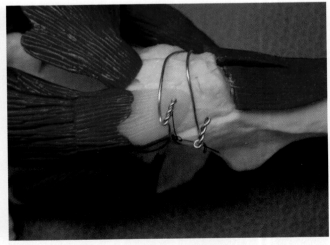

B

Figure 26. Repair of the trochanteric slide requires cerclage wires or cables and a secure repair of the external rotators through separate drill holes in the bone. Although not depicted in the photos above, the cerclage wires should be placed through separate drill holes in the lesser trochanter and the medial femoral shaft to prevent "bucket-handling" of the wires.

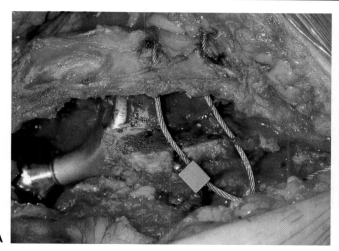

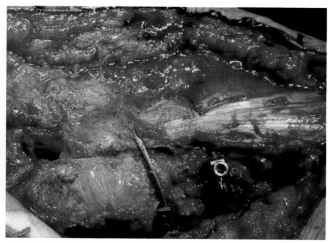

A   B

Figure 27. Following completion of the hip reconstruction, the trochanteric fragment is reapproximated with the use of two circumferential cables. These should be placed through separate drill holes in the lesser trochanter and femoral shaft. Placing drill holes in the fragment as seen in **A** may prevent an anatomic reduction unless corresponding holes are made anteriorly and posteriorly in the cortical margins of the host femur. The photo on the right **(B)** does not have the drill holes in the fragment, and note passage of the cables beneath the vastus lateralis and soft tissues. Should the trochanteric fragment not seat properly, the Midas Rex with an acorn-type burr may be necessary to contour the fragment appropriately. Following repair and before the cables or wires are finally secured, a full range of motion should be checked to make sure no anterior or posterior impingement exists.

tissue attachments to the osteotomized fragment of bone. As noted in the previous trochanteric exposures, the abductor-vastus sleeve remains intact. Once the component is removed, the femur can be reamed to accept a distally fixed prosthesis, and the trochanteric segment is machined to fit precisely back into place.

The indications for the extended trochanteric osteotomy include (a) removal of a well-fixed cemented or cementless femoral component, (b) proximal-medial bone loss in which cerclage cables/wires would abrade the femoral component directly, (c) osteoporotic or os-

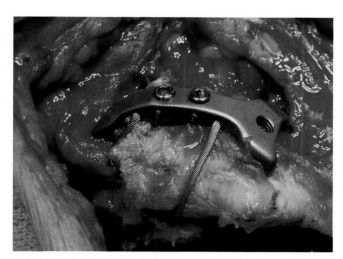

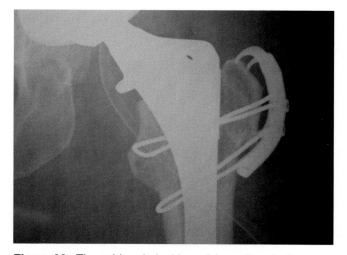

Figure 28. The use of a cable grip system is usually not necessary; however, should the fragment be compromised or the host bone bed be osteoporotic, this device may be of benefit in providing more secure fixation.

Figure 29. The cable grip in this revision arthroplasty was used to advance the trochanteric fragment. The proximal claws are designed to fit over the trochanter and not into the soft bone as shown. The curve on this particular design is not ideal in this case since the distal part of the claw is abutting against the femoral shaft. The claw should fit snugly on the fragment if possible.

teolytic trochanter that is not amenable to a trochanteric osteotomy or slide and would benefit from diaphyseal cerclage fixation, and (d) correction of any angular deformity of the proximal femur.

Clearly, this osteotomy popularized by W. Paprosky has taken the most difficult revision cases and made them manageable by the occasional revision surgeon. This osteotomy is a "must know" if removal of well-fixed femoral components is anticipated. Many times, what appears to be a loose femoral component, either by clinical exam or radiographically, one finds to be a well-fixed albeit subsided stem. Being prepared is a must.

Technique. The standard technique begins with a posterior approach; however, an anterolateral exposure can be done as well using the same principles described below. The osteotomy extends from the tip of the trochanter to a predetermined point distal to the vastus tubercle where the horizontal portion of the osteotomy is done. This distance is usually at least 5 cm from the trochanteric ridge, so that at least two cerclage wires/cables can be used to secure the diaphyseal portion of the osteotomized fragment. Using the posterior approach, the leg is held in internal rotation, exposing the vastus lateralis and external rotators. The external rotators are tagged with no. 2 Ticron sutures and retracted in a posterior direction, protecting the sciatic nerve from harm. The insertion of the gluteus maximus is released with the electrocautery. The hip capsule and scar tissue are excised, and the hip is dislocated in a posterior direction. Alternatively, the hip can remain located, and the osteotomy can be performed in a similar fashion with the stem in situ. The vastus lateralis is separated from its insertion on the linea aspera and held forward with a cobra retractor. Care should be taken not to strip the long trochanteric fragment of its soft tissue attachments, so depriving it of blood supply. Preoperative templating will assist in determining the extent of the osteotomy (see Fig. 30). One must make sure that 4 to 6 cm of host diaphysis remains intact so that a secure press fit can be obtained with the new revision prosthesis. In the unlikely event that the stem is loose and access to the canal is still required for cement removal, the femoral component can be utilized as a guide.

The osteotomy begins at the base of the trochanter and extends distally, and it is marked with the electrocautery staying just anterior to the linea aspera (see Figs. 31 and 32). A high-speed pencil tip burr (Midas Rex with TU-10) is used to make multiple perforations along the femoral shaft, and if possible, the anterolateral cortex is perforated as well (see Figs. 33–35). A short, thin kerf saw blade can also be used (see Fig. 36). A portion of bone representing at least one third of the femoral shaft is desired. Distally, the horizontal portion of the osteotomy is completed with the Midas Rex, taking care to round the corners to prevent a 90-degree stress riser (see Fig. 37). Multiple wide-curved or flat osteotomes are

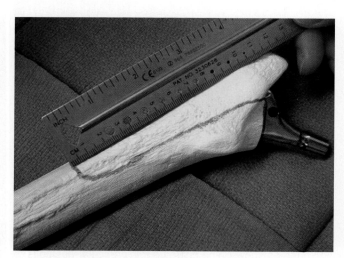

Figure 30. The length of the proposed osteotomy is measured off the preoperative radiograph from the tip of the trochanter distal.

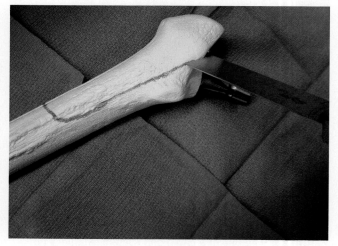

Figure 31. The proximal portion of the extended trochanteric osteotomy can be started with the oscillating saw.

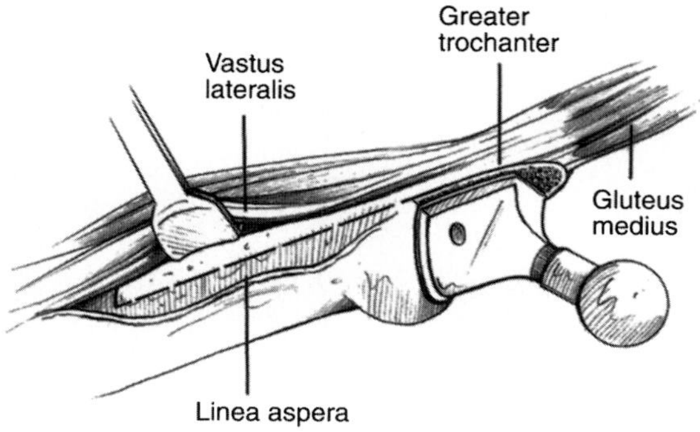

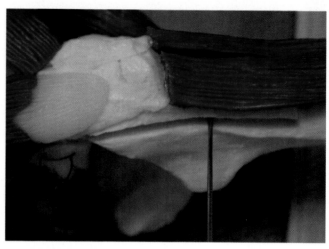

Figure 32. The extended trochanteric osteotomy begins with elevating the vastus lateralis off the shaft of the femur.

Figure 33. The anterior cortex should be perforated with multiple drill holes using either a 2.5-mm drill bit or the Midas Rex with a long TU-10 pencil tip and a short protective shroud.

passed posterior to anterior, and the anterolateral cortex is cracked at the previously placed perforations while hinging on the soft tissues (see Figs. 38 and 39). The proximal extent of the anterolateral cortex is usually cut with the saw as the burr rarely reaches that distance (Fig. 34). The gluteus medius, gluteus minimus, and vastus lateralis remain attached to the trochanter and lateral femoral osteotomy segment, which is now retracted in an anterior direction see (Figs. 40 and 41). Direct access to the femoral component interface and femoral canal is now possible. In performing this osteotomy in a patient with a well-fixed full-coat implant, a separate limited exposure anterolateral may be necessary to perforate the cortex. Care must be taken not to strip the vastus lateralis off the femur.

Following insertion of the revision prosthesis, the trochanteric fragment is fitted to the lateral shoulder of the implant. This is a crucial step, and the use of a high-speed acorn-type burr should be used to remove any impinging bone or retained cement. Multiple cable or monofilament wires (minimum two/maximum four) are used to secure the fragment to the proximal femur (see Figs. 42 and 43). The fragment is secured at shaft portion only if possible. Limited fixation around the trochanter proper may prevent complications that have

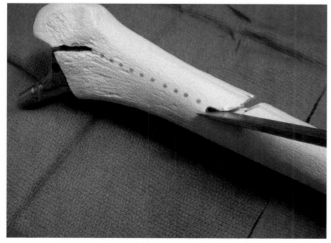

Figure 34. The anterior portion of the osteotomy is perforated with the Midas Rex (TU-10) or with a 3.2-mm-long drill bit. The osteotomy is slid from distal to proximal connecting the perforations.

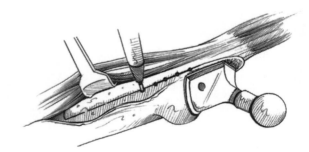

Figure 35. A high-speed burr is used to make multiple perforations from the base of the trochanter distally, staying just anterior to the linea aspera and perforating the anterolateral cortex.

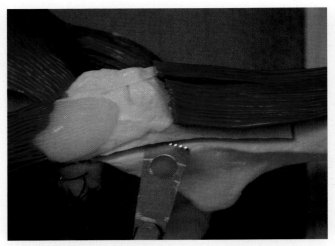

Figure 36. A thin kerf blade is used to perform the osteotomy posteriorly just above the linea aspera. If the retained femoral component in this case is only proximally coated, a short extended trochanteric osteotomy is performed.

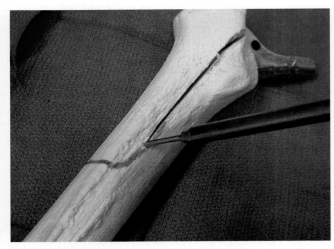

Figure 37. The Midas Rex is used to round the distal extent of the osteotomy, preventing a stress riser and a possible crack that could extend down the shaft of the femur.

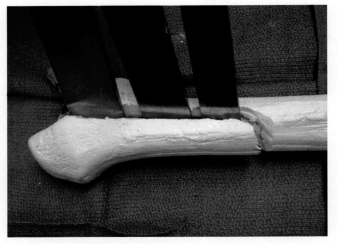

Figure 38. Multiple flat osteotomes are used to pry the osteotomy open.

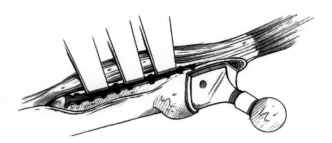

Figure 39. Wide osteotomes are now passed from posterior to anterior, cracking the perforated anterior cortex.

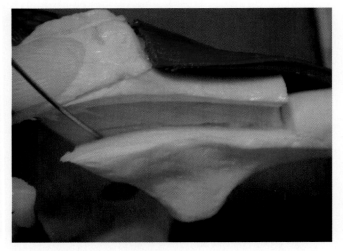

Figure 40. The trochanteric fragment along with its soft tissue attachments is now retracted anteriorly, gaining access to the proximal femoral canal.

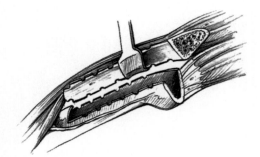

Figure 41. The gluteus medius, gluteus minimus, and vastus lateralis remain attached to the trochanter and osteotomy segment, which is retracted anteriorly as a separate unit.

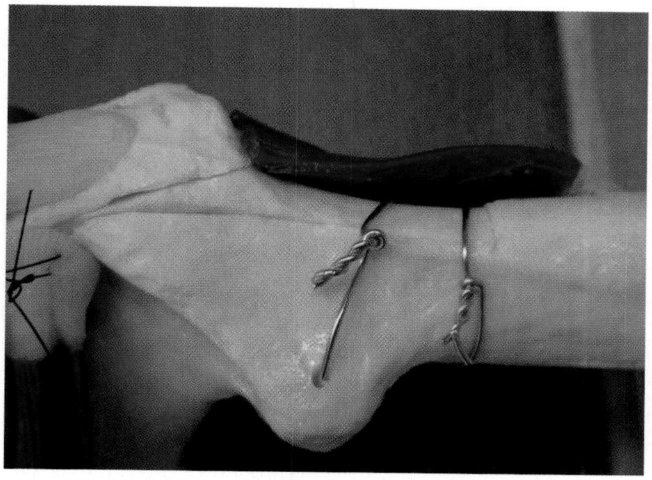

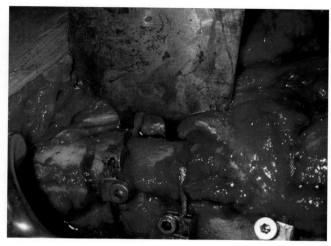

Figure 42. Repair is done with cerclage wires or cables around the shaft portion of the fragment with at least one cable/wire through a separate drill hole in the lesser trochanter. No fixation is generally necessary around the trochanter proper. Note repair of the external rotators back to their anatomic position. The use of a cable plate device is generally not required in these cases.

Figure 43. Cerclage cables secure this extended trochanteric osteotomy. The distal portion of the osteotomy fragment can be shortened if necessary to advance the abductor mechanism.

been reported with cables/wires that fray or break and migrate to the hip articulation. Prior to tightening the cables or wires, the hip should be relocated and placed through a complete range of motion. Any impingement of the trochanter will need to be addressed. The fragment can be shifted posteriorly or anteriorly if necessary. Should soft tissue tensioning be necessary, the distal portion of the osteotomy fragment can be trimmed, advancing the entire musculo-osseous sleeve distally. Cancellous bone graft can be placed along the posterior and distal osteotomy junction.

Should you elect to use a cemented revision stem, the technique is somewhat different. The trochanteric osteotomy should be secured in place prior to cementing of the stem. To prevent extrusion of the cement into the osteotomy site, Gelfoam can be utilized followed by standard fixation of the trochanteric fragment. A trial of the femoral stem should be performed, and impingement should be evaluated prior to cementing of the prosthesis.

Although this osteotomy was originally designed for a posterior approach, a similar technique can be performed from an anterolateral plane as well, taking great care to protect the sciatic nerve from injury. Caution should be exercised in trying this from an anterolateral or modified direct lateral approach as the incidence of trochanteric fracture and trochanteric escape has been reported to be higher than from the posterior approach.

Postoperatively, patients remain partial weight bearing for 8 to 12 weeks until the osteotomy site has healed. No abduction orthosis is necessary unless stability of the components is in question.

Fixation Options

The decision as to how to secure the trochanteric fragment has been the subject of much debate. The classic Charnley trochanteric osteotomy was secured with a variety of different wiring methods. No agreement could be reached on a reproducible method to secure the trochanter to its host bone bed, nor could a decision be made on whether to twist the wire or use a square knot. Every conceivable variation has been tried, and many authors have refined their particular technique (see *Master Techniques in Orthopaedic Surgery: The Hip*, 1st ed., Chapter 3). The introduction of cables and claw devices was thought to be a vast improvement over previous techniques. Designer series reports were impressive, although rarely reproducible. Although somewhat easier to use than monofilament wire, cable debris, cable breakage, and nonunion rates appeared to remain a major problem. Clearly, the message is as follows: There is a race between healing of the osteotomy site and breakage of the device. Larger grips, bigger cables, and thicker bolts do not guarantee union of the osteotomy. A large, healthy bleeding cancellous bed with a trochanteric fragment that is not under extreme tension is the best case scenario for healing. Even in this case, union rates are not 100%. Any compromise to the trochanteric fragment or cancellous bed will decrease union rates.

The type of fixation a surgeon chooses in securing the osteotomy should be based on several factors: (a) quality of the trochanteric fragment and host bone, (b) amount of tension on the trochanteric fragment, (c) structural integrity of the proximal femur, and (d) the surgeon's experience and expertise with fixation devices.

Fixation of the osteotomy types discussed in this chapter can be done with standard monofilament wire. Either 16- or 18-gauge cobalt chrome wire is appropriate. Stainless steel is not recommended any longer because of newer femoral components being manufactured from cobalt chrome alloys. In a fluid environment, this combination of metals creates concern. Doubling the wire increases the strength further. Twisting the wire without it breaking is somewhat of an art even with the use of various commercially available wire twisters. Although the use of a square knot is a stronger construct, it can be difficult to keep tension on the knot after the first throw. Any nicks or kinks in the wire can decrease the overall strength dramatically. Beaded monofilament wires may lessen the likelihood of the surgeon puncturing his or her glove or finger during wire placement. This is certainly of concern in light of the increasing numbers of high-risk patients with HIV or hepatitis B/C.

Should handling of the monofilament wire be problematic, then the use of cables is certainly acceptable. Should cables be used, certain precautions should be taken:

1. The cable tensioning devices can exert a tremendous amount of pressure around the fragment, and one has to be sure the cable does not cut through the proximal femur or fracture the trochanteric fragment.
2. The cables should not be placed where they may rub against the femoral stem since the debris generated would rapidly destroy the articulation.
3. The cable sleeves should be placed anterior or posterior since they have a tendency to cause a local bursitis.
4. The cables should be placed beneath the soft tissues and placed through drill holes in the lesser trochanter and medial cortical shaft.
5. The free ends of the cables should be cut nearly flush with the surface of the crimp sleeve to prevent any possibility of the cable ends fraying and breaking, sending the tiny fragments to the joint articulation.

Cable grip or claw devices have been used successfully over the past 15 years by many surgeons. The indications to use this type of device are not clear. Should you encounter a trochanteric fragment that has a poor host bed, is somewhat tenuous, and for which fixation is not possible with standard cerclage wiring, then a claw device may be an asset. If undue tension is encountered and you find that abduction of the leg is required to approximate the fragment to its host bed, then a cable grip may be required. Should you decide to use a claw, it is important to use drill holes through the lesser trochanter and proximal femur and keep a 45-degree distal angle for this. The cables should be separated by at least 2 to 3 cm to prevent "'bucket-handling" of the device. With the occasional patient for whom trochanteric advancement is necessary, a claw may provide additional stability. The early use of these devices has been fraught with complications, including cable breakage, fraying and fragmentation with small pieces of the cables traveling to the hip joint causing third-body wear, and early catastrophic failure of the arthroplasty.

Newer designed cable plates extend down the shaft of the femur and allow traverse cerclage cabling. In addition to providing femoral shaft fixation, more secure fixation of the fragment may help prevent nonunion and escape of the trochanteric fragment (see Fig. 44); however, most of these devices are bulky and may cause a certain amount of trochanteric bursitis. They ultimately may require removal. Again, the indication for the use of these claw type plates is unclear at this time.

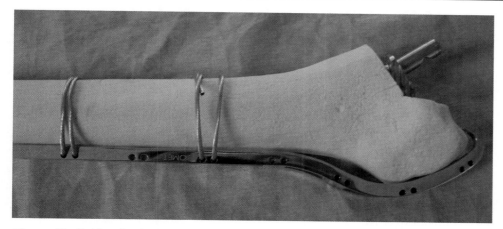

Figure 44. Cable grip plate. This prototype of a cable grip plate enabled traverse wires to be placed around the shaft of the femur securing the trochanteric fragment. Since this prototype was designed by the author, many variations are now available.

COMPLICATIONS

Nonunion remains the most common complication following trochanteric osteotomy. Should the nonunion result in trochanteric escape, a painful limp and possibly dislocation may occur. Nonunion rates range from about 5% to 30% in the revision setting. Although several authors have reported rates lower than this, most surgeons are unable to attain rates less than 5% even in the most experienced hands. For surgeons with less experience, the rate of nonunion is two to three times higher.

Although cables and cable devices remain very popular and offer several advantages over the use of monofilament wire, their history of problems cannot be ignored. Early designs had problems with cable debris that migrated to the joint and would cause accelerated wear of the arthroplasty. In addition, cable breakage and lysis around the lesser trochanter caused considerable alarm. Newer designed cables and cable cutters have virtually eliminated these problems. In addition, newer designed cable plates provide for additional transverse wire or cable placement along the shaft of the femur. However, no studies currently have shown that the newer designs of cables or cable plate devices have changed the rate of nonunion.

Trochanteric bursitis is probably the second most common complication following trochanteric osteotomy. Prominence of the hardware may be the cause in many of the cases; however, studies have shown that even after removal of the hardware, the pain persists. The use of newer, lower-profile cable plate devices may lessen the incidence of bursitis.

SUMMARY

The visualization afforded by removal of a portion or all of the trochanter is something of which every surgeon should avail himself or herself. It makes the most difficult cases more manageable and tolerable. Struggling through the difficult primary total hip or revision with poor visualization creates havoc for the surgeon and the patient. The general orthopaedic surgeon should have trochanteric osteotomy as part of his armamentarium. Complications relating to the fixation devices should not deter one from utilizing this technique in the appropriate setting.

RECOMMENDED READING

1. Archibeck MJ, Rosenberg AG, Berger RA, Silverton CD. Trochanteric osteotomy and fixation during total hip arthroplasty. *J Am Acad Orthop Surg* 11(3):163–173, 2003.

2. Aribindi R, Paprosky W, Nourbash P, et al. Extended proximal femoral osteotomy. *Instr Course Lect* 48:19–26, 1999.
3. Blackley HR, Rorabeck CH. Extensile exposures for revision hip arthroplasty. *Clin Orthop Relat Res* 381:77–87, 2000.
4. Charnley J. *Low Friction Arthroplasty*. Berlin: Springer Verlag, 1979.
5. Chen W, McAuley JP, Engh CA, et al. Extended slide trochanteric osteotomy for revision total hip arthroplasty. *J Bone Joint Surg* 82-A:1215–1219, 2000.
6. Dall D. Exposure of the hip by anterior osteotomy of the greater trochanter: a modified anterolateral approach. *J Bone Joint Surg* 68-B:382–386, 1986.
7. Debeyre J, Duliveux P. *Les Arthroplasties de la Hanche: Etude Critique a propos de 200 Cas Operes*. Paris: Editions Medicales Flammarion, 1954.
8. Della Valle CJ, Berger RA, Rosenberg AG, et al. Extended trochanteric osteotomy in complex total hip arthroplasty. *J Bone Joint Surg* 85-A:2385–2390, 2003.
9. English TA. The trochanteric approach to the hip for prosthetic replacement. *J Bone Joint Surg* 57A:1128–1132, 1975.
10. Fulkerson JP, Crelin ES, Keggi KJ. Anatomy and osteotomy of the greater trochanter. *Arch Surg* 114:19–21, 1979.
11. Head WC, Mallory TH, Berklacich FM, et al. Extensile exposure of the hip for revision arthroplasty. *J Arthroplasty* 2(4):265–273, 1987.
12. Langlais F, Lambotte JC, Collin P, et al. Trochanteric slide osteotomy in revision total hip arthroplasty for loosening. *J Bone Joint Surg* 85-B:510–516, 2003.
13. Masri BA, Campbell DG, Garbuz DS, Duncan CP. Seven specialized exposures for revision hip and knee replacement. *Orthop Clin North Am* 29:229–240, 1998.
14. Masterson EL, Masri BA, Duncan CP. Surgical approaches in revision hip replacement. *J Am Acad Orthop Surg* 6(2):84–92, 1998.
15. McFarland G, Osborne G. Approach to the hip: a suggested improvement on Kochers method. *J Bone Joint Surg* 36B:364, 1954.
16. McGory BJ, Bal SB, Harris WH. Trochanteric osteotomy for total hip arthroplasty: six variations and indications for their use. *J Am Acad Orthop Surg* 4(5):258–267, 1996.
17. Miner TM, Momberger NG, Chong D, Paprosky WL. The extended trochanteric osteotomy in revision hip arthroplasty: a critical review of 166 cases at mean 3-year, 9-month follow-up. *J Arthroplasty* 16:188–94, 2001.
18. Nezry N, Jeanrot C, Vinh TS, et al. Partial anterior trochanteric osteotomy in total hip arthroplasty: surgical technique and preliminary results of 127 cases. *J Arthroplasty* 18(3):333–337 2003.
19. Peter PC Jr, Head WC, Emerson RH Jr. An extended trochanteric osteotomy for revision total hip replacement. *J Bone Joint Surg* 75-B:158–159, 1993.
20. Silverton CD, Rosenberg AG. Management of the trochanter. In: *The Adult Hip*, Philadelphia: Lippincott Williams & Wilkins; 1998, 1269–1294.
21. Silverton CD, Jacobs JJ, Rosenberg AG, et al. Complications of a cable grip system. *J Arthroplasty* 11:400–404, 1996.
22. Sledge CB. *Master Techniques in Orthopaedic Surgery: The Hip*. 1st ed. Philadelphia: Lippincott Williams & Wilkins, 1998.
23. Younger TI, Bradford MS, Magnus RE, Paprosky WG. Extended proximal femoral osteotomy: a new technique for femoral revision arthroplasty. *J Arthroplasty* 10(3):329–338, 1995.

5

Retroperitoneal Approach for Revision Total Hip Arthroplasty

Sanaz Hariri and Harry E. Rubash

INDICATIONS

The proximity of pelvic and femoral nerves and vessels and urologic structures to the operative field during revision total hip arthroplasty (THA) may lead to rare but potentially serious complications. Vascular structures particularly at risk during revision THA include external iliac, common femoral, profundus femoris, obturator, superior and inferior gluteal, and internal pudendal arteries and veins. Neural structures at risk include sciatic, peroneal, femoral, and obturator nerves (1).

The locations of these structures can best be conceptualized using the acetabular quadrant system. Four quadrants are formed by drawing one line down from the anterior superior iliac spine (ASIS) that divides the acetabulum into equal halves; draw a second line perpendicular to the first at its midpoint. Areas of maximal danger for each structure are as follows: external iliac vessels in the anterior superior quadrant, the obturator nerves and vessels in the anterior inferior quadrant, the sciatic and superior gluteal nerve and vessels in the posterior superior quadrant, and inferior gluteal and internal pudendal structures in the posterior inferior quadrant (2).

In 1990, Shoenfeld et al. performed a Medline search to identify vascular injuries associated with THAs. In addition to their own 5 case studies, they found 63 more cases in the literature. Thirty-nine percent of the procedures were revision THAs. The most common injuries were to the external iliac and common femoral arteries. The injuries included 17 pseudoaneurysms, 31 thromboembolic complications, 18 vessel lacerations, and 2 traumatic arteriovenous fistulas. The most common causes of the injuries were as follows: 30 cement related, 12 due to retractor trauma, 7 due to excessive traction, and 5 due to intrapelvic migration of the acetabular component. Nearly half of these injuries necessitated emergent vascular surgery interventions. Seven percent of the patients died, 15% required major amputations, and 4% required minor amputations (3).

Giacchetto and Gallagher reviewed 56 case reports of vascular injuries following THAs. Seventeen of these cases were due to gradual intimal erosion by bone cement spicules in contact with major arteries. Fifteen of these cases were due to direct arterial injury from retractors. Six cases were due to protrusion of the prosthetic socket and subsequent impingement of the internal or external iliac arteries or external iliac vein. Other mechanisms included excess cement spilling over the anterior wall of the acetabulum or extruding into the pelvis via drill holes, fractures, or other medial wall deficiencies. Three patients developed claudication, one had persistent neuralgia of the great toe, three had resection arthroplasties, six required either below- or above-knee amputations, two had hip disarticulation, and four had related deaths (4).

The indications for an inguinal retroperitoneal approach to the pelvis in THAs are not well defined in the literature. In their own case study, Giacchetto and Gallagher found a pseudoaneurysm of the common femoral artery on arteriography in a patient after revision of a protrusio acetabulum component with a threaded socket. They used a combined inguinal and retroperitoneal approach to dissect the aneurysm (4). In contrast, al-Salman et al. advocated a "medial extraperitoneal exposure" for revision THA patients with a pelvic mass, pelvic pain, radiographic evidence of cement or the acetabular prosthesis in the pelvis, computed tomographic evidence of cement in the pelvis or proximity of the prosthesis to the iliac vessels, or an arteriography showing displacement or compression of the iliac vessels. In all of these cases, they obtained extraperitoneal medial exposure, mobilized and repaired the iliac vessels, and then revised the hip prosthesis (5).

Eftekhar and Nercessian incorporated the inguinal retroperitoneal approach in their two-stage approach to removing a prosthesis that has migrated into the pelvis (i.e., migration of the cup and cement medial to the iliopectineal line of the pelvis). In the first stage, they remove the femoral component and cement through a lateral transtrochanteric approach. Then, through an abdominal-retroperitoneal approach allowing exposure of the major intrapelvic structures, they remove the acetabular component and apply bone grafts to the pelvis. They found that intrapelvic visualization was particularly important, as in every patient severe scarring around the acetabular component was found. Invariably, the bladder, the ipsilateral ureter, and/or one or more nerves in the region (femoral, genitofemoral, or obturator) were adherent to the scar tissue. Between the two stages, the patient is first placed in traction and then allowed to walk but is made non–weight bearing on the operative limb. In the second stage, 9 to 12 months later, they perform the hip replacement (6). Currently, most surgeons perform this procedure in a single stage.

There are intraoperative (as opposed to preoperative) indications for a retroperitoneal approach to the pelvis reported in the literature. Scullin et al. reported on a patient with vigorous arterial bleeding during a revision THA. During the procedure, a large hematoma was evacuated. When they removed the Hohman retractor from the medial femoral neck, they could not locate and stop the vigorous arterial bleeding through the Watson-Jones approach. Even with clamping of the common femoral, profunda femoris, and superficial femoral arteries via a separate anterior approach, they were still unable to control the bleeding. Finally, they performed a retroperitoneal flank incision, the common iliac artery was bluntly dissected and clamped, and the bleeding immediately stopped. On examination, they found a 12-cm false aneurysm and defect of the external iliac artery with a small spicule of cement from the protruding acetabular component eroding into it (7).

Brentlinger and Hunter reported on a patient with acute hemorrhagic cystitis and abdominal pain 10 years after a THA. After various studies, it was thought that his protruded acetabular component was blocking the ureter. Intraoperatively, immediately after manipulation of the acetabular component, massive intrapelvic bleeding was encountered. While local pressure was applied to the socket to control the bleeding, a retroperitoneal approach was made to the abdomen, revealing a large erosion of the external iliac artery and a large pelvic hematoma. They evacuated the hematoma and removed both the acetabular component and cement without complications (8). Thus, while vascular injuries are uncommon, the surgeon should be familiar with the intrapelvic exposure to control a potentially life-threatening situation.

Described below is a one-stage retroperitoneal approach for revision THA both for patients deemed preoperatively to be at risk for vascular injury and for those who need rapid access to and control of vessels intraoperatively. Using a single-stage approach eliminates the morbidity and expense of a second exposure while also avoiding the scarring and limb shortening due to the interval period of pseudoarthrosis between the two stages.

During revision THAs, injury to the pelvic vasculature may result in devastating sequelae, including amputation and death. Accessing and gaining control of major vessels via an intrapelvic approach before turning one's attention to the prosthesis affords the surgeon the ability to expediently halt blood loss during the time it takes to begin a vascular repair. This chapter describes preoperative planning, surgical technique, postoperative care, and potential complications of a retroperitoneal approach for revision THA.

PREOPERATIVE PLANNING

If plain films demonstrate both (1) violation of the medial acetabular wall by cement, the prosthetic acetabular component, or screws and (2) no medial osseous rim separating these components from the intrapelvic contents, pelvic computed tomography (CT) should be considered (see Figs. 1 and 2). Review the scan to determine the location and amount of

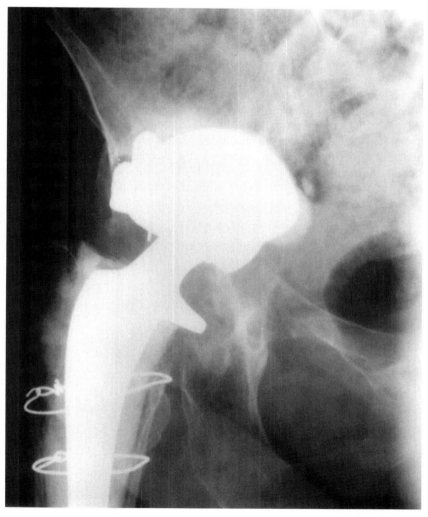

Figure 1. A preoperative anteroposterior plain film of a patient with medial migration of the acetabular component and no visualized medial quadrilateral plate. (From Petrera P, Trakru S, Mehta S, et al. Revision total hip arthroplasty with a retroperitoneal approach to the iliac vessels. *J Arthroplasty* 11:707, 1996, copyright 1996, with permission from Elsevier.)

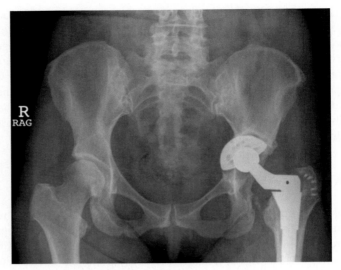

Figure 2. A protrusio left total hip arthroplasty is evident on this preoperative radiograph. There are radiolucencies almost circumferentially around the acetabular component.

intrapelvic cement, the proximity of the cement or screws to the iliac vessels and viscera, the extent of medial bone loss and protrusion, and the presence of anterior or posterior column deficiencies (see Fig. 3). The anteroposterior diameter of the acetabular bed can also be measured to allow for preoperative assessment of component sizing. In cases in which the CT demonstrates direct juxtaposition of cement, the acetabular component, or a screw with a vessel without an intervening osseous rim, a preoperative magnetic resonance angiogram and vascular surgery consult should be considered.

The external iliac vein and, more commonly, the external iliac artery are at particular risk for injury during revision as these vessels may have been shortened by contracture or tethered by scar. In patients with preexisting atherosclerotic disease, a thrombus or

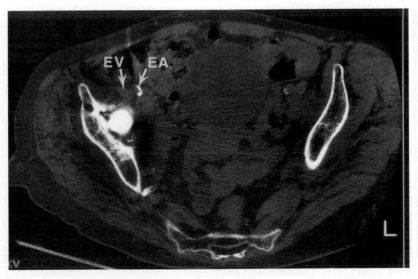

Figure 3. Computed tomography scan preoperatively shows a deficient right medial acetabular wall and anterior column. The external iliac artery *(EA)* and vein *(EV)* are just adjacent to the acetabular component. (From Petrera P, Trakru S, Mehta S, et al. Revision total hip arthroplasty with a retroperitoneal approach to the iliac vessels. *J Arthroplasty* 11:707, 1996, copyright 1996, with permission from Elsevier.)

embolus may lead to limb ischemia and infarction, respectively. In trying to avoid such a complication, patients with vascular disease should be assessed preoperatively with a Doppler. Those with pressure at the ankle of less than 50 mm Hg and those with clinical evidence of ischemia should see a vascular consultant preoperatively (1).

If parts of the urinary tract appear involved on imaging, a preoperative urology consult should also be requested.

SURGICAL TECHNIQUE

After induction of general anesthesia, the bladder is decompressed with a Foley catheter. Thigh-high thrombosis embolic deterrent stockings (TEDS) and a sequential compression device (SCD) are applied to the nonoperative side. The patient is rolled into a lateral decubitus position maintained with a beanbag and two padded kidney rests. The posterior kidney rest is then inched back just enough for a "floppy" lateral position. As usual, proper padding is essential to protect nerves and bony prominences on the dependent extremity.

The boundaries of the skin prep are 2 cm past the midumbilical line anteriorly, to the posterior superior iliac line posteriorly, to the thorax proximally, and distally far enough to include the entire operative extremity.

Start the curvilinear incision 3 cm medial to the anterior superior iliac spine (ASIS), leaving sufficient abdominal muscle for closure at the end of the case. Proceed medially to the femoral pulse just proximal to the inguinal ligament (see Fig. 4).

Divide the skin and subcutaneous tissue, then the external and internal obliques, and finally the transversus abdominis to enter the retroperitoneum (see Figs. 5 and 6). Dissect the external iliac vein and artery (vein lies posterior to the artery) free of the surrounding soft tissue. Expose, ligate, and divide the lateral branches of the iliac artery and vein that perforate the periacetabular area (see Fig. 7). Otherwise, these vessels are at risk for avulsion during implant or cement extraction.

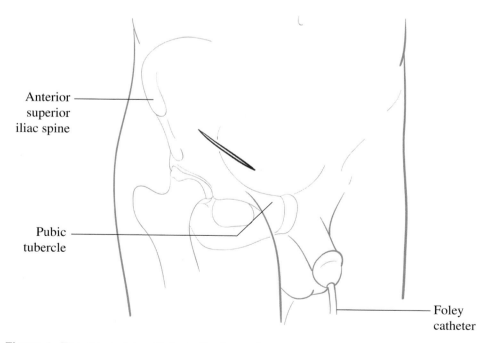

Figure 4. The skin incision. Palpate the femoral artery pulse to determine the incision's medial extent.

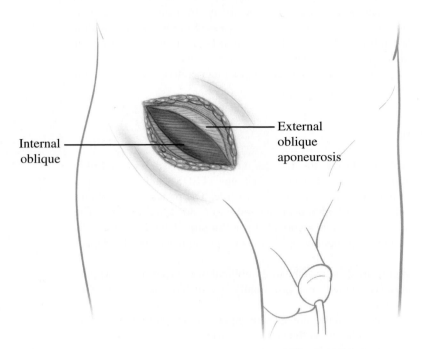

Figure 5. The external oblique aponeurosis has been incised revealing the internal oblique.

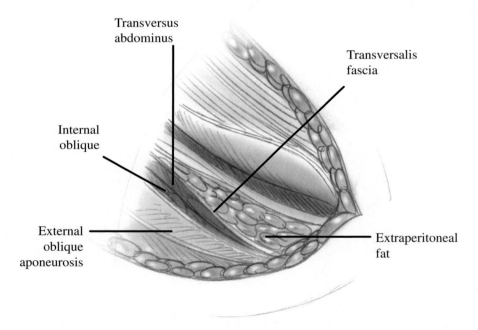

Figure 6. The extraperitoneal fat is exposed after sequential incisions through the external oblique, internal oblique, transversus abdominis, and finally the transversalis fascia.

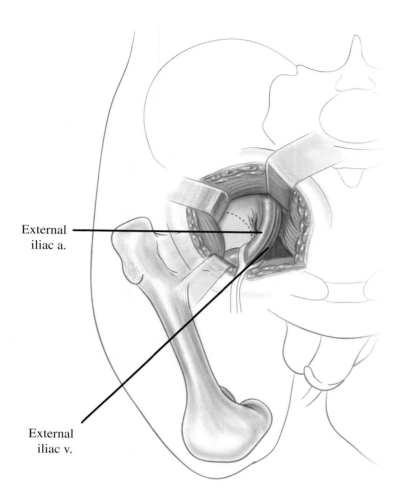

External
iliac a.

External
iliac v.

Figure 7. The external iliac artery and vein are dissected out and gently retracted medially to expose perforating vessels running posteriorly. These perforators may be substantial in size and are ligated.

Retract the iliac artery and vein out through the wound using silicone loops. A total of four silicone loops are used: one proximally and one distally on the iliac artery and one proximally and one distally on the iliac vein (see Figs. 8 and 9). Placing two loops on each vessel limits back-bleeding if that vessel is injured or transected. Fill the wound with an antibiotic saline-soaked abdominal pack. Temporarily approximate the skin with staples. The average time for this approach alone is about 1 hour and 15 minutes.

Roll the patient forward, and push the posterior kidney rest forward to support the patient in a direct lateral position (see Figs. 10 and 11). We use a modified Hardinge lateral approach for the hip revision, an uncemented acetabular component with screws if needed, and a cemented or cementless femoral component. Extreme care is taken during the acetabular exposure, preparation, and reaming. If serious hemorrhage ensues, the surgeon can tension the abdominal vessel loops and quickly open the abdominal incision. In most instances, ligation of avulsed perforators is necessary to halt the bleeding.

First, close the lateral incision. Then, remove the abdominal pack and vessel loops and close the abdominal incision in layers without a drain (see Fig. 12) (9).

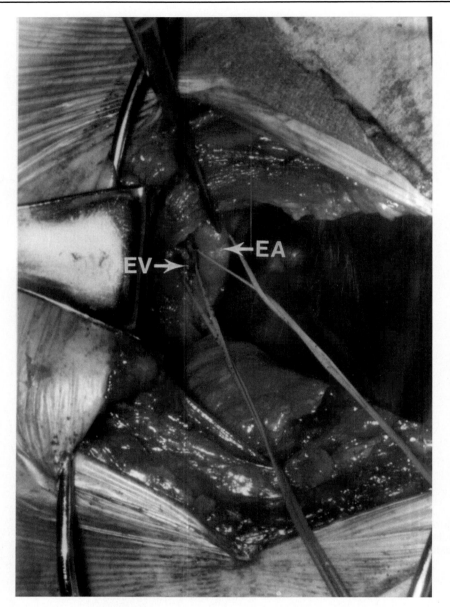

Figure 8. The external iliac artery *(EA)* and vein *(EV)* have been dissected out. Silicone loops have been placed around these structures as they travel distal to the inguinal ligament. (From Petrera P, Trakru S, Mehta S, et al. Revision total hip arthroplasty with a retroperitoneal approach to the iliac vessels. *J Arthroplasty* 11:707, 1996, copyright 1996, with permission from Elsevier.)

POSTOPERATIVE MANAGEMENT

Closely monitor the patients for ileus. Limit oral intake to clear fluids until bowel sounds return. Otherwise, management is the same as a revision THA of similar complexity. Weight bearing is determined by the stability of the components as assessed intraoperatively. Generally, with uncemented acetabular components, the patient is made partial weight bearing for 6 to 12 weeks until implant ingrowth is achieved. Patients should wear bilateral TEDS and SCDs during their whole hospital stay. On discharge, they should continue to wear the TEDS for a total of 6 weeks postoperatively. Use warfarin sodium for deep venous thrombosis prophylaxis for 4 weeks, monitoring it to maintain an international normalized ratio of 2 to 3.

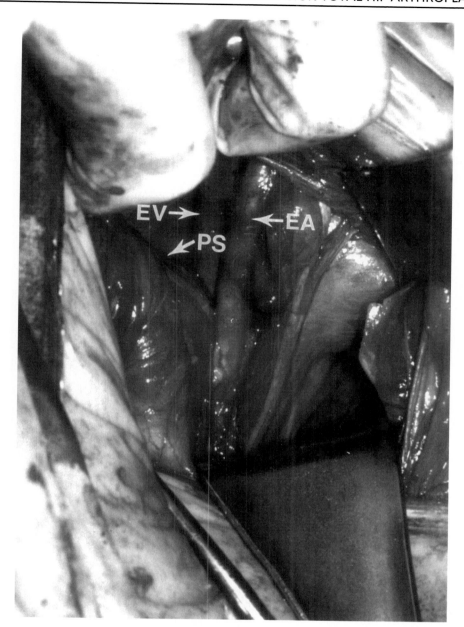

Figure 9. In this case, the external iliac artery *(EA)* is dissected free of the surrounding tissues. The external iliac venin *(EV)* is found to be adherent to the medial side of the acetabular component's pseudocapsule *(PS)*. (From Petrera P, Trakru S, Mehta S, et al. Revision total hip arthroplasty with a retroperitoneal approach to the iliac vessels. *J Arthroplasty* 11:706, 1996, copyright 1996, with permission from Elsevier.)

COMPLICATIONS

Vascular complications during the abdominal part of the procedure have been reported. Reiley et al. reported on a revision THA of a protrusion acetabular cup using an abdominal approach. They retracted the femoral nerve laterally and the femoral artery and vein medially. They reported removing the acetabular component "easily." However, 1 day after the procedure, the patient suffered an acute thrombosis of the external iliac artery, requiring a femoro-femoral bypass operation. Twelve hours later, compartment syndrome of the right calf developed, requiring fascial releases of all four compartments. Eventually, a large area of skin necrosis of the foot dorsum necessitated a below-knee amputation (10). Given this

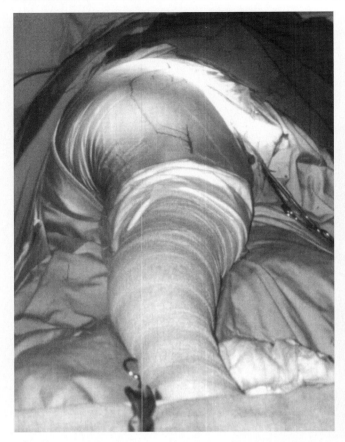

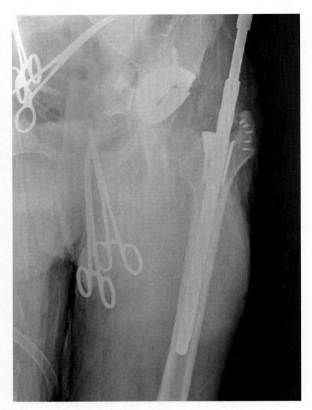

Figure 10. After the retroperitoneal approach in the floppy lateral position, the patient is positioned in left lateral decubitus for the revision THA. Note the surgical clamps anterior to the patient. These clamps are on the silicone loops around the iliac vein and artery. (Reproduced with permission from Petrera P, Trakru S, Mehta S, et al. Revision total hip arthroplasty with a retroperitoneal approach to the iliac vessels. *J Arthroplasty* 11:705, 1996, copyright 1996, with permission from Elsevier.)

Figure 11. This intraoperative radiograph includes the clamps holding the vessel loops. The vascular surgeon has completed the intrapelvic approach, and the revision THA is now in progress.

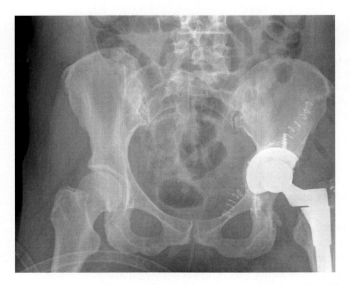

Figure 12. The staple line anteriorly closing the intrapelvic approach is evident on this postoperative radiograph.

possibility of serious vascular injury, one should consider having a vascular surgeon per-form the abdominal portion of the combined approach outlined above.

We have encountered violation of perforating vessels when using the curette for de-bridement. Immediate control of the bleeding was achieved by tensioning the loops on the iliac vessels. The vascular surgeon then provided definitive hemostasis via ligation of the perforator(s). Postoperatively, we encountered cases of ileus, which all resolved with con-servative treatment.

RECOMMENDED READING

1. Wasielewski RC, Crossett LS, Rubash HE. Neural and vascular injury in total hip arthroplasty. *Orthop Clin North Am* 23(2):219–235, 1992.
2. Wasielewski RC, Cooperstein LA, Kruger MP, Rubash HE. Acetabular anatomy and the transacetabular fixation of screws in total hip arthroplasty. *J Bone Joint Surg Am* 72(4):501–508, 1990.
3. Shoenfeld NA, Stuchin SA, Pearl R, Haveson S. The management of vascular injuries associated with total hip arthroplasty. *J Vasc Surg* 11(4):549–555, 1990.
4. Giacchetto J, Gallagher JJ. False aneurysm of the common femoral artery secondary to migration of a threaded acetabular component. a case report and review of the literature. *Clin Orthop Relat Res* 231:91–96, 1988.
5. al-Salman M, Taylor DC, Beauchamp CP, Duncan CP. Prevention of vascular injuries in revision total hip replacement. *Can J Surg* 35(3):261–264, 1992.
6. Eftekhar NS, Nercessian O. Intrapelvic migration of total hip prostheses. Operative treatment. *J Bone Joint Surg Am* 71(10):1480–1486, 1989.
7. Scullin JP, Nelson CL, Beven EG. False aneurysm of the left external iliac artery following total hip arthro-plasty. *Clin Orthop Relat Res* 113:145–149, 1975.
8. Brentlinger A, Hunter JR. Perforation of the external iliac artery and ureter presenting as acute hemorrhagic cystitis after total hip replacement. Report of a case. *J Bone Joint Surg Am* 69(4):620–622, 1987.
9. Petrera P, Trakru S, Mehta S, et al. Revision total hip arthroplasty with a retroperitoneal approach to the iliac vessels. *J Arthroplasty* 11(6):704—708, 1996.
10. Reiley MA, Bond D, Branick RI, Wilson EH. Vascular complications following total hip arthroplasty. A review of the literature and a report of two cases. *Clin Orthop Relat Res* 186:23–28, 1984.

6

Minimally Invasive Total Hip Arthroplasty

Richard Berger

Minimally invasive total hip replacement has the potential for minimizing surgical trauma, pain, and recovery time. To achieve the potential rapid recovery that these truly minimally invasive techniques allow, the entire traditional perioperative pathway needs to be expedited. When we combine a true minimally invasive total hip arthroplasty (THA), where no muscle or tendon is damaged as part of the surgery and with a new pathway that expedites that entire recovery process, outpatient total hip replacement is not only possible but also currently routinely performed at our institution.

These minimally invasive techniques in total hip replacement include single-incision and two-incision techniques. Most of the single-incision minimally invasive techniques for total hip replacement are a modification of traditional total hip replacement techniques. However, a new minimally invasive technique for total hip replacement was developed that uses two incisions. This new minimally invasive technique avoids transecting muscle or tendon, thereby minimizing morbidity and hastening recovery. This chapter describes this new minimally invasive hip replacement procedure performed with two incisions; one incision is for acetabular preparation and placement, and the other is for femoral preparation and placement. Unique instruments have been developed to facilitate this technique. Since the patient is supine with this technique, fluoroscopy can be used to aid in many steps in this process to ensure proper starting points for the incisions and accurate component position and alignment. Standard implants are used to maintain the present expectation of implant durability.

INDICATIONS/CONTRAINDICATIONS

As in most surgical procedures, female patients who are thin and not muscular with a small bone structure and atrophic changes are the easiest patients on whom to perform this procedure. These patients are the best to begin your experience. As experience is gained, the surgeon can progress to more challenging patient types. The most difficult patients are men who are heavy and muscular with a large bone structure and hypertrophic changes.

Allthough this procedure was found to be safe and practical for most patients who are candidates for traditional THA, there are conditions that are not amenable to the minimally invasive two-incision procedure at this time. Cadaveric work has shown that this two-incision procedure is very challenging in morbidly obese patients. Additionally, patients with very marked abnormal hip joint anatomy, significant prior surgical scarring, or complete hip dislocation may be better candidates for alternate THA approaches.

PREOPERATIVE PLANNING

The importance of preoperative planning and templating cannot be overemphasized. This is particularly true in the case of this minimally invasive THA approach since visualization of extra-articular landmarks is limited. The objective of preoperative planning is to enable you to gather anatomic parameters that will allow accurate intraoperative placement of the femoral and acetabular implants. Optimal femoral and acetabular component fit, the level of the femoral neck cut, the prosthetic neck length, and the femoral component offset can be evaluated through preoperative radiographic analysis. Preoperative planning also allows the surgeon to have the appropriate implants available at surgery.

Determining preoperative leg length is essential for restoration of the appropriate leg length during THA. As in all THAs, preoperative templating using an anteroposterior (AP) view of the pelvis is usually the most accurate method of determining proper leg length. Only in extremely unusual cases is a scanogram or computed tomographic (CT) evaluation of leg length helpful. From the clinical and radiographic information about leg lengths, determine the appropriate correction, if any, to be achieved during surgery.

Although rare, it may not be possible to restore offset in patients with an unusually large preoperative offset or with a severe varus deformity. In such cases, lengthening the limb can increase the tension in the abductor muscles. This method is especially useful when the involved hip is shorter than the contralateral hip. However, in these cases there is usually no choice but to lengthen the hip and leg. With lengthening, patient dissatisfaction may result; however, in some uncommon cases where stability and leg length cannot be optimized, it is more important to achieve hip stability than leg length equality.

The initial templating begins with the AP radiograph. Superimpose the acetabular templates sequentially on the pelvic x-ray film with the acetabular component in approximately 45 degrees of abduction. Assess several sizes to estimate which acetabular component will provide the best fit for maximum coverage. Mark the acetabular size and position and the center of the head on the x-ray films. Note the superior coverage of the acetabular component in 45 degrees of abduction; reproduce this during surgery to assure proper component abduction and avoid vertical positioning. Next, select the appropriate femoral template. To estimate the femoral implant size, assess both the distal stem size and the body size on the AP radiograph, and then check the stem size on the lateral radiograph. The stem of the femoral component should fill, or nearly fill, the medullary canal in the isthmus area on the AP x-ray film. Next, assess the fit of the stem body in the metaphyseal area. The medial portion of the body of the component should fill the proximal metaphysis as fully as possible.

After establishing the appropriate size of the femoral component, determine the height of its position in the proximal femur. If the leg length is to remain unchanged, the center of the head of the prosthesis should be at the same level as the center of the femoral head of the patient's hip. This should also correspond to the center of rotation of the acetabulum. To lengthen the limb, raise the template proximally. To shorten the limb, shift the template distally. Once the height has been determined, note the distance in millimeters from the collar or most proximal aspect of the porous surface to the top of the lesser trochanter.

SURGICAL APPROACH

The patient is placed in the supine position with a small bolster under the ischium on the affected side. This allows better visualization of the acetabulum as the femur falls posteriorly after the femoral head is resected. A radiolucent operating room table is used. The entire leg and hip are prepped and draped (see Fig. 1). The fluoroscope is used to define the femoral neck. A metallic instrument is used to mark the midline of the femoral neck from the junction of the head and neck distally to the intertrochanteric line (see Fig. 2). In addition, the interval between the sartorius medially and tensor fascia lata laterally should be palpated. Most of the incision should be lateral to this interval, avoiding the lateral femoral cutaneous nerve. The anterior incision is made directly over the femoral neck from the base of the femoral head distally about 1.5 in to the intertrochanteric line. The fascia of the sartorius is present in the proximal-medial incision, whereas the tensor fascia lata lies at the distal-lateral portion of the incision. The sartorius muscle and tensor fascia lata can be seen beneath the fascia. Just medial to the edge of the tensor fascia lata, the fascia is incised longitudinally, parallel to the sartorius muscle and tensor fascia lata. This lateral fascial incision avoids the lateral femoral cutaneous nerve, which is located superficial to the sartorius muscle. The sartorius is retracted medially, and the tensor fascia lata is retracted laterally, exposing the lateral border of the rectus femoris (see Fig. 3). The medial retractor is repositioned to retract the rectus muscle medially (see Fig. 4). This exposes the lateral circumflex vessels, which are coagulated with electrocautery. The pericapsular fat then is retracted medially and laterally, exposing the capsule over the femoral neck (see Fig. 5).

Two curved, lit Hohman retractors [part of the minimally invasive two-incision instrument set (Zimmer, Warsaw, Indiana)] are placed extracapsularly around the femoral neck, illuminating the capsule (Fig. 5). The capsule is incised in line with the femoral neck. This incision is made from the edge of the acetabulum distally to the intertrochanteric line. The two curved, lit Hohman retractors are repositioned intracapsularly, exposing the femoral head and neck from the acetabulum to the intertrochanteric line (see Figs. 6 and 7).

Since the muscles and tendons around the hip have not been disrupted, the hip cannot easily be dislocated. An in situ neck cut should be made. It is easier to remove the head in two pieces rather then one; therefore, two neck cuts are made. The initial neck osteotomy is made at the equator of the femoral head, as close to the acetabulum as possible, with an oscillating saw. A second cut is made 1 cm distal to this (see Fig. 8). The small 1-cm wafer of bone is removed using a threaded Steinmann pin. Next, a threaded Steinmann pin is placed into the femoral head, and the head is removed (see Fig. 9). If the ligamentum teres is intact, a curved osteotome is used to transect the ligamentum teres. Then, the final femoral neck osteotomy is made on the basis of preoperative templating. Appropriate femoral neck resection is confirmed with fluoroscopy (see Fig. 10) or by flexing and externally rotating the hip in a figure-of-four, which exposes the lesser trochanter.

Three curved, lit Hohman retractors are placed around the acetabulum, one anteriorly around the acetabulum, a second posteriorly around the acetabulum, and the third directly

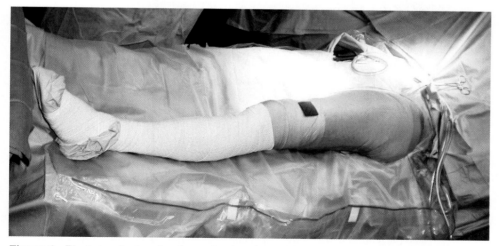

Figure 1. Photograph showing the entire leg draped for the two-incision minimally invasive THA. A small bolster under the ischium elevates the affected side of the pelvis.

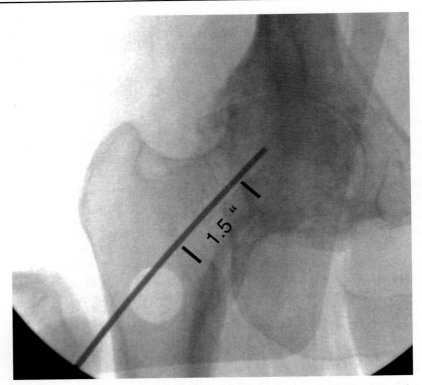

Figure 2. A fluoroscopic image shows the position of the incision over the femoral neck. The incision is made from the base of the head to the base of the femoral neck (approximately 1.5 inches).

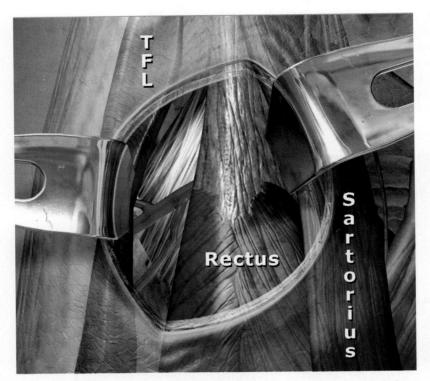

Figure 3. Illustration shows deep dissection of the anterior incision. The sartorius muscle is retracted medially, and the tensor fascia latae (TFL) are retracted laterally. The rectus femoris can be seen medially overlaying the capsule.

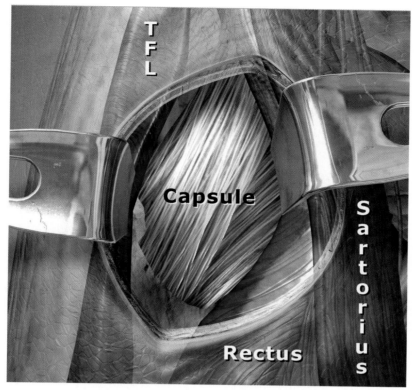

Figure 4. Illustration shows the capsule exposed by retracting the rectus femoris medially.

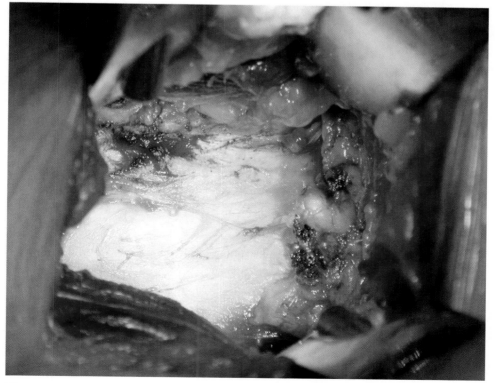

Figure 5. Photograph shows the lit Hohman retractors around the capsule providing excellent exposure.

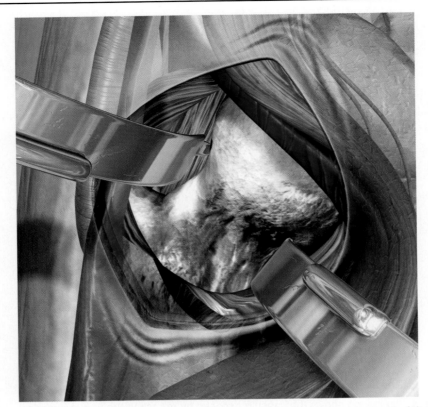

Figure 6. Illustration shows the femoral head and neck exposed by placement of the lit Hohman retractors intracapsularly around the femoral neck.

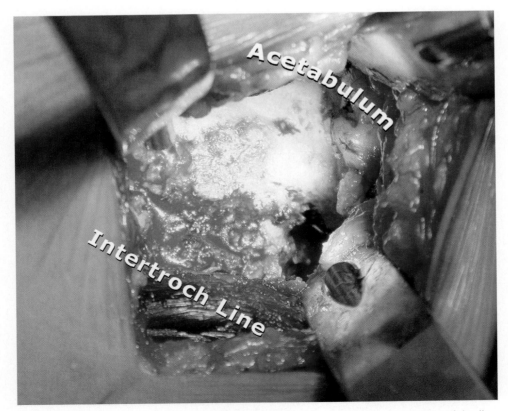

Figure 7. Photograph shows the femoral head and neck exposed by placement of the lit Hohman retractors intracapsularly around the femoral neck.

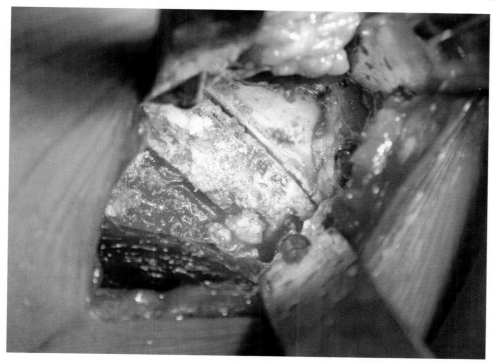

Figure 8. Photograph shows the initial two cuts in the femoral head and neck.

superiorly over the brim of the acetabulum. This retracts the capsule and allows excellent visualization of the acetabulum (see Fig. 11). The labrum is excised, exposing the entire peripheral bony rim of the acetabulum and the pulvinar.

The superior retractor is removed while the anterior and posterior retractors are left in place. Specially designed, low-profile reamers (part of the minimally invasive two-incision instrument set), which are cut out on the sides, are used to ream the acetabulum (see Fig. 12). These reamers are aggressive with square cutting teeth; therefore it is possible to start

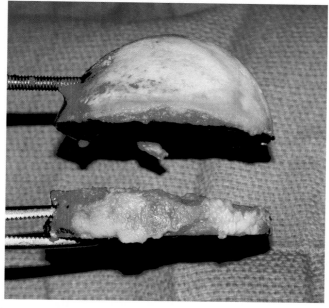

Figure 9. Photograph shows the femoral head and upper neck removed in two pieces.

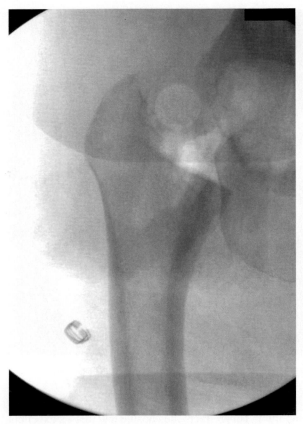

Figure 10. Fluoroscopic image shows the final femoral neck preparation.

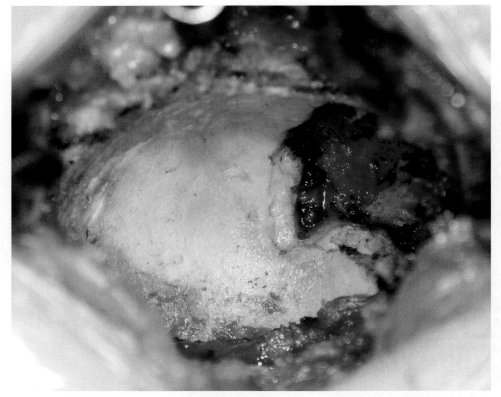

Figure 11. Photograph shows lit Hohman retractor placement and an excellent view of acetabulum.

with a reamer that is close in size to the intended final reamer to avoid inserting and extracting many reamers. Furthermore, the open design of these reamers allows visualization of the acetabulum during reaming. With gentle traction on the leg, the reamer is inserted in line with the femoral neck, with the cutouts of the reamer aligned with the two retractors. The cutout reamer is seated to the floor of the acetabulum (see Fig. 13). The acetabulum is reamed at 45 degrees of abduction and 20 degrees of anteversion. The fluoroscope can be used for visualization as the acetabulum is reamed. When the cutout reamers are rotating, they appear as solid reamers, so that the fit and fill of the acetabulum can be assessed (see Fig. 14). The acetabulum is sequentially reamed until a healthy bleeding bed of cancellous bone is present throughout. An acetabular component is selected that is 2 mm larger than the final reamer used.

A specialized dogleg acetabular inserter (part of the minimally invasive two-incision instrument set) with the supine positioner is used to place the chosen acetabulum shell. The anterior and posterior retractors are left in place as gentle traction is placed on the leg. The bolster beneath the ischium is removed so that the patient's pelvis is parallel to the bed and floor. This can be confirmed with fluoroscopy. The acetabular component is inserted as the retractors keep the capsule from invaginating (see Fig. 15). The acetabulum is viewed with the fluoroscope as the cup is positioned in 45 degrees of abduction and 20 degrees of anteversion, following the native acetabulum. The cup is then impacted in place (see Fig. 16). The inserter is then removed, and the final cup position is then confirmed (see Fig. 17). With the curved, lit acetabular retractor in place around the acetabulum, the stability of the shell is assessed. If desired, supplemental screws are placed in the posterosuperior quadrant of the shell. Finally, a small curved osteotome is used to remove any osteophytes around the rim of the acetabulum, and the polyethylene liner is impacted into the shell. All retractors are removed from the acetabulum, and attention is turned to the femur.

The leg is adducted and placed in neutral rotation. A 1- to 1.5-inch incision is made in the posterior lateral buttocks, just posterior to a line colinear to the femoral canal. A Charnley awl is guided through the posterior incision, posterior to the gluteus medius and minimus and anterior to the piriformis fossa down the femoral canal. Fluoroscopy can aid this starting point and can be used to visualize the leg in a frog lateral position to confirm the entry point. Specially designed side-cutting reamers (part of the minimally invasive two-incision instrument set) are used to enlarge this starting hole and position the starting point laterally against the trochanteric bed so that the stem is in a neutral position (see Fig. 18).

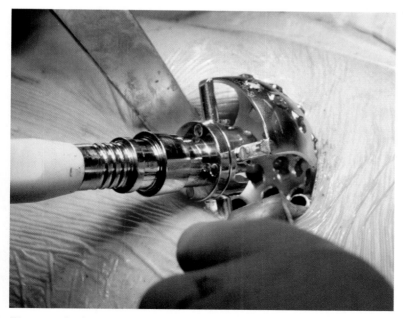

Figure 12. Photograph shows the acetabular reamer being placed into the anterior incision, between the two lit Hohman retractors.

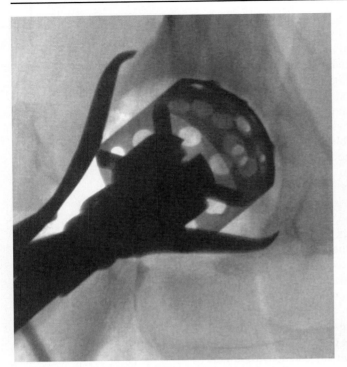

Figure 13. Fluoroscopic view shows the cutout reamer seated in the acetabulum between the two lit Hohman retractors prior to reaming.

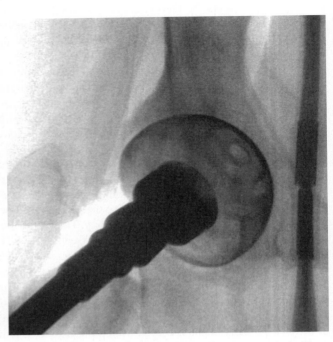

Figure 14. Fluoroscopic view shows the reamer seated in the acetabulum while reaming. During reaming, the cutout reaming appears hemispherical and provides excellent assessment of the position and size of the acetabulum.

These side-cutting reamers are used sequentially through the posterior incision within the same track as the Charnley awl. If a distally coated stem is to be used, flexible reamers are used to ream the canal until cortical chatter is obtained. Subsequently, straight reamers with a tissue-protecting sleeve then are used to ream the femoral diaphysis until good cortical chatter is obtained (see Fig. 19). If a proximally coated stem is to be used, proceed directly to broaching. (I recommend using a distally coated stem for this procedure.)

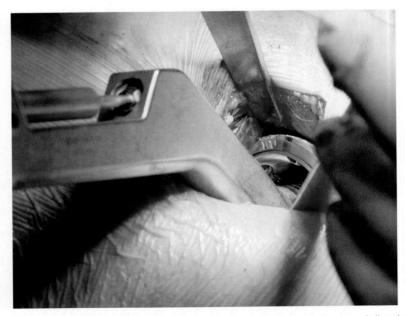

Figure 15. Photograph shows the acetabulum being inserted with the specialized supine positioner.

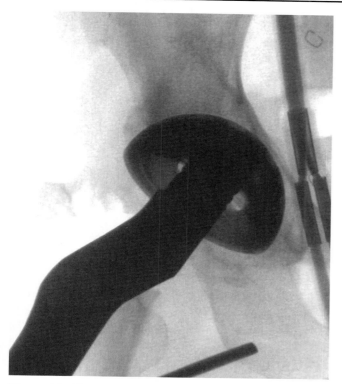

Figure 16. Fluoroscope view of acetabular component in place with the inserter still attached.

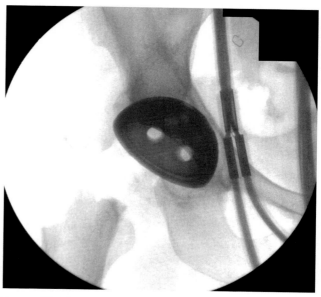

Figure 17. Fluoroscopic view of final acetabular component in place.

After reaming to the appropriate size, broaching is done. With visualization through the anterior wound, the rasp is rotationally aligned to the calcar. The rasp is fully seated. Rasps then are sequentially introduced and seated, finishing with the appropriate size (see Fig. 20). When the final rasp is seated, care must be taken to visualize the rotation of the rasp in the anterior wound to ensure alignment with the metaphysis.

A trial reduction may be performed. The trial neck and head are placed on the broach from the anterior wound. The hip is then put through a range of motion to assess stability. The hip should be stable in full extension with 90 degrees of external rotation and 90 degrees of

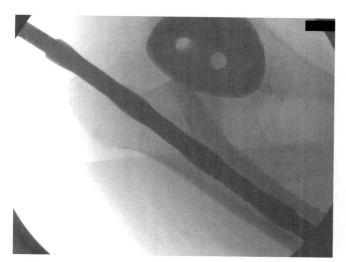

Figure 18. Fluoroscopic view shows the lateralization reamer reaming the trochanteric bed to achieve a neutral femoral alignment.

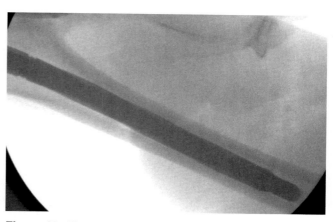

Figure 19. Fluoroscopic view shows the straight reamer reaming in a neutral femoral alignment.

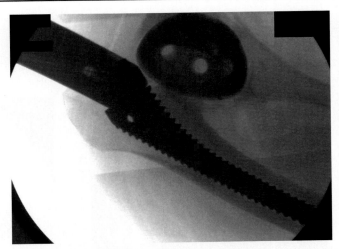

Figure 20. Fluoroscopic view shows the final femoral rasp seated.

flexion with 20 degrees of adduction and at least 50 degrees of internal rotation. The fluoroscope can be used to assess leg lengths by comparing the level of the lesser trochanters with the obturator foramen. In addition, with the patient in the supine position, the medial malleoli may be checked to assess leg length. When the trial reduction is complete, the head and neck are removed though the anterior incision, and the broach is removed through the posterior incision.

Two Hohman retractors are placed into the posterior wound, one anterior to the femoral neck and one posterior to the femoral neck. These retract the soft tissue as the stem is placed into the femoral canal. The stem then is introduced into the femoral canal from the posterior incision (see Fig. 21). Once down the canal, the stem is impacted into place as the rotation is controlled. Visualization through the anterior incision ensures no soft tissue entrapment between the calcar and the collar and assures correct stem version (see Fig. 22). The final stem is seated and confirmed with fluoroscopy (see Fig. 23).

With the actual component in place, repeat trial reduction is performed, placing the head from the anterior incision. The hip should be stable, and leg lengths should be equal. With the hip in external rotation and the bone hook around the neck, the actual metal head is then placed on the neck and gently impacted in place. The hip is located with gentle traction and internal rotation. The capsule is then closed. The fascia between the sartorius and the tensor fascia lata is closed, followed by closure of the anterior and posterior incisions. Two 2 × 2-inch bandages are used to cover the incisions (see Fig. 24). Figure 25 demonstrates

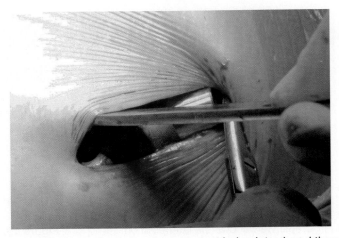

Figure 21. Photograph shows the femoral component being introduced through the posterior incision.

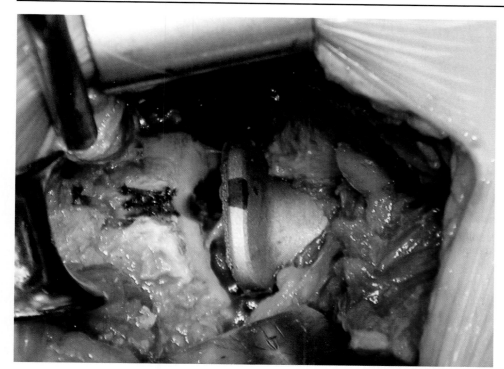

Figure 22. Photograph shows the femoral component's rotation in the anterior incision. The stem is a few millimeters from being seated. The apex of the calcar and the apex of the stem are marked, showing the stem in the correct version.

the postoperative radiographs of this case example. At 3 months, Figure 26 shows the anterior incision well healed.

POSTOPERATIVE MANAGEMENT

During the procedure and postoperatively, the patient is kept well hydrated to prevent postoperative hypotension and nausea. The Foley catheter is discontinued in all patients

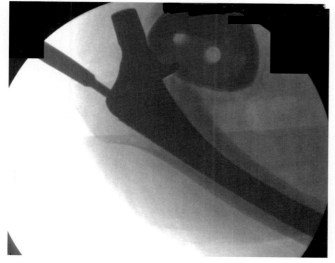

Figure 23. Fluoroscopic view shows the femoral component during insertion. The femoral component is seated in the final position.

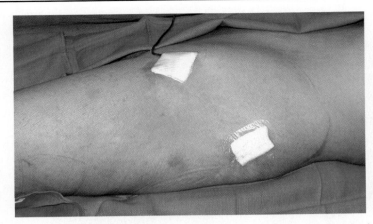

Figure 24. Photograph shows the final two 2 × 2-inch bandages covering the incisions on a patient who had a minimally invasive two-incision THA.

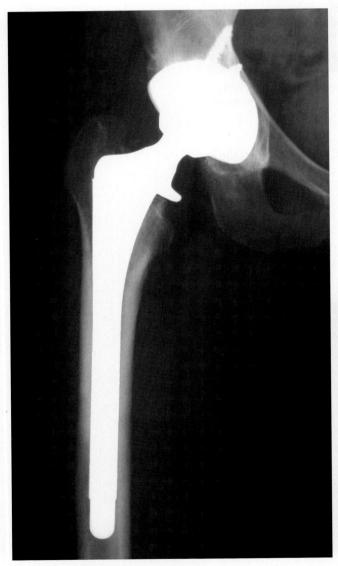

Figure 25. Postoperative radiographs show the minimally invasive two-incision THA reconstruction.

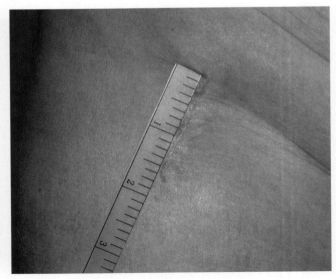

Figure 26. Photograph shows the anterior incision well healed at 3 months.

2 hours postoperatively. Twenty milligrams of oxycodone hydrochloride (OxyContin) are given orally 2 hours postoperatively, and the epidural is removed 4 hours postoperatively. The intravenous tubing is removed, and the intravenous catheter is maintained with a heparin lock 5 hours postoperatively.

Occupational and physical therapy are initiated at 5 to 6 hours postoperatively. Patients are weight bearing as tolerated on the surgically treated extremity. All patients are first taught bed and chair transfers. They receive teaching for ambulation: first with crutches, then with a cane, and finally without any assistive device the day of surgery. Last, patients are taught chair ascent and descent: first with crutches and then without any assistive. Patients are discharged from the hospital once strict criteria are met, including the ability to independently transfer out of and into bed from a standing position, rise to and from a chair to a standing position, ambulate 100 feet, and ascend and descend a full flight of stairs.

Upon discharge, patients continue taking celecoxib (Celebrex), 200 mg daily for at least 2 weeks and gradually decrease their dose of oxycodone hydrochloride as needed; hydrocodone is taken as needed for breakthrough pain. Starting the evening of surgery, all patients receive aspirin for deep venous thrombosis prophylaxis for 3 weeks.

Patients are encouraged to start activities as soon as tolerated. They are allowed to drive when off all narcotics. Home physical therapy is used until the patient can drive; then outpatient physical therapy is started. The patient and therapist are encouraged to advance as quickly as possible. No hip precautions are emphasized. Patients progress to a cane as tolerated. They are encouraged to use a cane until they can ambulate without a limp and then to discontinue use of the cane. Patients also are encouraged to resume activities as tolerated. Patients who work are encouraged to return to work as soon as they feel comfortable.

COMPLICATIONS

Complications of the minimally invasive two-incision total hip replacement are similar to those of traditional total hip replacement. The most common intraoperative complication is femoral fracture resulting from either varus alignment or excessive anteverting during femoral preparation or stem insertion. Outlined are commonly made mistakes and how to avoid them.

Anterior Incision

It is common to mark the anterior incision too medially. This is especially true on heavier patients. The incision should be centered over the tensor fascia lata (TFL) and extend just to the lateral border of the sartorius. The interval between the TFL and the sartorius can usually be palpated prior to the incision. Alternately, the incision should be made lateral to a line that extends from the anterior superior iliac spine (ASIS) to the center of the knee. Medial placement of the incision will cause the lateral aspect of the incision to be overstretched and possibly torn when preparing and placing the acetabulum. Furthermore, if the incision extends over the body of the sartorius, the lateral cutaneous nerve may be encountered and injured. Regarding the lateral cutaneous nerve, it is not advisable to explore or dissect the lateral cutaneous nerve; this may result in scarring of the nerve with subsequent hypoesthesia of the thigh.

Femoral Head Resection

First, a common mistake is to have the side edge of the saw either cut into the sartorius, the TFL, or the skin. This is avoided by proper retractor placement. Second, there is a tendency to not see the acetabulum prior to cutting the head. This results in a neck cut that is too low, making it very difficult to remove the femoral head since the resection will not be intracapsular. The femoral head should be exposed until the edge of the acetabulum is seen. Once the acetabulum is seen, the first neck cut is made as high on the head as possible, close to the edge of the acetabulum. Another common mistake is to not cleanly osteotomize the head, so that irregular edges remain, subsequently making head removal more difficult. After making the proximal cut, the second resection cut is made 1 cm distal to the proximal cut. It is common to use the saw so that the anterior aspect of the intercalary is thinner than the posterior aspect; this results in inability to remove the intercalary segment. The second femoral osteotomy must be made so that the anterior aspect of the intercalary piece is thicker than the posterior aspect; this allows the intercalary segment to be removed.

Acetabular Reaming

As the acetabulum is reamed in the correct version, the reamer can be levered on the femur, forcing the reamer anteriorly. This is especially true if a long neck remains. This anterior reaming of the acetabulum is not intuitive, as the anteversion of the reamer would usually cause the posterior acetabulum to be reamed more. This tendency to ream anteriorly can be counteracted by posterior pressure on the reamer during reaming.

Regarding acetabular positioning, it is common to overly antevert the acetabular component. Make sure the acetabular component is anatomic with the native acetabulum.

Posterior Incision

It is common to mark the posterior incision too anteriorly, colinear with the femoral canal. This will result in piercing and injuring the abductor. The posterior incision must be made posterior to a line colinear to the femoral canal. Then, the femoral awl is introduced posterior to the abductors.

Entering the Femoral Canal

Allowing the starting awl to enter the femoral canal too medially, into the cancellous bone of the osteotomy, is a common mistake. If this starting hole is placed medially, the side-cutting reamers will not ream laterally enough, resulting in a varus stem positioning or femoral fracture. This will be avoided if the femoral canal is initially entered at the most lateral aspect of the canal. With the laterally placed entry hole, the side-cutting reamers will then easily ream medially, to ensure a neutral alignment.

Broaching and Stem Placement

The broach and stem will initially seem retroverted when properly rotated. In other words, the common mistake is to overly antevert the broach and stem; this can result in femoral fracture.

Stem Insertion

In some cases, particularly with a larger stem or an extended offset stem, the femoral neck may get caught on the lateral edge of the acetabulum during insertion. This is caused by overly adducting the leg. Less adduction of the leg can alleviate this impingement. Alternately, bringing the leg into a neutral position and applying traction will deliver the neck through the capsule. In addition, if the capsule is entrapped between the collar and calcar, this maneuver, done when the stem is about 1 cm from fully seated, will free the capsule.

CONCLUSION

Minimally invasive surgery has the potential to minimize surgical trauma and pain while improving functional recovery in patients having total hip replacement. The minimally invasive two-incision total hip technique described here, where muscle and tendon trauma is minimized, shows substantial short-term pain and functional improvement over traditional hip replacement. In fact, of the last 200 of these procedures at Rush Hospital, all have been performed on an outpatient basis. Furthermore, unique instruments and fluoroscopic assistance enabled accurate component position and alignment.

While this minimally invasive two-incision technique shows great promise, this technique requires meticulous surgical technique, specialized instrumentation, and special instruction. As such, preclinical exercises, anatomy laboratories, cadaver training, and proctoring programs are strongly recommended for surgeons interested in this new technique to minimize complications and ensure the success of this new procedure.

RECOMMENDED READING

1. Berger RA. Total hip arthroplasty using the minimally invasive two-incision approach. *Clin Orthop Relat Res* 417:232–241, 2003.
2. Berger RA, Jacobs JJ, Meneghini MR, et al. Rapid rehabilitation and recovery with minimally invasive total hip arthroplasty. *Clin Orthop Relat Res* 429:239–247, 2004.
3. Berry DJ, Berger RA, Callaghan JJ, et al. Minimally invasive total hip arthroplasty. Development, early results, and a critical analysis. *J Bone Joint Surg Am* 85:2235–2246, 2003.

Nonarthroplasty Approaches

PART III

Nonarthroplasty Approaches

7

Femoral Osteotomy

Richard F. Santore and Thomas R. Turgeon

INDICATIONS/CONTRAINDICATIONS

The most validated indication for a valgus intertrochanteric osteotomy (ITO), also referred to as proximal femoral osteotomy, is for the treatment of femoral fracture nonunions. As originally espoused by Friedrich Pauwels (1), the inclination of the nonunion is reoriented to be more perpendicular to the forces which cross it, resulting in compression. The most common use for ITO is the correction of various posttraumatic and postsurgical deformities. Additional indications include the adult sequelae of Legg-Calvé-Perthe disease, developmental dysplasia, slipped capital femoral epiphysis, and rare cases of osteonecrosis. These indications share the common goals of normalization of hip biomechanics, correction of limb length inequality, and alleviation of impingement (2).

Varus and valgus angular reorientations of the proximal femur have unique features. For instance, varus osteotomies inherently shorten the length of the femur. This feature can be exploited to advantage in cases of ipsilateral long limb. When the converse is true, the shortening effect can be minimized by limiting the magnitude of the angular correction and avoiding the use of bone wedge resections. Valgus osteotomies, on the other hand, result in lengthening of the femoral shaft. This is a useful feature when deliberate lengthening is desired. When lengthening is not needed, wedge resections can assure maintenance of leg length equality. Both types of osteotomies may be performed in isolation or in combination with a corrective pelvic osteotomy.

Considerations in selection of candidates for osteotomy include young physiologic age, comfort in the intended position (abduction for varus and adduction for valgus), suitable radiographic improvement in the intended position, good hip mobility (a flexion arc of greater than 60 degrees), motivation by the patient to avoid premature total hip replacement, and pain interfering with life on a regular basis. As a general rule, osteotomy should not be performed as a prophylactic treatment in the absence of pain. Osteonecrosis is a suitable indication if the lesion is small in size, has a favorable location, is not associated with secondary arthritis, and can be partially extruded from the weight-bearing area of the sourcil by biplane osteotomy. Favorable location includes far lateral and superior for a valgus osteotomy and central or medial for varus. The primary direction of correction is anterior, via a flexion osteotomy. Flexion osteotomies should be done with anterior capsular release or resection to reduce tension in the anterior region of the hip joint. Pure flexion is done for anteromedial lesions, and flexion/valgus is done for superoanterolateral lesions. Collapse of the necrotic sector is not a strict contraindication, as long as the lesion size is small and the "position of comfort" test is favorable. Candidates must be well motivated to undergo the procedure and be able to understand benefits, limitations, and complications of intertrochanteric osteotomy.

There are several absolute contraindications to ITO. These include inflammatory arthritis, osteoporosis, active osteomyelitis, and severe stiffness. Relative contraindications include unrealistic expectations, depression, paradoxical "position of comfort" test, smoking, and inability to use crutches. Incongruency of the hip is a contraindication for varus, but not a contraindication for a salvage valgus osteotomy. Over time, rotational osteotomy of the acetabulum has supplanted angulation osteotomy of the proximal femur as the procedure of choice for adults with prearthritic and early arthritic changes from dysplasia. Occasionally, an intertrochanteric osteotomy is useful as an adjunct to the rotational osteotomy, as when a need exists for leg lengthening or derotation.

Overweight (body mass index [BMI] 25 to 30) and obese (BMI >30) patients should be approached with caution. Larger thigh girth can make the procedure difficult, and increased loads may test the limits of the fixation device prior to bone union. Heavy laborers may not have the lasting quality of outcome desired because of excessive loads applied to the remaining abnormal cartilage during daily work.

PREOPERATIVE PLANNING

Planning begins with good patient selection. One variable of importance is the "position of comfort" test. Comfort in hip adduction—including standing, walking, and supine on the exam table—supports the decision for a valgus osteotomy. Furthermore, a minimum of 15 degrees of passive adduction is necessary. Conversely, comfort in abduction is a favorable selection factor for a varus osteotomy, and 15 degrees of passive abduction is a prerequisite. Leg length needs to be assessed and incorporated into the decision-making process. If the ipsilateral leg is short, an opening-up, no-wedge resection technique can be used for a valgus osteotomy to equalize the lengths. This would be a relative contraindication to varus osteotomy because of the further shortening that would accrue from the varus angulation. If the leg lengths are equal, it is important to plan full wedge resection for a valgus osteotomy or a no-wedge technique for varus. If the ipsilateral leg is long, valgus osteotomy needs to be combined with both a full angular wedge resection and an intraoperatively determined full thickness bone segment resection. A varus osteotomy is very attractive in the circumstance of a long ipsilateral leg. Only in this circumstance should a full wedge be resected and only with confirmation of appropriate shortening on preoperative drawings or computer-based images. Varus of more than 20 degrees with full wedge resection can result in very significant shortening. This should only be done when the ipsilateral leg is significantly longer than the opposite limb or when identical bilateral procedures are planned, with the understanding of patient and family ahead of time. Management of the leg length status is one of the most important aspects of preoperative planning and operative technique. Just as in total hip replacement (THR), sudden, unanticipated change in leg length is one of the most poorly accepted consequences of surgery. Leg length status and the plans for its management should be a part of the preoperative discussion with the patient. The ability to make meaningful and purposeful changes in leg length is one of the true advantages of osteotomy of the hip on the femoral side. Even in cases of primary hip dysplasia, where a rotational osteotomy of the acetabulum is the primary procedure, adjunctive femoral osteotomy can be justified as a means of equalizing limb lengths when the discrepancy is significant (12 mm or more) and the type of osteotomy fits the overall plan. Even if no angulation of the proximal femur is needed, an ITO can be done with full thickness wedge resection for up to 3 inches of shortening to equalize limb lengths. Almost as important as the issue of leg length is the status of rotation of the limb. First, it is important to recognize that unintentional external rotation is one of the risks of the osteosynthesis, and this has to be taken into account in the preoperative planning and avoided at the time of surgery. Deliberate, purposeful derotation can be done in circumstances of axial malrotation that is developmental or posttraumatic in nature. It is important to observe and to document the orientation of the foot of the patient preoperatively in the supine position and in the walking position. In general, it is important to plan to orient the patella in the true anterior position at the time of osteosynthesis. Plain radiographic images should include standing anteroposterior (AP) pelvis, AP hip, AP hip in abduction (varus osteotomy) and/or adduction (valgus osteotomy), and frog lateral of the hip (see Fig. 1). False profile images, when performed properly, give a perfect lateral view of the proximal femur (Fig. 1C). This x-ray is taken with the patient standing perpendicular to a wall-mounted cassette with the ipsilateral hip against the cassette, the ipsilateral

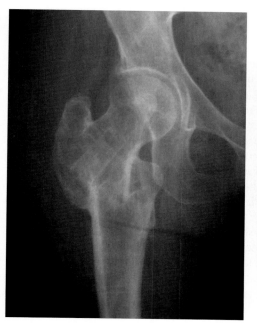

A

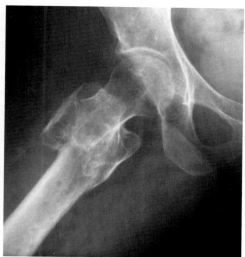

B

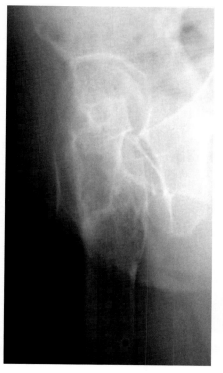

C

Figure 1. Case 1. A 53-year-old woman 19 months following fracture of right proximal femur, fixation with sliding screw construct, and malunion. **(A)** Anteroposterior (AP) view of the right hip. **(B)** Radiographic view of the right hip with hip abducted and externally rotated (frog lateral). **(C)** False profile view of the right hip. Note the medial and posterior displacement of femoral shaft relative to the proximal segment.

foot parallel to the x-ray cassette, and the contralateral hip rotated posteriorly enough to avoid superimposition of the two hips (approximately 20 degrees). Concentric reduction must be confirmed on the appropriate adduction or abduction view prior to consideration for reconstructive varus osteotomy surgery. Congruency is not a prerequisite for salvage valgus osteotomy. In this circumstance, relief of impingement in adduction or improvement of congruency, along with improved patient comfort, is the important consideration.

Once the x-rays have been completed and the type of osteotomy has been determined (i.e., valgus or varus, flexion or extension, or an appropriate combination of these), architectural drawings can be made to gauge the magnitude of correction that is appropriate and the consequences on other variables such as the length, displacement, and choice of fixation device. The AO manual is an excellent source of step-by-step planning and should be familiar to all who undertake osteotomy surgery (3). With the imaging complete, the following steps are taken to plan the osteotomy.

First, trace out the bony landmarks of the proximal femur and hemipelvis from the AP hip view as a single tracing and then make a second tracing with the proximal femur only. This can be done using tracing paper, a clear x-ray sheet, or any of a number of commercially available surgical-planning computer programs (see Fig. 2).

Next, overlay the proximal femur tracing over the combined femur and pelvis tracing. Keeping the femoral head in the center of rotation of the acetabulum, abduct (varus osteotomy) or adduct (valgus osteotomy) the femur, taking note of the changes in the neck-shaft angle, the relationship between the tip of the greater trochanter and the center of rotation of the femoral head, and the angles of the shafts of the two tracings. The target neck-shaft angle will vary depending on the clinical pathology and goals of the procedure. For example, in the case of a posttraumatic or iatrogenic varus, the goal should be a neck-shaft angle of 130 to 135 degrees. The neck-shaft angle of the patient's x-ray is measured, and the difference between that and 135 degrees is calculated. The femur tracing is rotated into adduction by that amount to assess the appearance of the neck-shaft segment. The amount of valgus should be quantified and rounded off to the nearest 5-degree value to make the intraoperative correlations easier. Next, a commercially available template of a blade plate is placed over the femur-only tracing and oriented to the head and neck segment with the side plate in a vertical orientation. The angle between the side plate and the rotated shaft of the tracing should equal

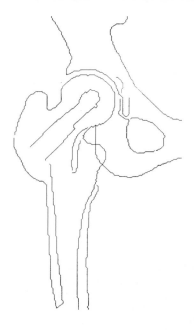

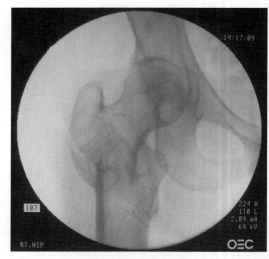

A   **B**

Figure 2. A: Preoperative plan tracing of bony anatomy of the right hip. **B:** Intraoperative fluoroscopic view corresponding to bony tracing of right hip.

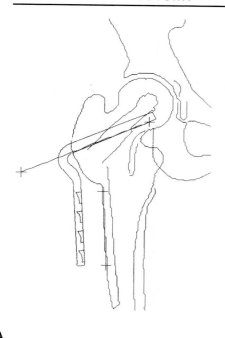

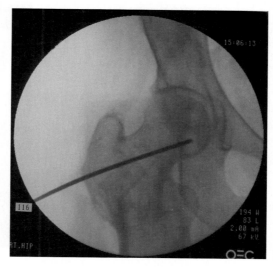

A   **B**

Figure 3. A: Preoperative plan with path of seating chisel marked out by the arrow and blade of blade plate. A 110-degree angled blade plate was selected on the basis of the morphology of the posttraumatic deformity. This required insertion of the K-wire at 70 degrees to the lateral cortex. Note that the plate is parallel to the lateral cortex of the femoral shaft, indicating that no varus or valgus correction is planned. **B:** Intraoperative path of seating chisel initially marked with a K-wire.

the previously determined magnitude of rotation. The blade plate position that is optimal transits the neck and enters the head in the center or just below the center of the head (see Fig. 3). Once the desired blade plate is identified and the amount of correction is ascertained (from 0 degrees to 40 degrees or more), there must be a plan for converting that into an intraoperative strategy. In this particular case, no frontal plane angular correction was needed, as the goals were shortening, derotation, and reversal of posttraumatic shaft displacement.

In another case (case 2), angular correction of 40 degrees was needed to reverse a postosteotomy nonunion with a 90-degree neck-shaft angle (see Figs. 4 and 5). High-angle blade plates are particularly useful in such circumstances. For instance, if a 130-degree plate for a 40-degree valgus correction of a nonunion is the result of the tracer or mathematical planning, the angle of the K-wire to be inserted into the proximal femur will be 90 degrees from the lateral shaft. When using high-angle blade plates, the difference between the angle of the plate and a 180-degree angle is the starting point. In our example, the difference is between 130 and 180 degrees for an angle of 50 degrees. This corresponds to the supplementary angle of plain geometry. To be perfectly clear, if one were to insert a 130-degree blade plate into a proximal femur at an angle to the shaft of 50 degrees, there would be no angular correction in the frontal plane after an osteotomy. This is the neutral insertion angle for this particular device. This would be the angle for a fracture fixation using a 130-degree angle blade plate without angular correction. Valgus corrections are calculated by adding the degrees of desired correction to the respective supplementary angle of the given blade plate. For the 40-degree correction with a 130-degree plate, the calculation is 50 degrees plus 40 degrees for a net of 90 degrees (see Figs. 6–9). In a theoretical example, using a 110-degree plate, what would be the correct angle of insertion of the K-wire and chisel to achieve a valgus correction of 20 degrees? First, calculate the supplementary angle of the 110-degree plate. That is 180 − 110 = 70 degrees. Next, add the desired valgus of 20 degrees to 70 degrees. Thus the chisel has to be inserted at an angle of 90 degrees to the shaft. To use a 110-degree plate for a shortening or pure extension or pure flexion osteotomy, with no frontal plane correction, the angle of insertion is the supplementary angle of 70 degrees.

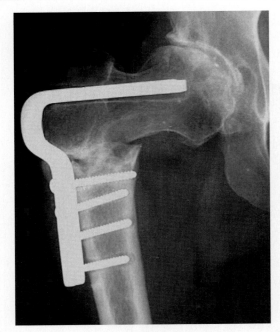

Figure 4. Case 2. AP radiograph of the right hip of a 34-year-old woman referred for hip replacement 10 months following varus proximal femoral osteotomy. The right leg is 2 cm short, and the patient has severe pain requiring two crutches to ambulate. Note the nonunion of the osteotomy, lifting of the plate from the lateral cortex, and widening of the medial blade tract due to motion.

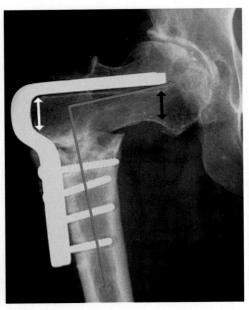

Figure 5. AP radiograph of proximal femoral nonunion with 90-degree neck-shaft angle marked in red. The adequate bone bridge for repeat blade plate fixation laterally is marked with a white double arrow. The adequate bone for blade fixation in the femoral head is marked with a black double arrow.

For femoral neck nonunions, the vertical nonunion angle is calculated, and the amount of valgus to make the nonunion more horizontal, without exceeding the 16-degree angle of compression of Pauwels, is calculated and rehearsed with the tracing paper. Valgus corrections of between 20 and 40 degrees may be selected. Often, there is preoperative shortening of the limb as well. Thus, the lengthening capability of valgus can be exploited by not taking any wedge. Up to 3 cm of lengthening can be achieved, depending on the width of the bone and the angle of valgus. This can be *approximated* by the planning. The final determination can only be made during surgery since it is influenced by factors in multiple

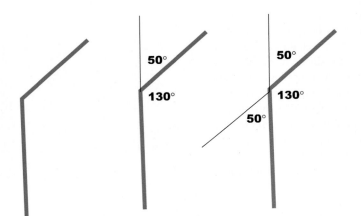

Figure 6. A 40-degree valgus correction with a 130-degree blade plate was determined from preoperative plans. The red line represents the 130-degree blade plate. Note that the supplementary angle is 50 degrees.

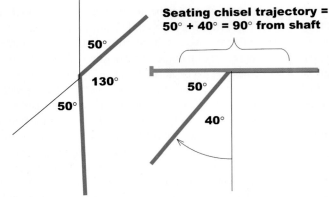

Figure 7. To achieve a 40-degree valgus correction, the seating chisel and subsequent blade plate must be inserted at an angle to the lateral cortex equal to the sum of the supplementary angle of the blade plate and the planned degree of correction. In this case, 50 + 40 = 90 degrees. The green line represents the seating chisel trajectory.

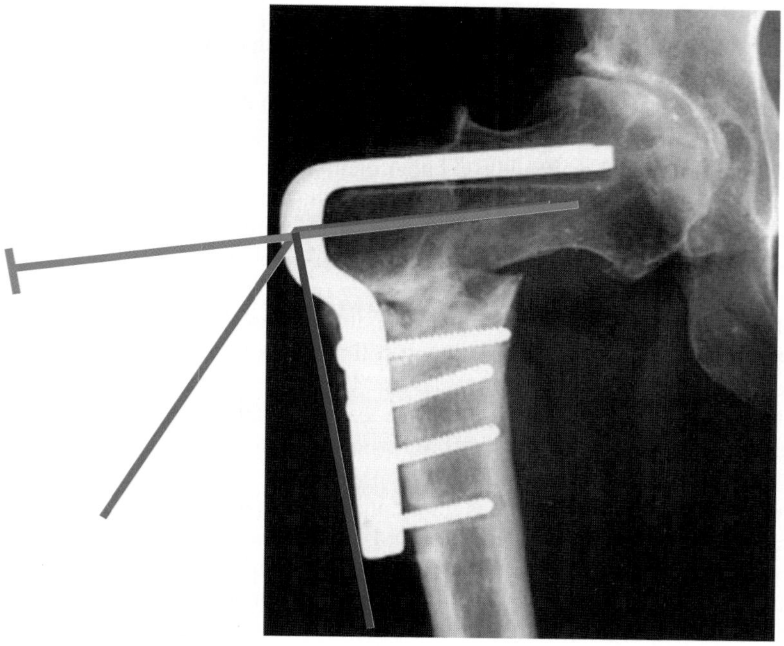

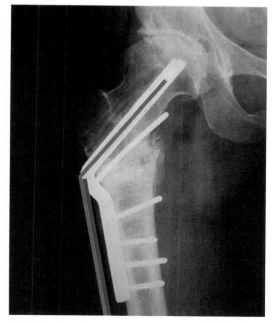

Figure 8. The seating chisel trajectory and the blade plate are superimposed on the pre-operative radiograph of the right hip in green and red, respectively. The blue line lies parallel to the lateral cortex of the femur.

planes and the degree of interfragmentary compression. Access to the other ankle to check leg length is important at the time of surgery.

Next, on the femur-only tracing, mark the point of insertion of the blade. In general, it should be close to the vastus tubercle, and a transverse osteotomy should exit on the medial side at the upper border of the lesser trochanter.

Figure 9. The blade plate *(red)* and the line parallel to the lateral cortex *(blue)* are superimposed on the postoperative hip radiograph following a 40-degree valgus osteotomy.

We now return to the first case, in which no angular correction was needed. In this particular case, the preferred transverse osteotomy cut would have resulted in a subtrochanteric cut on the medial side if the osteotomy was based simply on the distance from the vastus tubercle. Furthermore, a truly transverse osteotomy based at the proximal aspect of the lesser trochanter would result in an insufficient lateral bridge for the blade plate. Therefore, a slightly angled osteotomy was required rather than the standard transverse orientation (see Fig. 10). The distance between the osteotomy and the blade insertion must be a minimum of 15 mm. This is necessary to avoid the risk of fracture of the lateral bridge of bone between the chisel entry site and the osteotomy cut. In order to ensure such a bridge, the osteotomy may have to be moved distally, the entry site of the blade may have to be moved proximally, or a combination of the two. Depending on case-by-case morphologic variants, the bridge can be up to 24 mm in width and still conform to the geometry of the recess of the angled osteotomy plates of the AO design. The bone segment for resection to shorten the femur is outlined and includes most of the lesser trochanter (see Figs. 11 and 12).

Reduce the proximal femur fragment to the level of the osteotomy after removal of the bone segment (see Figs. 12B and 13).

It is preferable to use two strategies for planning and to make sure that there is complete final correspondence between the two methods. These include a "top-down" method, beginning with placement of the blade plate in the upper segment and calculating the angle to the shaft, as well as a "bottom-up" method calculating an angle from tracing and drawing the chisel insertion from the shaft. The two images should correspond.

Finally, a total hip template of appropriate magnification is superimposed on the femoral shaft distal to the osteotomy, and the displacement of the distal segment—i.e., frontal plane alignment—is set according to the ability of a stem to be inserted in the future. Preplanning of future THR should be an important principle of every proximal femoral osteotomy (see Fig. 14). Planning of the osteotomy at the upper border of the lesser trochanter is another principle that accommodates the geometric needs of future THR, as it preserves the anatomy below this level for cementless fixation of a stem (see Fig. 15).

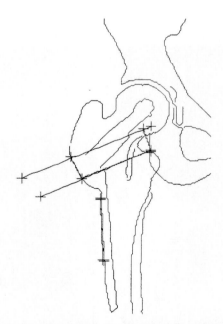

Figure 10. Preoperative plan of case 1 with ideal location of osteotomy marked at the proximal aspect of the lesser trochanter. Because of the posttraumatic deformity, a slightly oblique osteotomy line was required to preserve the lateral bony bridge. In this case, the osteotomy was planned parallel to the seating chisel with a lateral bony bridge of 20 mm between the seating chisel and the proposed osteotomy site.

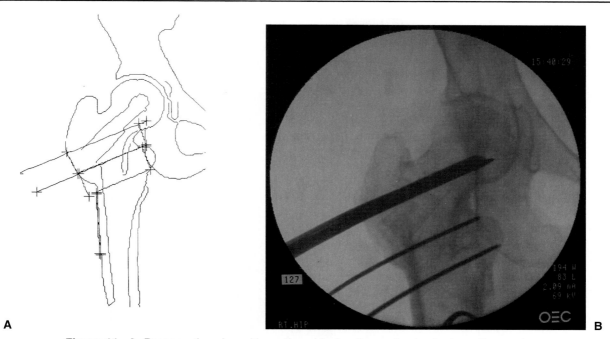

Figure 11. A: Preoperative plan with seating chisel path, proximal osteotomy line, and distal osteotomy line marked. In this case, all three are parallel for the desired correction with a planned full thickness bone segment resection. In the case of a no-wedge resection osteotomy, only one guide wire would be required. **B:** Intraoperative fluoroscopic view of the right hip with the seating chisel in place and two parallel K-wires marking out the proposed sites for osteotomies.

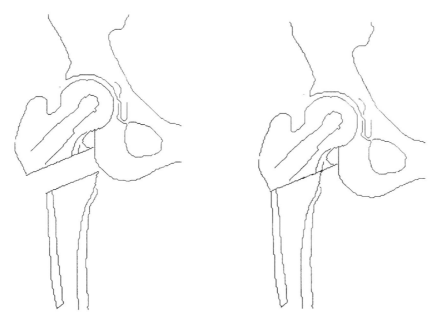

Figure 12. A: Preoperative plan with resected portion of bone removed and segments in their original positions. **B:** Preoperative plan with closure of the gap between the segments and lateralization of the femoral shaft.

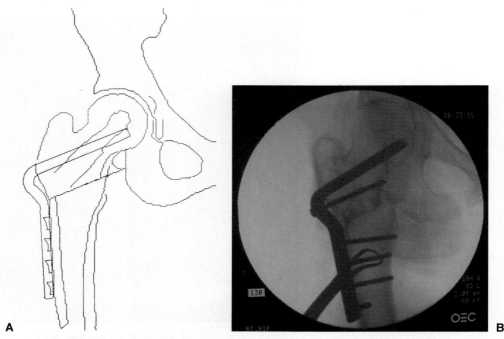

Figure 13. A: Preoperative plan with final bony alignment and blade plate in place. **B:** Intraoperative fluoroscopic view of the hip after definitive alignment and fixation of the femoral osteotomy. External rotation of the distal segment was done prior to fixation. Also note that the proximal screw in the upper fragment is inserted prior to any application of interfragmentary compression.

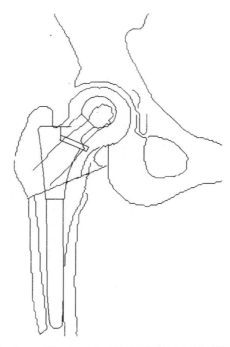

Figure 14. Preoperative plan with proposed bony resection and femoral lateralization with superimposed total hip replacement stem. An important principle of proximal femoral osteotomy surgery is to plan for possible future total hip replacement.

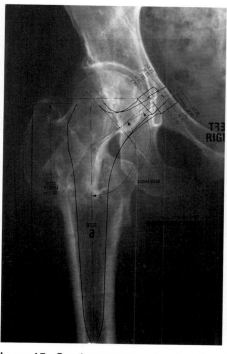
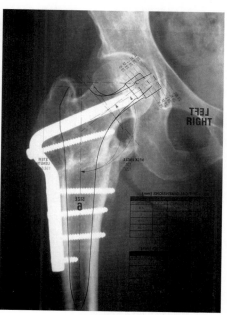

A   B

Figure 15. Contingency planning for future total hip replacement. **A:** Preoperative AP view radiograph of the right hip with superimposed hip arthroplasty template. Note that the deformity would not allow the use of a standard arthroplasty implant. **B:** Postoperative AP view radiograph of the right hip with superimposed cementless tapered wedge hip arthroplasty template. Note that the new bony anatomy allows for the use of a standard implant.

SURGERY

Patient Positioning

A radiolucent surgical table that allows for intraoperative fluoroscopic imaging of the affected hip is used. Following administration of a spinal anesthetic with adjunctive morphine crystals and optional general anesthetic, the patient is positioned in the supine position with the body shifted to the respective edge of the table until the soft tissue lateral to the proximal femur overhangs the edge of the bed (see Fig. 16). This shift accommodates both the surgical exposure, as the posterior tissues fall away from the surgical field during the procedure, and the need to perform fluoroscopic images of the K-wire, chisel, and blade plate in the frog lateral position during surgery. Care must be taken in this position to prevent the ipsilateral leg from falling off of the table either before or after draping. Once the position has been set, fluoroscopic views are taken of the entire pelvis to set the correct rotation, as well as AP and frog lateral views to make sure that the visualization needed during surgery is readily obtainable. Only then, after a time-out to verify patient identification and site and side of surgery, is the prepping and draping done. The entire leg is draped free, with easy access to the opposite ankle taken into account. Landmarks of the contralateral limb should be palpable through the drapes for assessment of leg lengths.

Technique[1]

A lateral incision is made over the proximal thigh, generally between 4 and 6 inches in length (10 to 15 cm), starting just distal to the tip of the greater trochanter and extending distally in a path parallel to the femoral shaft. The length of the incision may require adjust-

[1]All operative pictures correspond to case 1.

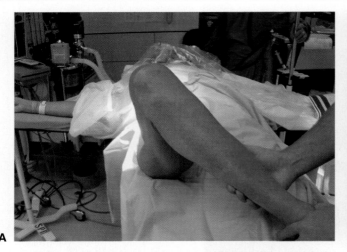

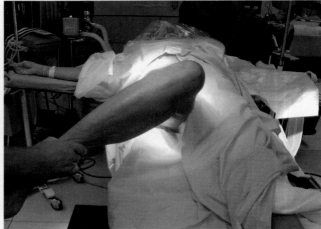

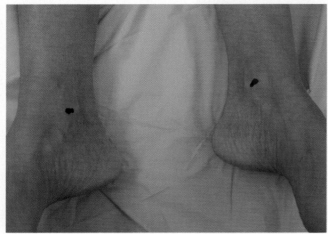

Figure 16. A: A 53-year-old woman with malunion of the right proximal femur at the time of surgery. Limited hip external rotation is seen with passive range of motion. Note that the patient is placed to the lateral edge of the surgical table to aid in retraction of the posterior tissues. **B:** Excessive hip internal rotation with passive range of motion. **C:** Note that the right (ipsilateral) leg is significantly longer than the left.

ment based on the thickness of the muscle or subcutaneous fat. The tensor fascia is split in line with its fibers (see Fig. 17). When intra-articular access for any reason is needed, the incision is extended anteriorly and proximally to permit dissection of the interval between the anterior edge of the abductors and the tensor fascia lata muscle to access the anterior capsule of the hip joint. The vastus lateralis is elevated off the lateral aspect of the femur. Care is taken to avoid excessive muscle stripping. Using fluoroscopic guidance, the lateral starting point for the proposed blade plate should be identified on the basis of the preoperative plan. The angle of insertion of the K-wire in the frontal plane is measured from the straight region of the lateral cortex, in accordance with the preoperative plan (see Fig. 3). In the case example, the angle was 70 degrees, to accommodate a 110-degree angled blade plate with no angular correction. It is just as important to verify the correct position of the wire in the orthogonal plane with the help of the frog lateral fluoroscopic image (see Fig. 18). With the K-wire in place to a depth of approximately 30 mm, the path can be confirmed on both the AP and lateral images and adjusted as needed. Once satisfied with the path, a second wire should be placed proximal to and in parallel with the first (see Fig. 19). This second wire will act as a guide for both the seating chisel and the definitive plate, and as such, should be of a diameter (7/64 in) that will not be easily bent. The proposed osteotomy site is then identified on the lateral cortex on the basis of the preoperative plan and confirmed on fluoroscopy. The minimum bridge of 15 mm of bone between the osteotomy and the blade insertion site must be maintained.

The path for the blade plate is created by drilling multiple 4.5-mm holes parallel to the first K-wire, using a guide for this purpose (see Fig. 20). If a flexion/extension component to the osteotomy is planned, then this must be accomplished prior to drilling the path for

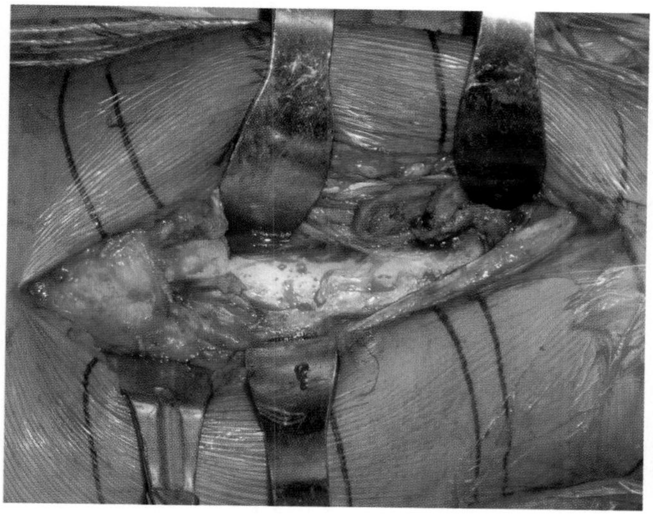

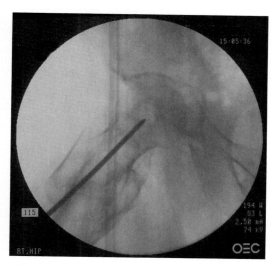

Figure 17. Incision over the lateral aspect of the proximal right thigh with exposure carried down to bone.

Figure 18. Intraoperative fluoroscopic view of the right hip in the frog lateral position. The proposed path for the blade of the blade plate is marked with a K-wire. The K-wire is centrally located within the femoral neck and head.

the blade plate. This is done by rotating the chisel the desired degrees of flexion (up to a maximum of 40 degrees) or extension (up to a maximum of 40 degrees). It is helpful to be familiar with the mathematical calculations of Bombelli, which integrate the frontal plane consequences of flexion and extension on the neck-shaft angle of the proximal femur on the frontal plane (4). Given the posterior position of the greater trochanter, extension results in increased varus in the frontal plane. When valgus osteotomies are combined with a significant extension component, additional degrees of valgus should be incorporated into the surgical plan. Conversely, in the case of a varus osteotomy, it is imperative to reduce the planned amount of varus if extension is needed. Otherwise, the varus effect in the frontal plane could be extreme. Using the remaining proximal wire as a guide, the seating chisel is

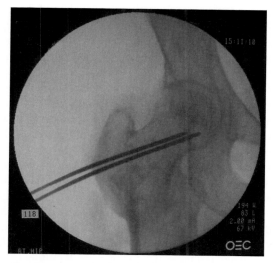

Figure 19. Intraoperative fluoroscopic view of the right hip with a second wire placed proximal to the proposed path for the blade plate in a parallel fashion. The proximal wire will serve as a reference during insertion of the seating chisel and definitive insertion of the blade plate. As such, it is important to place this wire proximal enough such that it is not deflected as the seating chisel is inserted.

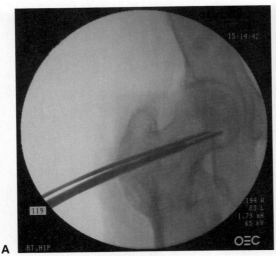
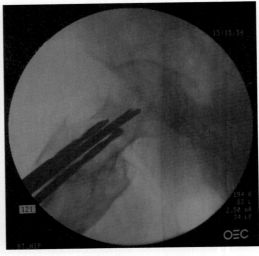

Figure 20. A: Intraoperative fluoroscopic view of the right hip while drilling the path for the seating chisel adjacent to the first K-wire. **B:** Intraoperative fluoroscopic view of the right hip in the frog lateral position with 4.5-mm drill bits at the anterior and posterior margins of the future seating chisel tract. This fluoroscopic view assures safe placement of the chisel within the borders of the femoral neck.

inserted under fluoroscopic guidance. This should be inserted to the depth of the planned blade plate. It is important to partially back out the chisel periodically during advancement to prevent incarceration (see Fig. 21). Once the chisel has been inserted to the final planned depth, the chisel is again partially backed out (approximately 15 mm) before making the osteotomy cut.

A new K-wire of smaller dimension is drilled across the femur at the proposed site of the osteotomy perpendicular to the axis of the bone with positioning confirmed by fluoroscopy. As mentioned previously, slight angulation may be required in special circumstances (see Figs. 11 and 22). The femur is then cut using the distal aspect of the K-wire as a guide. Prior to the cut, rotation control marks are made on the anterolateral surface, above and below the osteotomy site. The cut is made distal to the K-wire to ensure that no damage to the bridge of bone occurs proximally. Optional release of the iliopsoas tendon from the lesser trochanter is the next step. Indications for release include use of the lesser trochanter for a bone graft, avoidance of excessive stretch during deliberate lengthening or with lateral displacement of the distal fragment, or adherence to classic "muscle release" concepts of C. Voss, the architect of the "hanging hip" procedure for concentric arthritis in the pre-THR era. Any derotation is then done, *prior* to resection of any wedges. On the basis of the planned geometry of the correction, a wedge can be taken from the distal segment in one or two planes after controlling for rotation. If a two-plane wedge is planned, then this may be carried out as a single complex wedge or, less desirably, stepwise as two wedges. With the wedge(s) removed, mobility of the segments should be confirmed so that an adequate correction can be achieved.

With the definitive blade plate in hand, the seating chisel is removed, and the blade plate is inserted by hand along the tract using the proximal K-wire as a guide. The blade plate is then impacted into position to the intended depth. The distal plate is then provisionally reduced to the lateral cortex of the femur and held in place by a bone clamp (see Fig. 23). A cortical screw should then be placed into the most proximal screw hole of the plate prior to any interfragmentary compression. Rotation is carefully adjusted by relaxing any retraction around the proximal segment and then adjusting the patella into a direct anterior position, unless a deliberate derotation has already been done. In the latter case, this would be maintained. The bone clamp is then tightened. Leg lengths should then be compared. Fluoroscopic imaging should match the finished product of the preoperative plan (see Figs. 13A and 23). A dynamic compression device is used distally, and then definitive fixation is

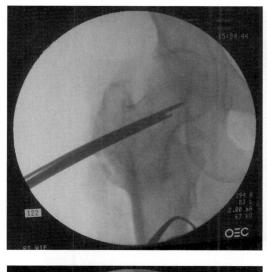

A

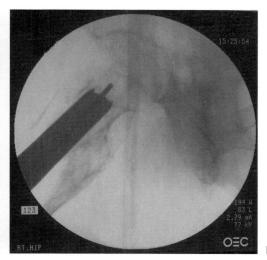

B

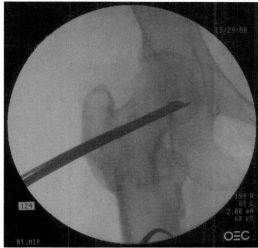

C

Figure 21. A: Intraoperative fluoroscopic view of the right hip with the seating chisel inserted through 80% of the planned pathway, using the proximal K-wire as a guide. **B:** Intraoperative fluoroscopic view of the right hip in the frog lateral position. Care is taken to avoid a breach of the femoral neck during seating chisel insertion. **C:** Intraoperative fluoroscopic view of the right hip with full insertion of the seating chisel.

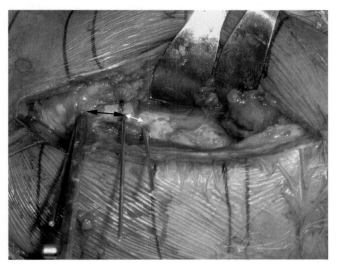

Figure 22. Intraoperative photograph of the wound with (from left to right) guide wire, seating chisel, K-wire marking proximal osteotomy, and K-wire marking distal osteotomy. This picture corresponds to the plan and fluoroscopic images of Figures 11A and B. The black double arrow represents the bony bridge between the seating chisel and the proximal osteotomy. The white double arrow represents the wedge of bone to be resected.

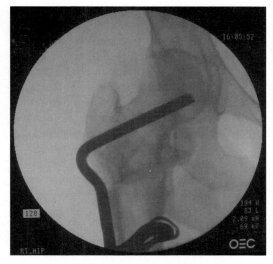

Figure 23. Intraoperative fluoroscopic view of the right hip with blade plate inserted and temporarily fixed to the femoral shaft with a clamp. No compression across the osteotomy site has occurred. At this point, the blade plate could be exchanged for one with a longer blade should greater lateralization of the femoral shaft be required.

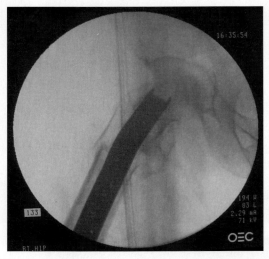

Figure 24. Intraoperative fluoroscopic view of the right hip in the frog lateral position after correction and definitive fixation.

achieved with additional cortical screws, inserted with neutral compression. Final intraoperative lateral fluoroscopic view reflects slight extension, as per R. Bombelli (see Fig. 24). Range of motion of the hip should be checked at several stages, i.e., after provisional fixation with the large clamp, after one or two screws, and then after soft tissue closure. Correct balance of internal and external rotation and equalization of leg lengths are demonstrated in this postoperative office visit of a successful osteotomy procedure (see Fig. 25). Malrota-

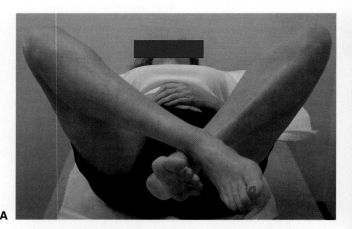

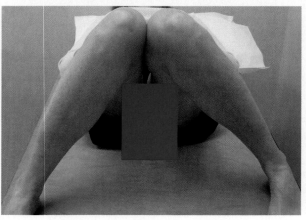

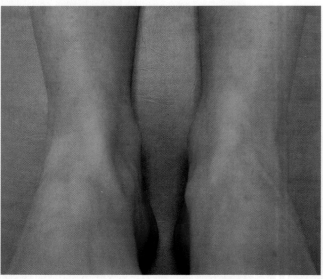

Figure 25. A: Postoperative clinical photograph at 16 weeks demonstrating improved external rotation with active range of motion equal to the opposite limb. **B:** Postoperative clinical photograph at 16 weeks demonstrating normalized internal rotation with active range of motion equal to the opposite limb. **C:** Postoperative clinical photograph at 16 weeks demonstrating equal leg lengths.

tion is one of the most frequent technical complications of intertrochanteric osteotomy and should be corrected if recognized after provisional or definitive osteosynthesis. An anatomic layer-by-layer closer is performed after irrigation.

POSTOPERATIVE MANAGEMENT

Patients should remain on touch-down weight-bearing precautions for 6 weeks following surgery followed by weight bearing to tolerance for 4 to 6 additional weeks. Full weight bearing should not begin until union across the osteotomy site is observed on radiographs (see Figs. 26 to 29). A cane or single crutch is used until there is no limp. We recommend routine hardware removal at 18 to 24 months following surgery for multiple reasons, including the frequency of hardware-related bursitis, the fatigue of metal over many years,

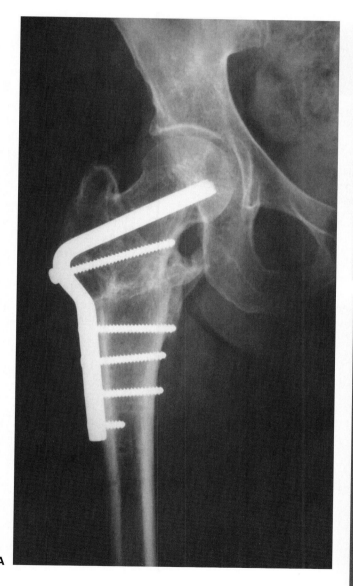

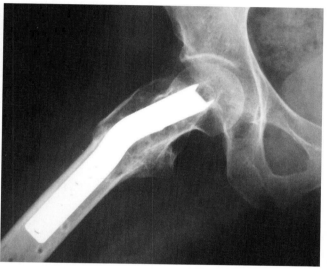

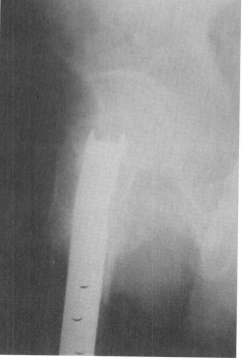

Figure 26. A 53-year-old woman with corrected proximal femoral malunion 7 months following osteotomy. **A:** AP view right hip. **B:** Frog lateral view right hip. **C:** False profile view right hip.

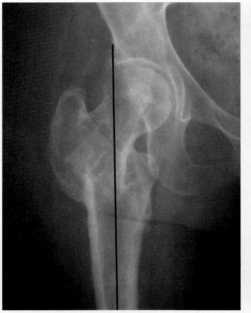
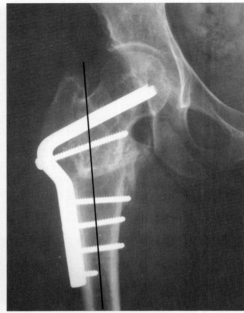

Figure 27. Comparison of preoperative **(A)** and postoperative **(B)** AP right hip views with femoral shaft axis marked. Note the lateralization of the femoral shaft relative to the preoperative view.

and the desirability of normal bone strength and absence of stress risers if THR is necessary in the future. This is performed on an outpatient basis and is followed by crutch-protected weight bearing for 4 to 6 weeks.

RESULTS

Valgus osteotomies have proven useful in the treatment of femoral neck nonunion in several studies. Marti et al. demonstrated a 94% union rate among 50 nonunions (5). Out of this series, only 7 had required total hip replacement by 7 years. Of 37 patients reviewed in detail, 22 had radiographic evidence of aseptic necrosis. Of these, only three had required

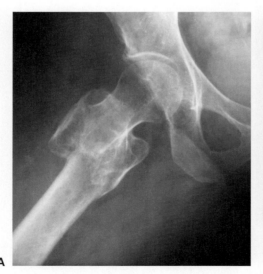
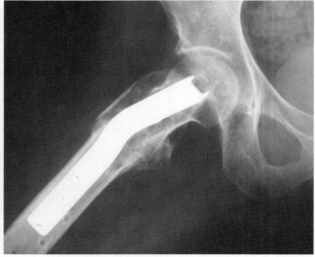

Figure 28. Comparison of preoperative **(A)** and postoperative **(B)** frog lateral right hip views. Note the correction of the deformity with the femoral shaft being translated anteriorly.

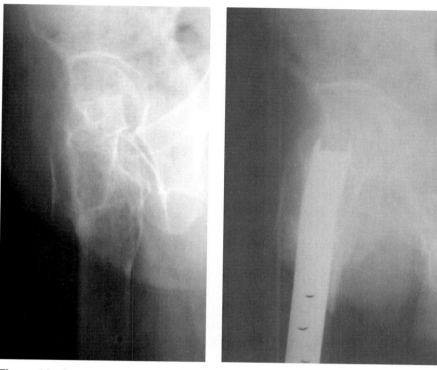

A

B

Figure 29. Comparison of preoperative **(A)** and postoperative **(B)** false profile right hip views. Note the correction of the deformity with the femoral shaft being translated anteriorly as was noted in Figure 28.

hip replacement. Thus, it was concluded that necrosis, prior to collapse, was not a contraindication to valgus osteotomy. Anglen found that all 13 of his patients experienced union, and 12 returned to normal daily function with no pain (6). Differences in union rates were noted by Weber and Cech, varying with the presence of aseptic necrosis of the femoral head (7). They found that of the 23 nonunions without aseptic necrosis, 91% healed and reported good to normal function. Of the 13 hips with a combination of nonunion and aseptic necrosis, only 54% healed, with the remaining 46% having a poor clinical outcome. Bartonicek et al. reported on a series of 11 malunited and 4 nonunited fractures (8). Healing occurred in 14 of the patients with an average improvement in leg lengths of 2 cm. Hip flexion was greater than 90 degrees in all patients at final follow-up. In managing the deformity of slipped capital femoral epiphysis in adults with triplane osteotomy, Imhauser reported only one case of severe arthritis and pain at a minimum of 11 years of follow-up of 68 hips treated with valgus ITO (9). Fifty-five patients were clinically assessed, and of these, 25% had early degenerative changes. Five patients had significantly limited ranges of motion.

Limited success has been reported for the use of valgus and valgus-flexion osteotomies in aseptic necrosis. Maistrelli et al. reported only 58% good and excellent results at 8 years in 106 cases (10). With an average of 10.4 years of follow-up, Drescher et al. found that 27% of 70 cases of flexion ITO had undergone THR with a mean time to replacement of 8.7 years (11). Early results were more favorable with 90% survival at 5 years. Specific subgroups had improved results from the average. These included patients less than 55 years of age, good preoperative range of motion, patients with no evidence of collapse, less than 200-degree necrotic (Kerboul) angle, and posttraumatic or idiopathic etiology (10–12). Steroid- and alcohol-induced cases tended to have poorer outcomes (10).

Use of a valgus-extension ITO for treatment of osteoarthritis in dysplastic hips has been demonstrated as effective, but with pain relief less than that provided by THR. Langlais et al. reported on 150 cases and found that pain relief was durable at an average of 6 years of follow-up for 81% to 88% of patients, depending on the underlying pathology (13). The joint space was also found to be improved in 60% of cases. Maistrelli et al.'s series of 277 cases found that 67% had good to excellent results more than 11 years out from surgery (14). This increased to 76% when assessing only those patients less than 40 years of age. Preoperative flexion of greater than 60 degrees was associated with success in 68% of cases versus 31% with limited flexion. Mechanical etiology was associated with a 71% success rate versus 42% in "primary" osteoarthritis. It is clear that salvage osteotomy is an unusual option at this point in the evolution of THR; however, it cannot be completely abandoned in young patients who have good morphologic indications.

Varus osteotomy for the treatment of sequelae of developmental dysplasia of the hip has been declining in popularity with the success of the rotational pelvic osteotomies. Morscher reported on 179 cases performed in cases with lateral joint space narrowing, sclerosis, and congruency in abduction (15). He also reported using valgus osteotomies in an additional 84 cases with pronounced head deformity and congruency in adduction. Good to excellent results were reported in 88% in the total study at final follow-up. Iwase et al. found 89% and 87% successful results among 52 cases at 10 and 15 years, respectively (16). The higher success rates reported in this series are likely related to a younger patient age (mean of 25 years) at the time of surgery.

COMPLICATIONS

Nonunion of the femoral osteotomy is uncommon but does occur. When it occurs, it is associated with screw and hardware breakage, as well as loss of the position achieved at the original surgery. Prosthetic options should rarely be considered, as treatment of the nonunion with refixation and bone grafting is usually successful. There are several techniques that can minimize this risk, beginning with patient selection. Tobacco smoking is a potent inhibitor of bone healing and must be addressed. Patients should abstain from smoking for a minimum of 2 weeks prior to and 12 weeks after surgery (ideally never resuming). Incapacity for compliance with restricted weight bearing (i.e., crutch usage) should be considered a contraindication, as should obesity (BMI >30), because of the potential loss of fixation with the increased forces transmitted across the osteotomy. We avoid nonsteroidal anti-inflammatory drug use after the third day postoperatively. Every osteotomy is a race between bone union and hardware/fixation failure. Efforts should be made to shift the balance in favor of union.

Malrotation, especially excessive external rotation of the distal fragments; unplanned or excessive shortening or lengthening of the limb; fracture of the bone bridge between the chisel site and the osteotomy level; and bursitis over the hardware are other recognized complications.

Ultimately, progression of arthritis is a common occurrence in these patients. The goal is to have many years of comfort and function before any additional surgery is required. A patient who undergoes an osteotomy only to require a hip replacement 2 years later would, in retrospect, have been better served by an arthroplasty as the index procedure. Middle-aged patients with progressively increasing hip pain of recent duration may be in a phase of rapid arthritic progression. Osteotomy in these patients should be considered with caution.

Nerve palsy can result as a consequence of osteotomy surgery. Gentle retraction with relaxation when not required reduces the stretch on nerves. Protection of the soft tissues when making the bone cuts is important. Planned lengthening of more that 2.5 cm should be done with caution.

Fracture of the femur can occur after hardware removal but is very rare. This risk can be minimized by advising patients of the risk and requesting that they use crutches until able to walk with no limp (approximately 4 to 6 weeks) and avoid impact and contact recreational activities for several months following implant removal.

Deep venous thrombosis and pulmonary embolism can also occur. We routinely use the same anticoagulation protocol for these patients as is recommended for total hip replacement patients. The investment of time and thought that is given to the selection, planning, and postoperative care is rewarded by the high degree of patient satisfaction with joint preservation surgery.

RECOMMENDED READING

1. Pauwels F. *Atlas of Biomechanics of the Healthy and Diseased Hip.* New York: Springer-Verlag, 1975.
2. Barr RJ, Santore RF. Osteotomies about the hip—adults. In: Chapman MW, Szabo RM, Marder R, et al., eds. *Chapman's Orthopaedic Surgery.* 3rd ed. Philadelphia: Lippincott Williams & Wilkins, 2001:2723–2768.
3. Ganz R. Proximal femur. In: Allgower M, ed. *Manual of Internal Fixation.* New York: Springer-Verlag, 1991: 524–525.
4. Bombelli R. *Osteoarthritis of the Hip: Pathogenesis and Consequent Therapy.* New York: Springer-Verlag, 1976.
5. Marti RK, Schuller HM, Raaymakers EL. Intertrochanteric osteotomy for non-union of the femoral neck. *J Bone Joint Surg Br* 71:782–787, 1989.
6. Anglen JO. Intertrochanteric osteotomy for failed internal fixation of femoral neck fracture. *Clin Orthop Relat Res* 341:175–182, 1997.
7. Weber BG, Cech O. *Pseudarthrosis: Pathophysiology, Biomechanics, Therapy, Results.* New York: Grune & Stratton, 1976.
8. Bartonicek J, Skala-Rosenbaum J, Dousa P. Valgus intertrochanteric osteotomy for malunion and nonunion of trochanteric fractures. *J Orthop Trauma* 17:606–612, 2003.
9. Imhauser G. [Late results of Imhauser's osteotomy for slipped capital femoral epiphysis]. *Z Orthop Ihre Grenzgeb* 115:716–725, 1977.
10. Maistrelli G, Fusco U, Avai A, et al. Osteonecrosis of the hip treated by intertrochanteric osteotomy. A 4- to 15-year follow-up. *J Bone Joint Surg Br* 70:761–766, 1988.
11. Drescher W, Furst M, Hahne HJ, et al. Survival analysis of hips treated with flexion osteotomy for femoral head necrosis. *J Bone Joint Surg Br* 85:969–974, 2003.
12. Dinulescu I, Stanculescu D, Nicolescu M, et al. Long-term follow-up after intertrochanteric osteotomies for avascular necrosis of the femoral head. *Bull Hosp Jt Dis* 57:84–87, 1998.
13. Langlais F, Roure JL, Maquet P. Valgus osteotomy in severe osteoarthritis of the hip. *J Bone Joint Surg Br* 61:424–431, 1979.
14. Maistrelli GL, Gerundini M, Fusco U, et al. Valgus-extension osteotomy for osteoarthritis of the hip. Indications and long-term results. *J Bone Joint Surg Br* 72:653–657, 1990.
15. Morscher E. Intertrochanteric osteotomy in osteoarthritis of the hip. In: Riley LH Jr, ed. *The Hip: Proceedings of the Eighth Open Scientific Meeting of the Hip Society.* St. Louis, Mo: Mosby, 1980: 24–26.
16. Iwase T, Hasegawa Y, Kawamoto K, et al. Twenty years' followup of intertrochanteric osteotomy for treatment of the dysplastic hip. *Clin Orthop Relat Res* 331:245–255, 1996.

8

Periacetabular Osteotomy

Robert T. Trousdale

INDICATIONS/CONTRAINDICATIONS AND PREOPERATIVE PLANNING

The Bernese periacetabular osteotomy has become the procedure of choice in many centers for the treatment of young patients with symptomatic hip dysplasia in the absence of severe secondary arthritis. Younger patients with hip dysplasia without marked degenerative joint disease should still rely on nonarthroplasty options to help control pain and hopefully retard the progress of arthritic changes. Multiple different types of osteotomies have been developed to improve symptoms and joint mechanics in young patients with symptomatic hip dysplasia. In 1992, we began using the Bernese periacetabular osteotomy because of its balance between minimal exposure, acceptable complication rate, and the ability to provide optimal correction of the dysplastic hip (see Fig. 1). Its advantages are multiple and have been well described. It can be performed through one incision without major violation of the abductors; the pelvic ring and outlet are not disrupted, which allows for early mobilization; there is no need for postoperative immobilization; and it allows for future vaginal delivery without complication in women. Furthermore, it allows optimal correction both medially and laterally and version changes as needed. One can also perform a capsulotomy to both assess and treat impingement and labral pathology without markedly compromising acetabular blood supply.

In our mind, the ideal patient for a reconstructive pelvic osteotomy is one who is relatively young, has minimal secondary arthritic changes, and has a poorly covered femoral head. The socket and femoral head should be relatively round with the ability to obtain a congruent hip after correction.

SURGICAL TECHNIQUE

Most of our patients have this procedure done under regional epidural anesthesia. We have abandoned the use of preoperative autologous blood donation since intraoperative cell saver appears very helpful in minimizing the need for allogenic blood. Presently, our allogenic transfusion rate is less than one in five patients.

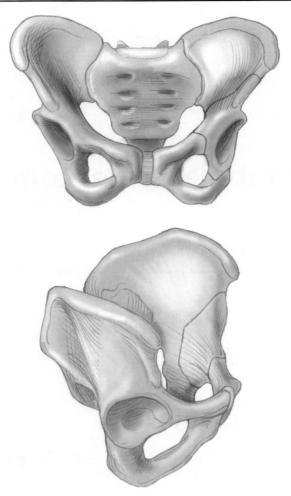

Figure 1. Diagrams showing location of osteotomies.

The patient is placed on an image table. A Foley catheter is inserted. We use intraoperative electromyography (EMG) monitoring of the sciatic nerve and femoral nerve to minimize the chance of permanent neurologic injury (see Fig. 2). In 1992, we began performing the procedure using an anterior incision with exposure of both the inner and outer tables of the pelvis. In 1996, we began utilizing the same skin incision, performing the osteotomy only through the inner aspect of the pelvis, leaving the abductors intact on the outer aspect of the ilium. We feel that this has dramatically improved the rate of healing, the time allowable to weight bearing, and the resolution of the postoperative limp. The incision typically begins along the border of the iliac crest, proceeds along the anterior superior iliac spine, and continues distally, ending approximately 3 cm distal and anterior to the greater trochanter (see Fig. 3). The plane between the tensor fascia lata and sartorius is developed, incising the deep fascia over the tensor fascia lata, avoiding direct injury to the lateral femoral cutaneous nerve. The sartorius origin is reflected from the anterior superior iliac spine, the hip is flexed and adducted, and the inner table of the pelvis is exposed to the sciatic notch. The pubis is then exposed by retracting the iliopsoas tendon medially, and a Hohmann retractor is placed in the pubic bone. The direct head of the rectus is reflected distally from the anterior inferior iliac spine, exposing the anterior hip capsule. Using blunt dissection, one proceeds distally and medially, and under an image intensifier, a scissors is used to palpate the ischium and obturator foramen.

Performing the osteotomies has become relatively routine with the aid of an image intensifier. We use the image intensifier at four critical points during the performance of the osteotomies. We perform the ischial osteotomy initially, and an anteroposterior image is

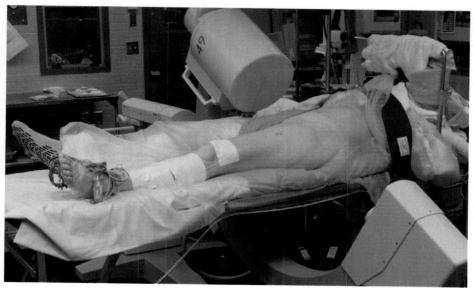

Figure 2. Intraoperative photograph showing EMG monitor and fluoroscopy in place. This patient's left hip is the operated side.

used to assure that the osteotomy is distal and medial enough and oriented in the proper direction (see Fig. 4). The ischial osteotome is left in place as a guide when performing the last osteotomy (the posterior iliac osteotomy). Often, one can palpate this osteotome medially and distally over the quadrilateral surface. We then expose the pubic bone using the Hohmann retractor, checking with the image intensifier to make sure that we are medial enough, which will prevent entry of the osteotomy into the joint. The pubic osteotomy is performed in an oblique fashion, proximal-medial to distal-lateral, which facilitates mobilization of the fragment. The iliac cut is typically performed just at the level just distal to the anterior superior iliac spine, but an anteroposterior image is obtained to make sure one is high enough above the joint to allow satisfactory fixation of the distal fragment. It is often helpful to orientate the iliac cut slightly distal to make sure that when the iliac cut is turned to connect with the ischial cut, one is distal to the top of the sciatic notch. The image intensifier really becomes helpful with the last osteotomy (see Fig. 5). We get a 45-degree oblique x-ray showing the posterior column of the acetabulum, and one can make sure that

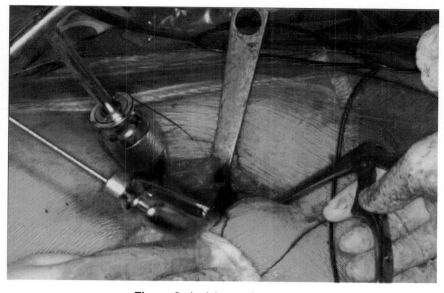

Figure 3. Incision and exposure.

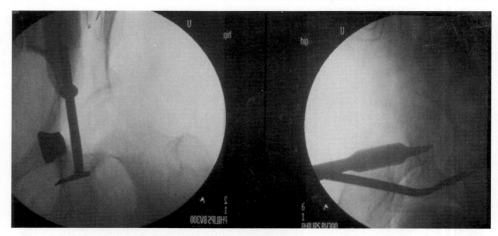

Figure 4. Intraoperative fluoroscopy showing placement of ischial osteotome. A Hohman retractor is in the lateral aspect of the pubic bone.

the posterior osteotomy is extra-articular, as well as that one has not violated the posterior column of the pelvis. Once the cuts are made, the fragment is mobilized. Occasionally, the "corners" of the cuts can impinge or catch, limiting mobilization. One has to be careful not to hinge the fragment with correction. This error is easily detected both by palpation as well as radiographically. The acetabular teardrop should flip radiographically, proving that the fragment is not hinging. If one is hinging posteriorly and inferiorly, this corner of the fragment can be trimmed with an osteotome or rongeur, and this will facilitate mobility of the fragment. When all three osteotomies are completed in the proper location, the posterior column should be left intact, and the acetabular fragment should be free and mobile.

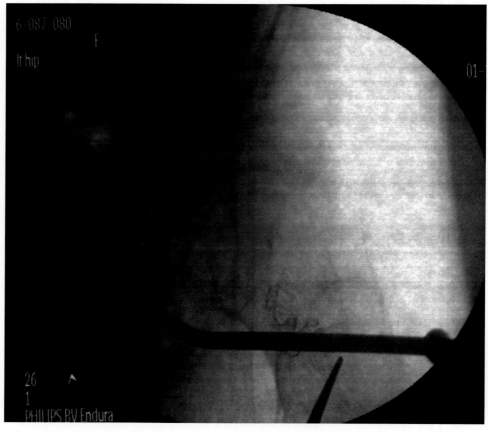

Figure 5. Intraoperative fluoroscopy showing the posterior iliac cut joining the ischial cut.

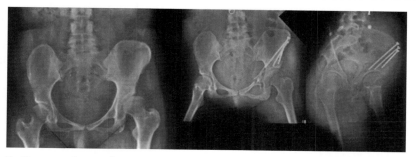

Figure 6. Preoperative and postoperative radiographs of a dysplastic left hip with satisfactory correction in all planes.

The most difficult part of the operation is obtaining proper correction. Figure 6 shows a well-corrected osteotomy. We presently think of the proper correction in four different steps: proper medialization of the hip center of rotation, proper acetabular version, proper lateral coverage, and proper anteroposterior coverage of the femoral head. In reality, there is only one perfect correction for each dysplastic hip, and errors in correction in any one of the above-mentioned planes can lead to suboptimal coverage, decreased contact area of the hip joint, increased contact forces, impingement, or secondary subluxation of the joint. When assessing correction, we get a true anteroposterior pelvic radiograph with temporary fixation of the osteotomized fragment. Making sure the pelvis is not tilted in any direction will facilitate proper assessment of acetabular version and medialization. A true antero-posterior radiograph should have symmetrical obturator foramens with the coccyx ending approximately 1 cm proximal to the symphysis pubis. Medialization of the fragment allows one to decrease the joint contact forces by decreasing the body weight lever arm. In most dysplastic hips, the hip center is abnormally lateralized. If the contralateral hip is normal, one can use that as a guide for proper medialization. In cases of bilateral dysplasia, we place the medial aspect of the femoral head just lateral (0 to 5 mm) to the ilioischial line. Proper lateral correction is best assessed by normalizing the weight-bearing acetabular surface of the acetabulum and making the weight-bearing surface between 0 and 10 degrees off horizontal. It is important not to overcorrect laterally, as this can lead to impingement and may potentially bring the fovea into the weight-bearing surface. If the Tönnis angle (angle of acetabular sourcil) has been normalized and the Wieberg angle is still less than optimal, consideration then should be given to performing a varus femoral osteotomy. Intraoperative functional views with fluoroscopy can help in that decision-making process. Anterior correction and anteversion are critical, as it is very easy to overcorrect the fragment anteriorly, which will lead to anterior impingement of the femoral head-neck junction on the anterior rim of the acetabulum with secondary limitation of hip flexion and potential pain. In extreme cases, anterior overcorrection can lead to posterior subluxation of the femoral head and anterior impingement. On a true anteroposterior radiograph of the pelvis, the relationship of the anterior and posterior acetabular rims relative to the lateral edge of the weight-bearing surface will give an indication of anteversion. We like the anterior wall to cover approximately one third of the femoral head and the posterior wall to cover about one half of the femoral head, and both those walls should meet at the lateral aspect of the acetabular sourcil. If the anterior wall covers less of the femoral head than the posterior wall, and they meet at the lateral aspect of the sourcil on a true anteroposterior pelvic radiograph, then the socket is adequately anteverted. If the posterior wall meets the sourcil medial to the anterior wall, then the socket has been retroverted. Once correction in all planes is deemed satisfactory, temporary smooth pins are removed and replaced with three 4.5-mm fully threaded cortical screws (Fig. 6). The hip capsule is then opened to assess the labrum. If the labrum is detached from the rim and repairable, it is fixed with sutures. If it is frayed and nonrepairable, we will perform an elliptical excision. We also check to make sure we can flex the hip up to 110 to 115 degrees without impingement of the head-neck junction on the acetabular rim. If there is impingement, we make sure we have not retroverted the socket. If socket anteversion is felt to be appropriate, we will improve the head-neck ratio by doing an osteochondroplasty at the anterior head-neck junction.

POSTOPERATIVE MANAGEMENT AND REHABILITATION

The patient is mobilized on ambulatory aids the day after surgery. Intravenous antibiotics are used for 24 hours. Drains are removed the day after surgery. We leave the epidural and Foley catheter in place for 24 to 48 hours. Aspirin is used for 6 weeks for deep venous thrombosis prophylaxis. Weight bearing as tolerated is begun at 6 weeks with adduction exercises, water therapy, and stationary bike exercises at 4 weeks.

COMPLICATIONS

Potential complications of this operation are multiple. Over the past 13 years, the operative time in our hands has significantly decreased, as has the blood loss (average operative time is now about 122 min, and blood loss is 480 cc). Heterotopic ossification, symptomatic hardware, infection, and wound problems are relatively rare. We have had 3 known cases of deep venous thrombosis in the first 300 patients. One of these patients had an asymptomatic pulmonary embolus.

Major neurologic problems are relatively uncommon in our hands with the use of the intraoperative EMG monitoring. We have noted that approximately 25% of patients are at potential risk for nerve damage, but only 0.7% had peroneal palsy at greater than 1 year from the procedure. We have not had any femoral or tibial nerve problems. Numbness in the lateral femoral cutaneous nerve distribution is common (>50%), but at 1 year from surgery, most patients have had their numbness resolved (<10%). We continue to use intraoperative cell saver but no longer have patients donate autologous blood. The average blood loss is approximately 400 cc.

Iliac osteotomy union is the routine. We have an approximate 8% rate of pubic nonunions, but we have not operated on any of these patients. The iliac osteotomy has healed in all patients. We have had two ischial nonunions, one of which required bone grafting. The rate of pubic nonunion appears directly related to the severity of the dysplasia. The larger the correction that is required, the larger the gap between the pubic bones and the higher chance of pubic nonunion.

Although the learning curve for this procedure in our hands has been relatively long, a well-done osteotomy in the properly selected patient is a relatively reliable and successful procedure for the patient with symptomatic hip dysplasia.

RECOMMENDED READING

1. Clohisy JC, Barrett JE, Gordon E, et al. Periacetabular osteotomy for the treatment of severe acetabular dysplasia. *J Bone Joint Surg Am* 87:254–259, 2005.
2. Crockarell J, Trousdale RT, Cabanela ME, Berry DJ. Early experience and results with the periacetabular osteotomy. The Mayo Clinic experience. *Clin Orthop Relat Res* 363:45–53, 1999.
3. Davey JP, Santore RF. Complications of periacetabular osteotomy. *Clin Orthop Relat Res* 353:33–37, 1999.
4. Ganz R, Klaue K, Vinh TS, Mast JW. A new periacetabular osteotomy for the treatment of hip dysplasias. Technique and preliminary results. *Clin Orthop Relat Res* 232:26–36, 1988.
5. Hussell JG, Mast JW, Mayo KA, et al. A comparison of different surgical approaches for the periacetabular osteotomy. *Clin Orthop Relat Res* 363:64–72, 1999.
6. Murphy SB, Millis MB. Periacetabular osteotomy without abductor dissection using direct anterior exposure. *Clin Orthop Relat Res* 364:92–98, 1999.
7. Myers SR, Eijer H, Ganz R. Anterior femoroacetabular impingement after periacetabular osteotomy. *Clin Orthop Relat Res* 363:93–99, 1999.
8. Pring ME, Trousdale RT, Cabanela ME, Harper CM. Intraoperative electromyographic monitoring during periacetabular osteotomy. *Clin Orthop Relat Res* 400:158–164, 2002.
9. Siebenrock KA, Schöll E, Lottenbach M, Ganz R. Bernese periacetabular osteotomy. *Clin Orthop Relat Res* 363:9–20, 1999.
10. Trousdale RT, Ekkernkamp A, Ganz R. Periacetabular osteotomy for the dysplastic hip with osteoarthritis. *J Bone Joint Surg Am* 77:73–85, 1995.

9

Arthroscopy

Joseph C. McCarthy and Jo-ann Lee

INDICATIONS

Advances in technology and technique have facilitated comprehensive access to the hip arthroscopically. This has allowed minimally invasive treatment of an evolving series of conditions in and about the hip joint. Labral tears most often present with mechanical symptoms such as buckling, clicking, or catching and painful, restricted range of joint motion. Labral tears most frequently occur on the articular nonvascular white zone and will not heal with conservative treatment.

Chondral lesions are one of the most elusive sources of hip joint pain. These lesions are most frequently found in association with a labral tear but may also occur with loose bodies, posterior dislocation, osteonecrosis, slipped capital femoral epiphysis, dysplasia, and degenerative arthritis (see Fig. 1). The extent or thickness of the cartilage injury is the most decisive predictor of surgical outcome. Dysplasia may produce hyperplasia of the labrum, which can make it more susceptible to an injury or tear. Hyperplasia may result in impingement, which produces mechanical symptoms such as locking, catching, or buckling. Arthroscopic debridement of the labrum may alleviate mechanical symptoms.

Calcified loose bodies are readily identified by radiographic studies. If not evident on plain films, computed tomography (CT) or magnetic resonance (MR) scanning, with or without contrast, can be more sensitive. Mechanical symptoms such as locking or catching can corroborate clinical suspicion. Arthroscopy establishes the diagnosis, as well as provides simultaneous treatment using a minimally invasive technique. Loose bodies may occur as an isolated fragment, or they may be multiple (2 to 300) as seen in synovial chondromatosis. In synovial chondromatosis, the bodies typically aggregate together in grapelike clusters and often adhere to the synovium about the fovea.

Arthroscopy has a limited role in osteonecrosis and should be reserved for those patients in early stages with mechanical symptoms. Arthroscopy can be performed simultaneously with a core decompression in order to more thoroughly evaluate the chondral surfaces. A patient with osteonecrosis can be left symptomatic from an untreated chondral lesion. Arthroscopy allows a comprehensive mapping of the femoral head and acetabular joint surfaces, the labrum and the synovium, but has no role in end-stage disease with a collapsed femoral head.

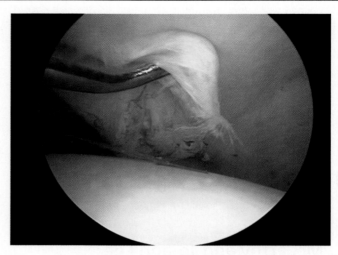

Figure 1. Arthroscopic photo showing a labral tear with adjacent acetabular chondral lesion. The femoral head is shown at the bottom of the photo.

Most patients with a painful total hip replacement do not require arthroscopic evaluation, but when unexplained symptoms persist despite appropriate conservative treatment and a workup that is unrevealing, arthroscopy can be valuable. In suspected sepsis with negative joint aspirations, arthroscopy can establish a diagnosis with joint fluid analysis and synovial biopsy. At the same time, debridement of exudates and impinging granulation tissue is performed along with copious lavage and appropriate intravenous antibiotic therapy. Intra-articular third bodies such as broken trochanteric wire or porous beads can often be successfully removed arthroscopically. An acetabular screw that showed progressive backing out on x-ray has been successfully removed. A diagnosis was established on a patient with a metal-on-metal articulating surface who had a large inguinal cyst with repeated negative joint aspirations. There was metal-on-metal corrosion at the head-neck articulation as well as numerous porous beads throughout the joint, including at the metal-metal bearing interface.

Posttraumatic hematomas can be evacuated, chondral loose bodies can be removed, and labral injuries (often posterior with trauma) can be repaired arthroscopically. Dislocations and fracture dislocations can also produce shear damage to the chondral surfaces of the femoral head or acetabulum not often seen by magnetic resonance imaging (MRI). Intra-articular foreign bodies, such as bullet fragments with or without an associated fracture, can affect the hip and can be removed arthroscopically.

CONTRAINDICATIONS

Absolute contraindications include hip pain referred from other sources such as a compression fracture of the lumbar spine. Osteonecrosis or synovitis in the absence of mechanical symptoms do not warrant arthroscopy. Acute skin lesions or ulceration, especially in the vicinity of portal placement, or sepsis with accompanying osteomyelitis or abscess formation would exclude arthroscopy. Advanced osteoarthritis, Grade III or IV heterotopic bone, joint ankylosis, and significant protrusio are all contraindications.

Morbid obesity is a relative contraindication for arthroscopy, not only because of distraction limitations but also because of the requisite length of instruments necessary to access and maneuver within the deeply recessed joint. Moderate dysplasia needs to be judiciously evaluated prior to arthroscopic intervention. If there is evidence of instability, femoral head translation, or an upsloping acetabular sourcil, then arthroscopy is not warranted.

PREOPERATIVE PLANNING

Judicious patient selection is a key factor in predicting successful surgical outcomes. This includes only those patients with mechanical symptoms (catching, locking, or buckling) that persist despite normal radiographic findings and failed conservative therapy. Positive exam findings include positive McCarthy sign; inguinal pain with flexion, adduction, and internal rotation; and inguinal pain with resisted straight leg-raising. Arthroscopy is not a substitute for clinical acumen. Occasionally an intra-articular joint injection with a steroid and marcaine, done under fluoroscopic control, may help to clarify whether the source of pain is intra-articular.

Radiologic studies including plain radiographs, arthrography, bone scintigraphy, CT, and MRI often have poor diagnostic yield for intra-articular lesions. While the addition of contrast agents in conjunction with CT and MRI may increase the diagnostic yield of intra-articular hip pathology, arthrography may increase diagnostic yield (see Fig. 2).

Labral tears may contribute to the progression of degenerative arthritis. Patients at increased risk are those with developmental dysplasia, those with tears associated with full thickness chondral lesions, and those with tears present for greater than 5 years. The key point to be emphasized is that surgical outcomes are significantly correlated with the extent of the articular surface involvement and the degree of damage.

SURGICAL TECHNIQUE

The lateral approach requires that the patient be positioned in the lateral decubitus position with the affected hip up. Most intra-articular lesions occur in the anterior, superior quadrant of the hip and can be treated easily via the two primary portals of the lateral approach. Surgeons may use a modified fracture table or a dedicated hip distractor that is available through Innomed Corp. (Savannah, Georgia) (see Fig. 3). This device can be positioned on a regular operating room table and is adjustable in multiple planes. Adequate distraction is required to lift the femoral head away from the acetabulum to allow passage of instruments into the recesses of the joint. It is important not only for visualization but also to prevent scuffing of chondral surfaces. A well-padded perineal post is positioned and adjusted prior to applying

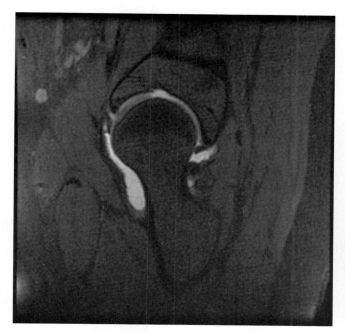

Figure 2. An MRI gadolinium-enhanced image showing an anterior labral tear.

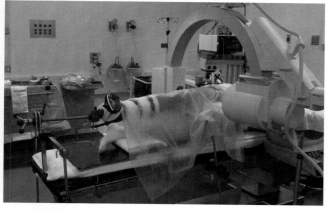

Figure 3. This shows the room setup with the patient positioned in the lateral decubitus position with the leg in the distractor.

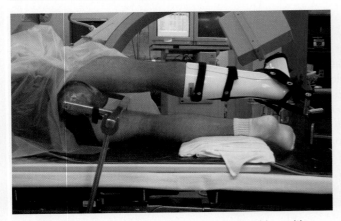

Figure 4. This shows the patient in lateral position with a well-padded peroneal post.

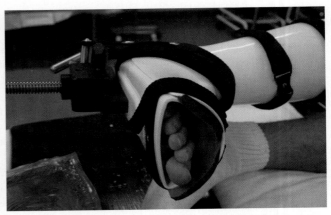

Figure 5. The foot is carefully padded prior to being securely placed in the boot.

traction (see Fig. 4). Axial traction is applied via a carefully padded foot boot with the heel firmly seated and secured (see Fig. 5). The traction device is adjusted such that the foot can be maintained in neutral position regarding eversion and/or inversion of the hind foot, thereby avoiding undue stress to the ligamentous structures on one side or the other of the ankle. Distraction is applied with the leg abducted between 0° and 20°, depending on the patient's neck shaft angle and the depth of the acetabulum. The hip then is placed in slight forward flexion of approximately 10° to 20° (see Fig. 6). General anesthesia with adequate skeletal

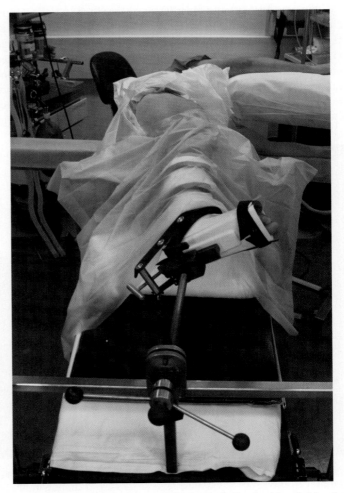

Figure 6. The leg is placed in slight forward flexion with the foot in slight external rotation.

muscle relaxation also reduces the force required to distract the hip. A tensiometer on the hip distraction device may be a significant help in preventing overzealous distraction. Adequate distraction should be 8 to 10 mm for ease of instrument entrance. With this technique, the majority of hip arthroscopies can be done with distraction forces between 25 and 100 lbs of direct axial traction. Avoid continuous traction for more than 1.5 hours at a time. Inadvertent loss of traction while instruments are in the joint may result in harm to the articular cartilage or instrument breakage within the joint.

Fluoroscopic images determine the relative distraction of the femoral head from the acetabulum (see Fig. 7). The negative intra-articular pressure that results from the distraction force is released using a 6-inch, 18-gauge spinal needle with a Nitinol wire and an image intensifier if necessary. The needle is placed superior to the greater trochanter and tangential to the acetabulum, and a "give" sensation is felt upon capsule entry. A second 6-inch, 18-gauge spinal needle is then advanced into the hip capsule, and then the joint is injected with approximately 30 to 40 cc of normal saline. Flow from the second spinal needle confirms intra-articular placement of both needles (see Fig. 8).

The entire weight-bearing articular surface of the acetabulum and femoral head can be visualized using paratrochanteric portals with a 30° scope. The paratrochanteric portals pass through fewer muscle planes, avoid potential injury to the lateral femoral cutaneous nerve, and puncture the superior hip capsule, which is slightly thinner. The skin incisions are superficial, not penetrating deeper than the subcutaneous adipose tissue. Then, tapered blunt trocars are used to pass through the adipose, fascia, and muscle tissue. This technique protects all interceding neurovascular structures and muscle from sharp equipment and repetitive trauma during the exchange of instruments. The pressure required varies by patient and by capsular location. The hip capsule becomes palpable as a firm but not solid structure. When entering the joint, a firm but gentle "pop" should be encountered, followed by easy advancement of the trocar and sheath. Confirmation of positioning with image intensification should be done.

Anterior Trochanteric Portal

This portal is located 2 cm anterior and 1 cm proximal to the greater trochanter. The cannula is aimed toward the center of the acetabulum at the fovea while keeping it as close to the femoral head as possible. This portal transgresses the anterior musculotendinous junc-

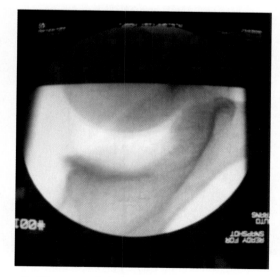

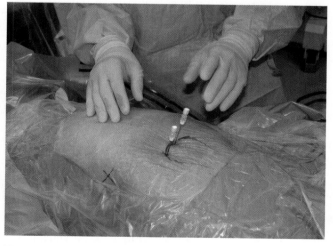

Figure 7. Fluoroscopic images show the distraction of the femoral head. At least 8 to 11 mm of distraction is needed. The thickness of the cartilage of the femoral head and the labrum should be taken into consideration when aiming the spinal needles toward the fovea.

Figure 8. The skin is marked at the superior ridge of the greater trochanter and anterior superior iliac spine (ASIS). The spinal needles are then directed cephalad toward the fovea.

tion of the gluteus medius, the tendinous region of the gluteus minimus, and the anterior hip capsule before entering the joint. The neurovascular structure that is at potential risk with this portal is the superior gluteal nerve. It is located 4 to 6 cm above the tip of the greater trochanter. This portal provides excellent visualization of the femoral head, anterior neck, anterior labrum, and synovial tissues beneath the zona orbicularis. In combination with the posterior superior trochanteric portal, it is an extremely useful portal for instrumentation and treatment of anterior labral lesions and acetabular chondral lesions.

Proximal Trochanteric Portal

The entry point for this portal is placed at the junction of the posterior and middle one third of the superior trochanteric ridge, essentially mirroring the anterior paratrochanteric portal. Correct positioning of the posterior trochanteric portal passes through the posterior margin of the musculotendinous junction of the gluteus medius muscle. The initial trocar placement is slightly superior and slightly anterior to avoid deflection posteriorly and potential injury to the sciatic nerve. Positioning of the hip in flexion greater than 20° can translate the sciatic nerve anteriorly, bringing this structure into jeopardy. Likewise, external rotation of the femur posteriorly translates the greater trochanter and increases the likelihood of posterior deflection of the trocar, which may potentiate injury to the sciatic nerve. It is for this reason that the leg must be placed in neutral or slight internal rotation when passing the needle or trocar for this portal. The posterior paratrochanteric portal is used to view the posterior capsule, posterior labrum, and the posterior femoral head. An important point with the posterolateral portal is that the "pop" that is encountered when entering the joint must be felt before bone is encountered. If bone is felt without the sensation of traversing the capsule, the trocar is too high and the outer wall of the acetabulum is encountered, or if it is too low, it may be the head of the femur that is encountered. Image intensification is helpful to alter the position of the portal pathway. The posterolateral portal is considered a very safe portal. Placing this portal under direct visualization facilitates its intra-articular position. This is commonly done by placing the camera in the anterolateral portal first (see Fig. 9).

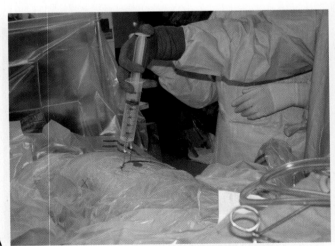
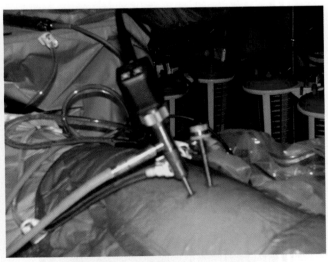

A   B

Figure 9. A: The spinal needles are flushed with normal saline to confirm intra-articular placement. **B:** The placement of the anterior and posterior trochanteric portals is shown. The anterior portal is placed at the anterior third of the trochanter, and the posterior portal is the mirror image, being placed at the posterior third of the trochanter. Both portals are aimed at the fovea. If an additional portal is needed, it is placed directly under the ASIS at the trochanteric level and directed into the joint with arthroscopic visualization.

Techniques and Pearls

The labrum is an important anatomic structure in the hip joint with many functions; therefore the least intrusive means of resecting or stabilizing a labral tear should be emphasized and overresection of labral tissue should be avoided. Chondral flaps are addressed with a microfracture technique using either mechanical or electrothermal resection. If the chondral lesion is full-thickness, microfracture using a specialized chondral pick is performed. Loose bodies that are large or adherent may have to be morcellized to facilitate extraction.

Instrumentation

The intra-articular structures in the hip joint can most often be visualized with a standard 30-degree arthroscope; however, there are times when a 70-degree lens may be needed. This is particularly true for loose bodies at the base of the fovea, Pipkin fracture fragments, and lesions of the labrum adjacent to the transverse acetabular ligament. The arthroscope can be exchanged among the portals to facilitate visualization of the existing pathology. Instruments should always be passed through long tapered cannulae to protect the surrounding tissues for safe entry into the joint. Telescoping cannulae are extremely helpful for removal of large loose bodies or to accommodate angled punches. A variety of probes and hooks are first used to evaluate the intra-articular structures (see Fig. 10). Loose bodies or tissue flaps such as labral tears can be resected and simultaneously aspirated with a variety of long suction punches designed specifically for hip arthroscopy. Extralength mechanical shavers can also be useful for debridement of labral tears (see Fig. 11). Curved shaver blades with either convex or concave surfaces improve navigation of the convex surface of the femoral head. Flexible thermal devices with precise control of temperature and coagulation are extremely useful in debriding chondral flaps and the torn labral rim (see Fig. 12). These tools, while beneficial, must be used judiciously to avoid overresection of tissue or thermal injury to bone. Inflamed, redundant synovial tissue can also be resected and coagulated.

POSTOPERATIVE MANAGEMENT

Hip arthroscopy is outpatient surgery. Most patients require crutches from 2 to 7 days. Patients may progress to full weight bearing as soon as comfort allows. Most patients are able to drive within 24 to 48 hours of the surgery.

Activity is gradually increased as comfort permits. This includes walking (not on a treadmill), riding a stationary bike, or swimming once the stitches are removed. Twisting and pivoting motions should be avoided for the first 6 weeks as they may produce sharp pain until postoperative swelling has subsided. Patients may rarely experience numbness in the perineum (including vagina or penis) or foot that can last from a few days up to a few weeks. This distraction neuropraxia, like a knee tourniquet neuropraxia, resolves with time. Other activities to be avoided are skiing and stair-climbing machines, and deep squats. Depending upon the job and type of physical labor required, most patients return to work in 4 to 7 days. Aspirin is prescribed as an anticoagulant for the first 4 weeks after surgery.

Most people with even mild acetabular dysplasia experience clicking, but the pain associated with the clicking and the episodes of locking or buckling should be resolved. Patients are told that further hip surgery is difficult to predict because of the many variables involved; however, the extent of chondral damage cannot be overstated as a predictor of the surgical outcome.

REHABILITATION

Formal physical therapy is not encouraged for the first 6 weeks after surgery while joint effusion persists. Patients may walk, swim, or ride a stationary bike as comfort allows dur-

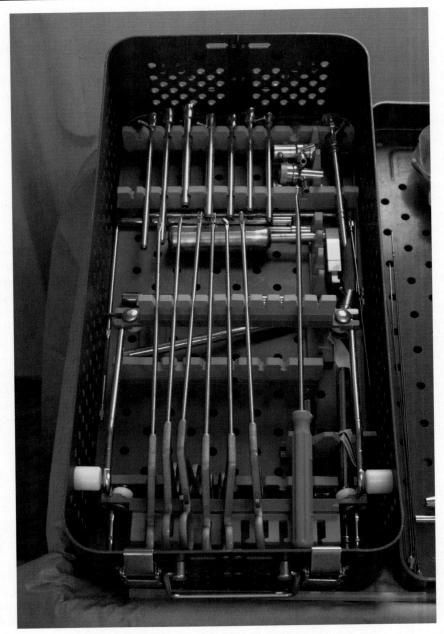

Figure 10. A tray of hip-specific operating instruments is shown, including long graspers, punches, and telescoping cannulas.

ing the first 6 weeks. Therapy protocols for patients with high demand such as competitive athletes also begin after the first 6 weeks. They begin with general conditioning and lower body resistance training, then progress to more sport-specific activities (Arthrex Corporation, Naples, FL).

RESULTS

Again, it cannot be overstated that surgical outcomes are directly dependent on the extent of articular surface involvement. Over 90% of patients will have an excellent result if the labral tear is addressed and the femoral and acetabular chondral surfaces are intact. If there is a grade I or II chondral lesion of either the adjacent acetabular chondral surface or

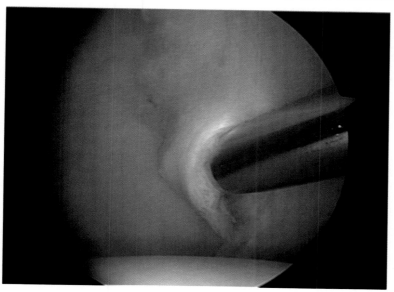

Figure 11. This is an intraoperative photo of a mechanical shaver being used to resect a labral lesion with an adjacent chondral flap lesion.

femoral head, 70% to 80% will have a good to excellent result. Conversely, if the articular cartilage involvement is full thickness and diffuse on the femoral head and acetabulum, 70% to 80% are associated with a poor result in follow-up, and 40% to 50% will require total joint arthroplasty within 2 years of arthroscopy.

COMPLICATIONS

Arthroscopy complications can be described as permanent or transient. Sciatic or femoral palsy, avascular necrosis, compartment syndrome, and broken instruments have all been reported. Transient peroneal or pudendal nerve effects as well as chondral scuffing have been associated with difficult or prolonged distraction. Table 1 summarizes the reported complications with the author's corresponding complication rate. Complications are best avoided with sufficient distraction (7 to 10 mm), dedicated hip instruments, and precise surgical skills. Hip arthroscopy involves a high learning curve. Meticulous attention to positioning, distraction time, and portal placement are essential. Technical challenges that

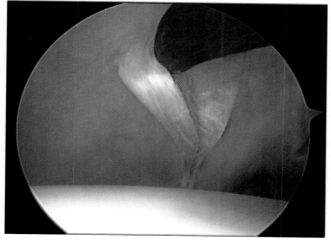

Figure 12. This is an intraoperative photo of a thermal device being used for chondroplasty of a watershed lesion (lesion at the labrochondral junction).

Table 1. *Complications**

Complication	Frequency
Infections	0
DVT	0
PE	0
Heterotopic bone	0
Avasclar necrosis	0
Major nerve or vessel injury	Sciatic 0
	Femoral 0
	LFC 2 transient
Compartment syndrome	0
Broken instruments	0
Fluid extravasation	0
Ankle strain	20 (1.3%)
Pudendal or peroneal hypoesthesia (transient)	25 (1.7%)
Mild chondral scuffing	14 (1%)

*DVT, deep vein thrombosis; LFC, lateral femoral cutaneous; PE, pulmonary embolism.

previously limited hip joint access have been overcome; therefore, the indications for arthroscopic surgery continue to expand.

RECOMMENDED READING

1. Byrd JW. Hip arthroscopy: patient assessment and indications. *Inst Course Lect* 52:711–719, 2003.
2. Byrd JW, Jones KS. Prospective analysis of hip arthroscopy with 2 year follow-up. *Arthroscopy* 16(6):578–587, 2000.
3. Glick JM. Hip arthroscopy using the lateral approach. *Instr Course Lect* 37:223–231, 1988.
4. McCarthy JC, ed. *Early Hip Disorders: Advances in Detection and Minimally Invasive Treatment.* New York: Springer-Verlag, 2003.
5. McCarthy JC, Noble PC, Schuck MR, et al. The Otto E. Aufranc Award: the role of labral lesions to development of early degenerative hip disease. *Clin Orthop Relat Res* 393:25–37, 2001.
6. McCarthy JC, Lee JA. Acetabular dysplasia: a paradigm of arthroscopic examination of chondral injuries. *Clin Orthop Relat Res* 405:122–128, 2002.

10

Arthrodesis: The Vancouver Technique

Clive P. Duncan, Robert W. McGraw,
and Christopher P. Beauchamp

INDICATIONS/CONTRAINDICATIONS

Arthrodesis is one of the alternatives to hip arthroplasty. Though infrequently advocated and even less frequently accepted by patients, it remains a valuable operative solution for treating a variety of conditions affecting the young hip. Regardless of improvements in prosthetic design and arthroplasty technique, the joint replacement option should be considered with caution in the young in view of the ongoing problems with loosening, breakage, disassembly, and osteolysis.

Arthrodesis of the hip is ideally indicated in the young, heavy set, unskilled male manual laborer with monarticular hip disease. Contraindications to this operation are low back pain and ipsilateral knee disease. Contralateral hip disease is a relative contraindication as well, on the grounds that arthrodesis on one side may lead to increased functional demands on the other during basic activities of daily living and recreational activities.

The Vancouver technique for hip arthrodesis is simple and precise. Immediate mobilization and early protected weight bearing are permitted. Close-fitting male/female reamers are used to achieve maximum coaptation, and a cobra plate is used to achieve rigid internal fixation. An additional anterior neutralization plate can be added to add further rigidity to the construct. Medialization is achieved by reaming the floor of the acetabulum, or a little beyond, thereby avoiding the need for the additional pelvic osteotomy described in the Schneider technique. Trochanteric osteotomy with anatomic relocation preserves the abductors for future conversion to a total joint arthroplasty—a request now encountered with increasing frequency. Supplementary immobilization such as a hip spica is not necessary, except in the unreliable patient.

PREOPERATIVE PLANNING

Appropriate clinical and laboratory investigation should be carried out to ensure that the hip disease is monarticular and no significant pathology exists in the lower spine, ipsilateral knee, or contralateral hip. It is important to measure leg lengths carefully and inform the patient of changes that will occur as a result of the procedure.

The radiographs should be carefully evaluated to recognize potential intraoperative difficulties. Inadequate bone stock to permit stable coaptation and fixation of the femoral head to the acetabulum would be a contraindication to the procedure, without the use of more specialized techniques. Retained fixation hardware around the acetabulum or in the femur may require removal to successfully complete the technique. Extensive osteonecrosis of the femoral head, after debridement of unstable collapsing bone, may result in a greater leg length discrepancy. The patient would need to be aware of this before operation.

Ongoing infection, in most cases, would require debridement and control before the definitive procedure. Rotational or angular malunion of the femur would require appropriate modification of the position of arthrodesis to ensure that the final position of the limb is satisfactory, or less commonly, an osteotomy of the femur as well with simultaneous fixation of this and the fusion site using the cobra plate.

Otherwise, the clinical and laboratory workup is quite standard and similar to that used for any major reconstructive orthopaedic procedure.

SURGERY

Patient Positioning

The patient is positioned laterally on the operating room table with the affected side up and secured with two deflated bean bags (see Fig. 1). A cross-table anteroposterior radio-

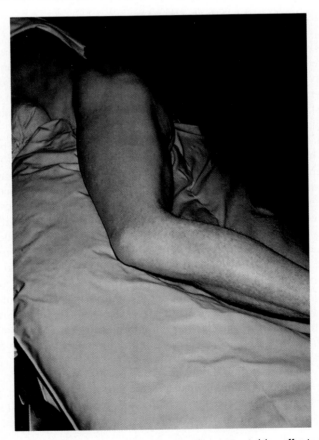

Figure 1. Patient in lateral position on operating room table, affected side up.

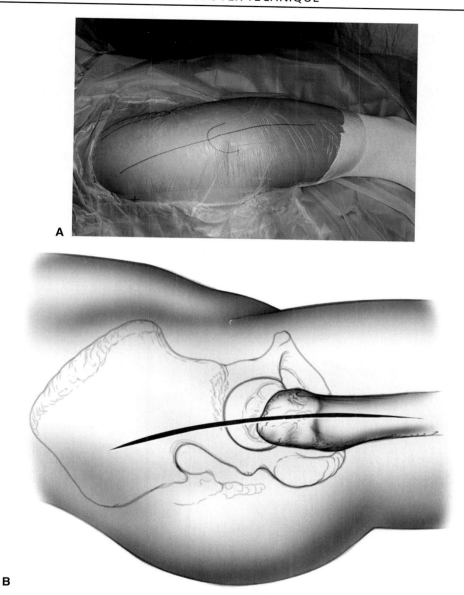

Figure 2. The incision is lateral, centered over the greater trochanter, extending somewhat posteriorly in its upper half.

graph is obtained to confirm the exact position of the pelvis. The underlying leg is placed in flexion to help reduce the degree of lumbar lordosis. The overlying leg is placed in 20-degree flexion and at least 10-degree adduction. The latter will be corrected as compression is applied to the cobra plate. Patient positioning is crucial. The leg is prepped and draped free, leaving the knee and as much of the leg exposed as possible.

A straight lateral incision that curves slightly posteriorly in its proximal extent is made (see Fig. 2). The fascia lata is divided, and the vastus lateralis is reflected (see Fig. 3). The greater trochanter is osteotomized, and the abductor mass is elevated and retracted proximally (see Fig. 4). Great care is taken to protect the superior gluteal bundle. A generous anterior capsulectomy is carried out, and the hip is dislocated anteriorly (see Fig. 5). The posterior soft tissues are left intact (external rotators and capsule) to preserve that route of blood supply to the femoral head. The acetabulum is then exposed. Medialization of the arthrodesis site is obtained by removing the medial acetabular bone to the inner wall of the pelvis (see Fig. 6). If the femoral head is enlarged, this may be dealt with first to facilitate exposure of the acetabulum. Otherwise, the femoral head is shaped with a variety of instruments to remove osteophytes, and an oversized female reamer is used to shape the

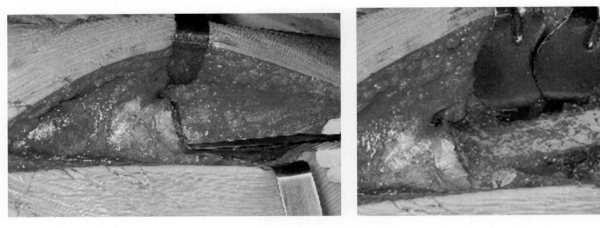

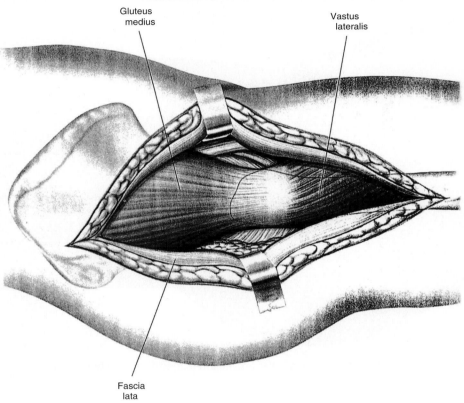

Figure 3. The femoral shaft is exposed by elevating the vasti.

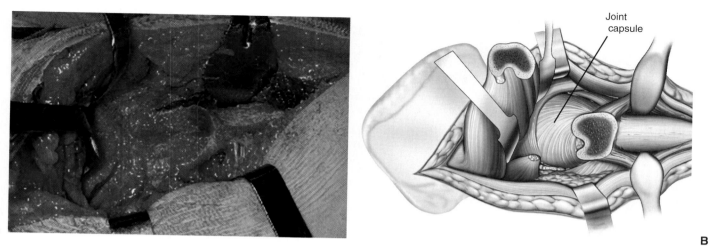

A

B

Joint capsule

Figure 4. A standard trochanteric osteotomy is completed.

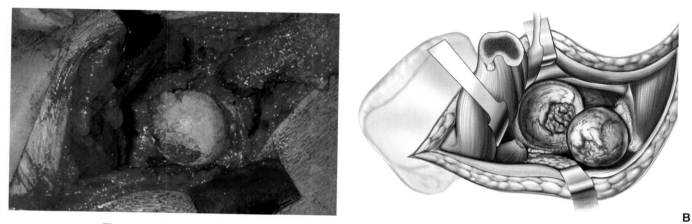

A

B

Figure 5. After a generous capsulectomy, the hip is dislocated anteriorly. The leg is placed in a drape bag over the side of the table.

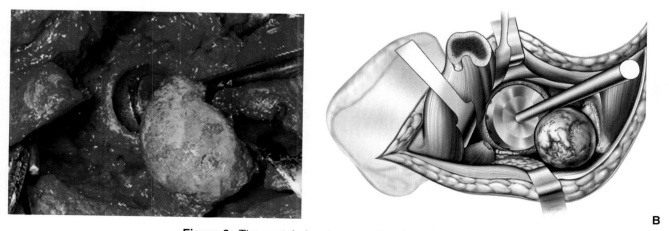

A

B

Figure 6. The acetabulum is reamed and medialized.

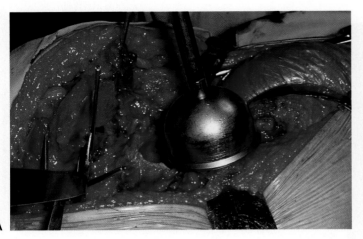
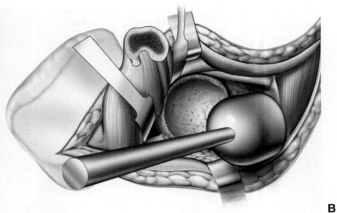

Figure 7. The femoral head is reamed with a matching concave reamer.

femoral head (see Fig. 7). The reaming devices are selected in this manner in order to create a spherically congruent arthrodesis site (see Fig. 8). The hip is reduced, and the contact area is assessed. Usually, this will result in a very tight cancellous-to-cancellous approximation (see Fig. 9).

The leg is then carefully positioned, and the cobra plate is affixed in the described fashion with one screw proximally. The desired final position of fusion is 20-degree flexion, 5-degree external rotation, and neutral duction (normally, the femur is in 5 to 10 degrees of adduction with reference to the pelvis). As the application of compression tends to abduct the femur slightly, the plate is initially applied with the leg adducted 10 degrees more than the desired final position (see Fig. 10). The application of the compression plate begins with the central proximal screw through the roof of the acetabulum and distal compression screw in the femoral shaft. Initial compression is applied, and a check radiograph is taken to confirm that the femur is in the desired degree of adduction. This should measure 10 to 20 degrees so as to achieve the desirable final position when compression is complete. If the position in all three planes (flexion, duction, and rotation) is not satisfactory, modification at this part of the procedure is important and simple to achieve. If satisfactory, the remaining proximal screws are inserted, compression is completed, and the remaining screws are inserted into the femoral shaft. If there is any concern about position, another check radiograph is performed before the final screws are inserted. It is crucial to ensure that the correct degree of flexion is present before the proximal screws are inserted and the correct degree of rotation has been achieved before the distal screws are placed. Bone removed

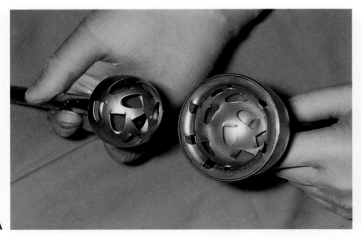
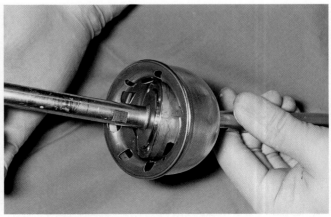

Figure 8. Matching reamers, formerly used for resurfacing arthroplasty of the hip joint.

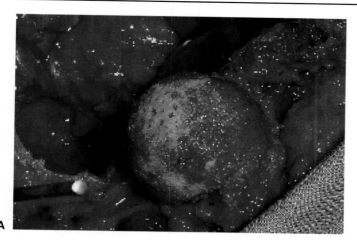

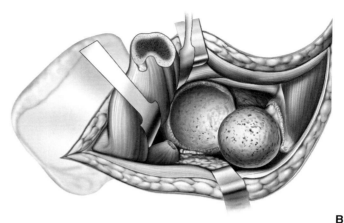

A

B

Figure 9. Prepared surfaces result in a very tight cancellous-to-cancellous approximation.

from the acetabulum and any additional bone from the greater trochanteric region that was trimmed is used as a bone graft. The greater trochanter is reattached in its normal position to preserve abductor muscle length (see Fig. 11). The techniques that have been described to insert a vascularized bone graft across the hip joint, using the anterior iliac crest (with abductors attached) or the greater trochanter (with the abductors attached), are not required and are undesirable. Damage to the abductors will compromise the outcome after conversion to a hip replacement at a future date. A repeat radiograph is obtained (see Fig. 12). The wound is closed in a routine manner.

POSTOPERATIVE MANAGEMENT

The patient is transferred to a standard orthopaedic bed and made comfortable with pillows. Mobilization begins on the first postoperative day. The drains, if used, are removed between 24 and 48 hours following surgery. Feather-touch weight bearing is permitted from the outset. A fiberglass pantaloon spica should be considered if there is any concern regarding the rigidity of fixation or the compliance of the patient. The patient is discharged from hospital 3 to 5 days following surgery.

The patient is advised to use crutches at all times for 3 months following the surgery. With excellent coaptation and rigid internal fixation, protected weight bearing can begin at

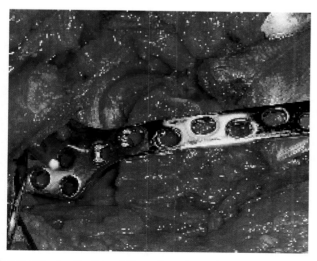

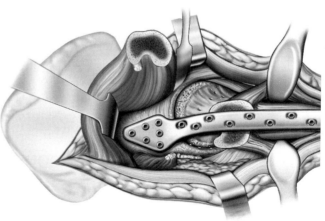

A

B

Figure 10. Application of the cobra plate after it has molded to the shape of the acetabulum and femur, and initial fixation with one proximal and the distal outrigger compression screw.

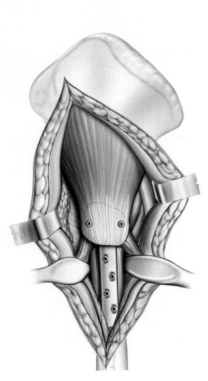

Figure 11. Replacement of the greater trochanter in the anatomic position.

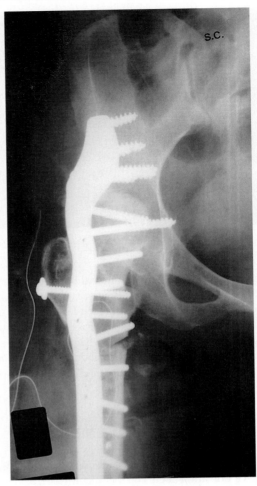

Figure 12. Final intraoperative radiograph of hip fusion and simultaneous subtrochanteric osteotomy to correct severe deformity.

6 weeks and gradually increase to full weight bearing by 12 weeks. The average time to independent, full weight bearing is 12 weeks.

In the straightforward case, union is expected at 3 to 4 months. The patient is followed up at 6 to 12 weeks. The persistence of pain, the presence of motion, and the failure of the joint space to become obliterated on the radiographs at 6 months would strongly suggest nonunion. This is particularly so if the screws are loose or if there is a halo of osteolysis around the screw tips.

If the patient received adequate education before the procedure and the technique is completed with precision, complete relief of hip pain is expected in every patient, and a satisfactory level of function is expected in the majority. Before the operation, it is wise to have the patient meet previous patients functioning well on a hip arthrodesis. Return to work can be expected 6 to 12 months after the operation.

COMPLICATIONS

Malposition

Malposition can be avoided if the technique is followed precisely. Intraoperative radiographic monitoring will detect malpositioning, especially in difficult cases such as a previous femoral osteotomy.

Nonunion

Nonunion is very uncommon. Nonunion following this technique has been treated successfully by a precise repetition of the technique with bone graft and supplementary internal fixation.

Patient Dissatisfaction

Patient dissatisfaction may occur in spite of a successful arthrodesis. This outcome can be avoided by astute patient selection and appropriate preoperative education of the patient and family.

Unrelieved Pain

Continued pain in an apparently successful arthrodesis may necessitate the later removal of the internal fixation device.

RECOMMENDED READING

1. Barmada R, Abraham E, Ray RD. Hip fusion utilizing the cobra head plate. *J Bone Joint Surg* 58(4):541–544, 1976.
2. Beauchamp CP, Duncan CP, McGraw RW. Don't throw away the reamers—a new technique of hip arthrodesis. *J Bone Joint Surg* 67-B(2):330, 1985.
3. Callaghan J, Brand R, Pedersen D. Hip arthrodesis: a long-term followup. *J Bone Joint Surg* 67a:1328–1334, 1985.
4. Duncan CP, Spangehl M, Beauchamp C, McGraw R. Hip arthrodesis: an important option for advanced disease in the young adult. *Can J Surg* 38(suppl 1):39–45, 1995.
5. Fulkerson JP. Arthrodesis for disabling hip pain in children and adolescents. *Clin Orthop Relat Res* 128:296–302, 1977.
6. Kostuik J, Alexander D. Arthrodesis for failed arthroplasty of the hip. *Clin Orthop Relat Res* 188:173–182, 1984.
7. Panagiotopoulos KP, Robbins GM, Masri BA, Duncan CP. Conversion of hip arthrodesis to total hip arthroplasty. *Instruct Course Lect* 50:297–305, 2001.
8. Schneider R. Hip arthrodesis with the cobra head plate and pelvic osteotomy. *Reconstr Surg Traumatol* 14:1–37, 1974.
9. Sponseller PD, McBeath AA, Perpich M. Hip arthrodesis in young patients: a long-term follow-up study, *J Bone Joint Surg* 66:853–859, 1984.

PART IV

Surgery for Avascular Necrosis

11

Hemiarthroplasty

Thomas Schmalzried and John Antoniades

INDICATIONS AND CONTRAINDICATIONS

The indications for hemiresurfacing arthroplasty are young patients with Ficat stage III and early stage IV osteonecrosis of the femoral head (1). Contraindications include stage IV osteonecrosis with obvious acetabular involvement, active infection, open physeal plates, and lack of sufficient femoral head to allow femoral component fixation. Extensive cystic degeneration could compromise component fixation and lead to early loosening.

PREOPERATIVE PLANNING

The radiographic exam should include a low anteroposterior pelvis with the beam centered on the pubis, a frog lateral of the involved hip, and a cross-table lateral (2). These views are used to template component size, taking into account magnification and the fact that about half of the cartilage space belongs to the femur. In our experience, the templating is accurate to plus or minus one component size.

SURGICAL TECHNIQUE

This surgical technique is not tailored to a specific instrumentation system but rather is intended as a guideline for the principles of hemiresurfacing. It is anticipated that the instrumentation will evolve and that there will be differences among manufacturers.

Patient Positioning

We prefer the lateral decubitus and secure the patient with commonly available positioners. We prefer a "low-profile" support directly on the pubis and a second support more proximal on the sternum with a posterior support low on the sacrum. The femoral neurovascular structures can be compressed when the hip is flexed and adducted during the exposure. A misplaced anterior support could compromise the neurovascular structures.

The contralateral leg is extended to allow the operative extremity to drop in adduction. Preoperative antibiotics are given, and the extremity is draped (see Fig. 1).

Exposure

A posterior approach is used to avoid abductor muscle compromise. The proximal portion of the incision is angled slightly more posteriorly to accommodate the dislocated femoral head (see Fig. 2). The tensor fascia is incised posterior to the greater trochanter, and the gluteus maximus muscle is split in line with its fibers. The limb is positioned in about 30 degrees of internal rotation. A cobra retractor is used to protect the abductors (see Fig. 3). The short external rotators are transected near their attachment to facilitate subsequent repair. It is usually not necessary to take more than half of the quadratus femoris, and the gluteus maximus tendon can usually be left intact. Place a blunt Hohman retractor, inferiorly, between the capsule and the detached external rotators (see Fig. 4).

A horizontal incision is made in the capsule roughly along a line corresponding to the inferior border of the piriformis. The capsule is then released off the femoral neck posteriorly and anteriorly to the midcoronal plane (see Fig. 5). This is generally enough capsular release to allow the head to dislocate with flexion, adduction, and internal rotation. If the labrum is intact, do not disturb it. A torn or degenerated labrum can be resected.

The "working position" for femoral resurfacing is about 80 degrees of hip flexion, 30 degrees of adduction, and 100 degrees of internal rotation. Place an elevator under the femoral neck, paying careful attention to this posterior retractor placement and position so as to not injure the sciatic nerve. Place another cobra retractor around the inferior neck. The cobra under the abductors remains in place (see Fig. 6).

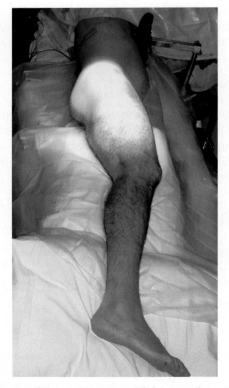

Figure 1. Positioning for a surface replacement. Make sure the extremity can be flexed beyond 90 degrees. The operative extremity can also be adducted without impinging the other leg or table.

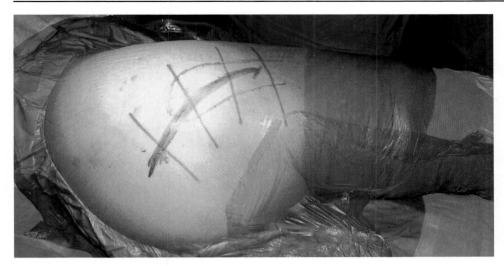

Figure 2. Incision for the hemiarthroplasty. The patient is lateral decubitus with the right side up. The foot is to the right of the figure, and the head is to the left. The proximal limb curves more posteriorly than a standard posterior approach.

Femoral Sizing

Ring gauges or a caliper can be used to assess the diameter of the femoral head. Within the range of available component sizes, pick the implant diameter that approximates the head diameter. Some consideration may be given to selecting the smaller of the available components. In the event of persistent pain with a well-fixed femoral component, the smaller femoral component would facilitate conversion to a total resurfacing since a correspondingly smaller acetabular component would be needed. To our knowledge, there are no clinical data showing any relationship between the accuracy of the size match of the component to the femoral head and the outcome of the hemiresurfacing, given that the match has generally been within plus or minus 2 mm.

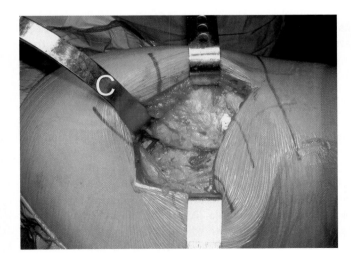

Figure 3. Internally rotate the leg to expose the posterior part of the greater trochanter. Incise the tensor fascia and gluteus maximus fascia in line with the incision. Find the posterior part of the gluteus medius by finger dissection. Place a cobra retractor (*C*) underneath. Identify the piriformis tendon. Dissect anteriorly with a Cobb elevator under the gluteus minimus and above the capsule. Reposition the cobra retractor under the retractors.

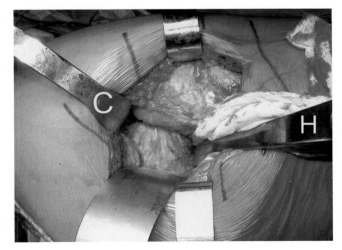

Figure 4. Release the piriformis tendon as near the insertion as possible. Moving distally, release the rest of the external rotators. A blunt Hohman retractor *(H)* maintains the exposure of the inferior part of the capsule. The superior cobra retractor *(C)* stays in place.

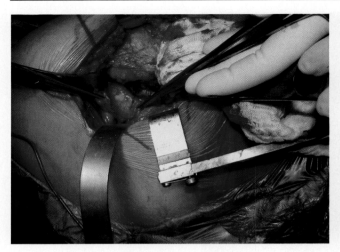

Figure 5. Make a capsulotomy from the acetabular rim posteriorly to the base of the femoral neck. Release the inferior limb of the capsule with cautery. Reposition the Hohman retractor inside the inferior limb of the capsule. Hold the superior limb with a Kocher clamp and incise the capsule off the neck from posterior to anterior. The capsule needs to be released to the midcoronal plane to dislocate the hip.

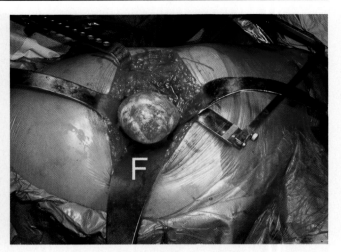

Figure 6. Dislocate the hip by internal rotation and flexion. Adduct the leg and place a femoral neck elevator *(F)* posteriorly. This allows the neck to be presented out of the wound. The inferior Hohman retractor is removed, and another cobra retractor is placed around the inferior neck.

Femoral Head Preparation

There are several techniques to prepare the femoral head, but the principles are the same. The generic goals of hemiresurfacing are to remove a "shell" of bone from the circumference of the femoral head of roughly uniform thickness without injuring the femoral neck. We recommend that the synovium on the neck be left intact. The orientation of the bone preparation should be in 130 to 140 degrees valgus and "physiologic anteversion" (10 to 15 degrees) in order to load the cement–bone interface in compression.

Begin with a cylindrical reamer two to three sizes larger than that for the component that will be used. Ream generally along the described axis of 130 to 140 degrees valgus and 10 to 15 degrees of anteversion. Since most hips with avascular necrosis have normal proximal femoral morphology, this axis will closely approximate the axis of the femoral neck. The goal of the initial reamer is to "shave" only a couple of millimeters of bone from around the hemisphere. The cylindrical reamer can be used for guide pin insertion. Place a guide pin through the reamer, and then orient that composite as desired. A large goniometer is helpful to achieve the desired valgus orientation. Progressively smaller cylindrical reamers are then used until the selected size is reached. If the "shell" of reamed bone is eccentric, a second guide pin can be inserted in a new entry point that corrects the eccentricity but maintains the same valgus and anteverted orientation. The final cylindrical reamer (for the selected size) is used having optimized the axis.

Although there may be slight differences in the next steps, depending on the specific instrumentation used, bone is removed from the top of the femoral head that is roughly equal to the thickness of the femoral component. Several systems also have a chamfer reamer. If there is a short stem on the prosthesis, the central hole needs to be drilled to the appropriate depth and diameter. There is currently debate as to whether or not cementing the central stem is desirable. Cementing the stem may provide additional fixation in compromised bone, as is often the case with avascular necrosis.

Femoral component trials are helpful to assure uniform bone resection and full component seating (see Fig. 7). The trial should move freely around the head. There is currently debate regarding the optimal fit between the prepared bone and the femoral component. It is important to know how tight or loose the fit is, since this has implications for cement viscosity and the timing of component insertion. When the fit is tight, it may be difficult to fully seat the prosthesis when the cement is viscous.

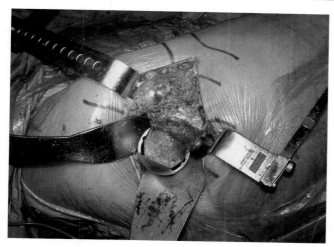

Figure 7. After the femoral head is prepared, a trial component can be used to check the "fit." The trial should seat fully and move around the head with minimal effort.

Cement Technique

Sclerotic bone is drilled with a one-eighth-inch drill bit to a depth of about 5 mm (see Fig. 8). The same drill bit is used to drill into the prominence of the lesser trochanter, directed slightly superiorly, to a depth of about 1 to 2 cm. A small cannula, such as one used for outflow in knee arthroscopy, is then inserted to a similar depth. When attached to the operating room wall suction, this draws in blood from the proximal femur and provides a bloodless interface. If the suction is strong or the bone is quite porous, it may also pull cement into the prepared femoral bone (see Fig. 9).

Mix the cement. While the cement is being mixed, the femoral head is irrigated with pulsatile lavage. Drying is accomplished with lap sponges and suction from the lesser trochanteric cannula. An additional suction cannula can be used in the central hole.

The cement can be poured in a low-viscosity state into the femoral head, filling only one third of the sphere. Gently "swirl" the component to get the cement on the sidewalls. Cement bonds best to metal when it is "wet" (3,4). When the cement becomes more viscous and does not stick to the surgeon's gloves, finger-pressurize cement into the prepared bone, concentrating on the cylindrical portion. Most components have parallel sidewalls, which

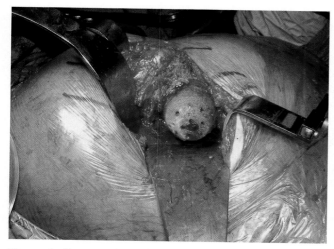

Figure 8. Remove the trial, and place evenly spaced drill holes on the distal and chamfer cuts. This ensures an optimal cement–bone interface.

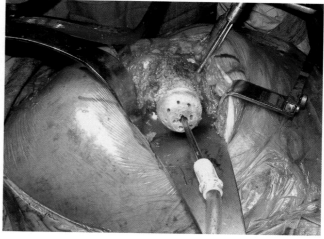

Figure 9. Place suction in the central hole and in the lesser trochanter. This prevents blood from interfering with cement mantle.

generate little compressive force for cement penetration into the cylindrical region. During component insertion, there are relatively high compressive forces in the dome and chamfer regions, which drive cement intrusion in those regions.

Finger-pack cement into the central hole, if desired. Then place the femoral component onto the femoral head. The amount of force required to fully seat the component is variable. Place a lap sponge over the component and use a soft impactor (so as not to scratch the surface) and a mallet to assure full seating, if necessary. Remove excess cement with a small curette and allow the cement to harden before reducing in the acetabulum. Carefully check for any overhanging or loose cement, especially anteriorly, where it is hard to see. Irrigate and clear the acetabulum and reduce the hip.

Closure

Close the posterior capsule with interrupted sutures. Approximate the piriformis tendon and other short external rotators to their soft "stumps" near the greater trochanter. Close the fascia over a drain. Close the deep subcutaneous layer with polyglactic acid suture (Vicryl) and the skin with staples.

POSTOPERATIVE MANAGEMENT

Intravenous antibiotics are given for 24 hours. We give indomethacin 25 mg three times a day for 5 days for prophylaxis against heterotopic bone (5). The patient can be mobilized immediately with 50% weight bearing (two crutches) and progress to full weight bearing by 6 weeks. We encourage early range of motion but limit flexion to 120 degrees with the posterior arthrotomy. The drain is pulled on postoperative day one. We use injectable agents for deep venous thrombosis prophylaxis, initiated 24 hours after surgery and given for 3 weeks (6).

RESULTS

Patients recover relatively quickly postoperatively. Pain relief with hemiarthroplasty is not as predictable as with a total hip replacement. About 80% to 85% of patients have satisfactory pain relief. Decisions regarding further operative management of those with pain should be deferred for 6 months. Some hips do improve with time. The functional results are less than that of a total resurfacing. Range of motion is not an issue.

COMPLICATIONS

Wear of acetabular cartilage is the most common mode of failure in the long term. Following a pain-free period, insidious and progressive groin pain can occur. X-rays show reduction in cartilage space. The options at this point are a conversion to a total hip replacement or conversion to a corresponding acetabular component.

Femoral component loosening is rare. We have never seen osteolysis with a hemiresurfacing. We have never had a dislocation or a femoral neck fracture.

RECOMMENDED READING

1. Ficat RP, Arlet J. *Ischemia and Necrosis of Bone*. Baltimore: Williams & Wilkins; 1980.
2. Balinger P, Frank E, eds. *Merrill's Atlas of Radiographic Positions and Radiologic Procedures*. Vol 1. St Louis: Mosby; 1998: 370–372.
3. James S, Schmalzreid TP, McGarry FJ, Harris W. Extensive porosity at the cement-femoral interface: a preliminary study. *J Biomed Mater Res* 27:71–78, 1993.
4. Shepard M, Kabo JM, Lieberman JR. Influence of cement technique on the interface strength of femoral components. *Clin Orthop Relat Res* 381:26–35, 2000.
5. Amstutz HC, Fowble VA, Schmalzreid TP, Dorey FJ. Short-course indomethacin prevents heterotopic ossification in a high risk population following total hip arthroplasty. *J Arthroplasty* 12(2):126–32, 1997.
6. Kearon C. Duration of venous thromboembolism prophylaxis after surgery. *Chest* 124(6 suppl):386S–392S, 2003.

12

Core Decompression and Nonvascularized Bone Grafting

Hari P. Bezwada, Phillip S. Ragland, Craig M. Thomas, and Michael A. Mont

INDICATIONS/CONTRAINDICATIONS

Osteonecrosis of the femoral head is a disease primarily affecting younger patients that often leads to disabling arthritis and might finally require total hip arthroplasty. The ultimate treatment goal is simply pain relief. Ideally, in the early stages of the disease, a surgeon may attempt to maintain a congruent hip joint and thereby potentially delay or even avoid the need for a total hip arthroplasty. As this is a disease of primarily younger patients, it is our philosophy to use procedures aimed at saving the femoral head, even though further intervention might eventually be necessary. Treatment should be based on a combined evaluation of clinical, roentgenographic, and intraoperative factors. We believe that most of the treatment determination can be based on the roentgenographic evaluation with the use of additional patient-specific factors and operative findings for refinement. This chapter will demonstrate specific operative techniques for both core decompression and nonvascularized bone grafting.

Decision making in the treatment of osteonecrosis can be systematic and based on disease stage as manifested by radiographic findings. Treatment options will, in part, be influenced by the surgeon's familiarity with various procedures. As certain treatment modalities have better results for different disease stages, it is important that the treating surgeon show flexibility and use modalities appropriate for the extent of disease. Patient-related factors, including general health, activity level, and age, may also guide the decision-making process. The possibility of the need for future procedures should also influence treatment. It is not uncommon that the patient with osteonecrosis of the femoral head will require multiple procedures in his or her lifetime.

PREOPERATIVE PLANNING

The majority of patients have a presenting complaint of groin pain, although approximately 10% of patients may have nonspecific symptoms. Often, a patient with occultly diagnosed osteonecrosis may have nonspecific hip, trochanteric, or buttock symptoms that are from another pathological entity. The proposed treatment plan should be catered to the patient's age, activity level, and general health. The presence of a severe systemic illness or a limited life expectancy might preclude a major surgical procedure. Further, similar lesions may not be treated in the same way in two patients of different ages and activity levels. For example, a hip with femoral head collapse without acetabular involvement might be best treated with a bone-grafting procedure or limited femoral-resurfacing arthroplasty in a healthy 18-year-old patient. Similar radiographic changes in a 68-year-old patient would more likely be treated with a total hip arthroplasty. The role of various clinical factors in terms of treatment outcomes has been debated. Although age has not been directly implicated in various studies as a prognostic factor, many physicians will treat a patient less than 30 years of age differently than a patient that presents with osteonecrosis who is greater than 60 years of age. For older patients, it might be more appropriate to perform a total hip arthroplasty when the life expectancy is less than that of a teenager, with less activity demands, and chances of success with a head-sparing procedure such as bone grafting would also appear to be less likely.

Additionally, a surgeon should consider that this disease is often bilateral, and when planning treatment, the surgeon may attempt to treat both hips at the same time, rather than subject the patient to two separate anesthetic exposures. However, staging procedures by 6 to 12 weeks might be preferred if the postoperative rehabilitation requires non–weight bearing. This may be further influenced by the symptomatology and the level of collapse of the hip.

In formulating a treatment plan, we use four essential roentgenographic findings that have been shown in multiple studies to have prognostic value. First, the lesion should be classified with regard to collapse: Is it a pre- or postcollapse lesion? Precollapse lesions obviously have the best prognosis. Second, the size of the necrotic segment should be assessed as small lesions have the most favorable results. The next feature of importance is the amount of head depression, as lesions with less than 2 mm of head depression tend to have a more favorable outcome. Finally, acetabular involvement should be characterized as any sign of osteoarthritis will limit treatment options.

In addition to the clinical and radiographic factors just discussed, intraoperative findings are helpful in directing treatment. Intraoperative findings are a valuable tool in confirming the stage of osteonecrosis previously discovered on imaging studies. For example, one might plan a bone-grafting procedure on the basis of radiographic findings; however, intraoperatively, if substantial changes to the articular cartilage of the femoral head were found and precluded grafting, then this would override the preoperative radiographic staging, and the patient might undergo a resurfacing arthroplasty. A recommended treatment algorithm based on preoperative and operative staging is given in Figure 1. It is essential to understand this algorithm in order to understand the appropriate use of core decompression and nonvascularized bone-grafting procedures as well as other procedures contemplated for this disease.

CORE DECOMPRESSION

Indications

In both small- and medium-sized precollapse lesions, where the femoral head contour is smooth, the results of core decompression are generally good. This is true for both lesions that have sclerotic and cystic areas on plain roentgenograms and those symptomatic lesions with only magnetic resonance imaging findings. The rationale for core decompression is that it decreases intraosseous pressure in the femoral head and may immediately relieve the associated pain.

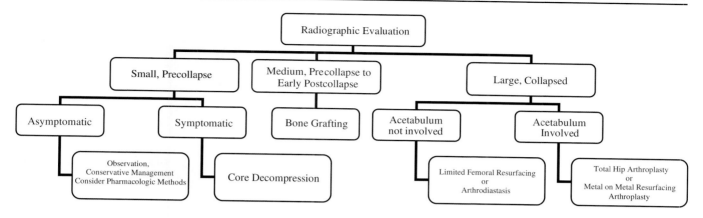

Figure 1. The authors' treatment algorithm based on radiographic assessment and clinical presentation.

Surgery

Patient Positioning. The patient is positioned supine on a radiolucent operating room table or a standard operating room table with a radiolucent extension. If that is not available, then a fracture table can also be used. Fluoroscopy is used to adequately visualize the acetabulum, femoral head, neck, and proximal femur. The leg is prepped and draped free so that the leg can be rotated and flexed (see Fig. 2).

Surgical Technique. The hip is placed in extension and internal rotation to compensate for femoral neck anteversion. Under fluoroscopic guidance, a 1/8-inch Steinman pin is inserted percutaneously through the lateral cortex in the metaphyseal region (see Fig. 3). The starting point should be superior to the cortical (diaphyseal) portion of the femur in order to minimize the subtrochanteric fracture risk. The pin is then advanced through the femoral neck into the lesion, as previously determined from earlier imaging studies, under fluoroscopic guidance. The drill is removed from the pin, and the hip is then flexed and externally rotated to evaluate the anterior to posterior position of the pin. If this position is satisfactory, the hip is extended and internally rotated (see Fig. 4). The pin is drilled to the appropriate depth with care to avoid penetrating the chondral surface. We perform two passes

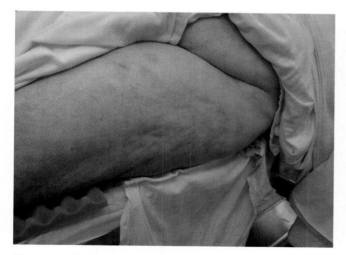

Figure 2. Supine patient positioning for core decompression on a radiolucent bed extension.

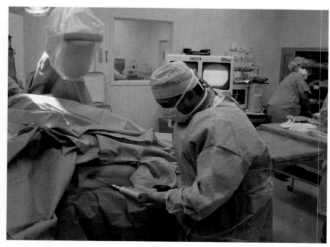

Figure 3. The Steinman pin placed percutaneously to the lateral cortex.

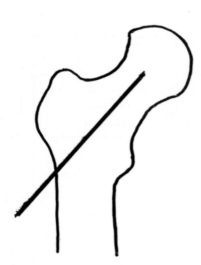

Figure 4. Diagram illustrating the technique for multiple small-diameter drilling.

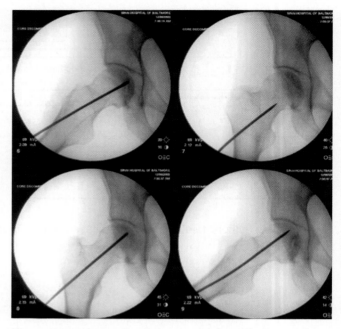

Figure 5. Intraoperative fluoroscopic views demonstrating appropriate pin placement in both anterior-posterior and lateral views.

into smaller lesions and three passes into larger lesions using a single entry point (see Fig. 5). The skin may need a single suture; we often use an absorbable monofilament suture followed by a small dressing, or even a small adhesive bandage (see Fig. 6).

Postoperative Management

Patients are discharged home the same day on protected weight bearing (approximately 50%) for a period of 6 weeks postoperatively, after which they are advanced to full weight bearing without impact loading for the first year following surgery.

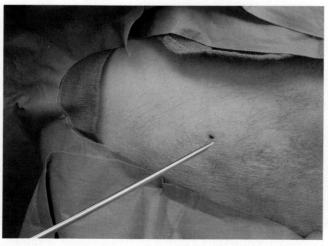

Figure 6. Photograph demonstrating the small percutaneous wound.

Results

In a recent review of 54 hips at a minimum follow-up of 10 years, either clinical or radiographic failure occurred in only 4 of 13 hips without plain radiographic changes and in none of the 7 hips with sclerotic changes (1). In that same study, larger lesions and precollapse lesions with cystic changes fared worse. In another study, 128 hips were followed for a mean of 11 years after core decompression, and successful clinical results were reported in 22 of 25 (88%) hips with normal roentgenograms (2). In that same study, core decompression was successful in 36 of 51 (71%) hips with precollapse lesions. In a review of 24 studies of core decompression, Mont et al. (3) found satisfactory clinical results in 741 of 1,166 hips (63.5%). In addition, they found only 182 of 819 hips (22.7%) to be successful that were managed nonoperatively (3). Furthermore, precollapse lesions had a 71% success rate when managed with core decompression compared with a 34.5% success rate when managed nonoperatively.

Trephines, drills, or cannulas on the order of 8 to 10 mm in diameter are commonly used to perform a core decompression. This method requires insertion under fluoroscopic guidance in order to penetrate the lesion. This technique with multiple drillings may lead to complications when the use of these large diameter trephines weakens the femoral head or if the trephine penetrates the femoral head and thus injures the articular cartilage and enters the joint space. In addition, if the entry site is made too low (in the diaphyseal region) a subtrochanteric hip fracture can occur. Recently, a multiple-small-diameter-drilling technique has been described as a method similar to core decompression. Kim et al. (4) compared 35 hips that underwent a multiple-small-diameter-drilling technique to 30 hips that underwent a standard core decompression, at a mean follow-up of 60.3 months. The hips that underwent multiple drilling had a significantly longer time to collapse—mean 42.3 months versus 22.6 months—and a lower rate of collapse—55% versus 85.7%—than hips that underwent standard core decompression. Mont et al. (5) also used multiple percutaneous small-diameter drillings. Thirty-two of 45 hips (71%) had good or excellent results at a mean 2-year follow-up. However, Ficat Stage I hips (24 of 30 hips, 80%) were more successful than Ficat Stage II hips (8 of 15 hips, 57%).

In summary, core decompression can lead to satisfactory results in small- and medium-sized precollapse lesions. The overall results of core decompression are not promising in more advanced stages. We believe that core decompression should not be performed in large-sized lesions or when collapse is present, except as a possible short-term palliative treatment method.

NONVASCULARIZED BONE GRAFTING

Indications

Bone grafting has numerous theoretical advantages in precollapse and early postcollapse lesions. Bone grafting allows for removal of weak necrotic bone, decompression of the femoral head, and stimulation of both repair and remodeling of subchondral bone. It also provides for maintenance of articular congruity and prevention of collapse. Both cancellous bone and cortical bone may be used in these procedures.

In general, there are three methods that have been utilized for nonvascularized bone grafting of the femoral head: cortical strut grafting through a core track in the femoral head and neck, bone grafting through the articular cartilage (the trapdoor procedure), and bone grafting through the femoral neck or femoral head neck junction ("lightbulb" procedure).

Cortical Strut Grafting. Cortical strut grafts can be placed through a core track made in the femoral neck and head (see Fig. 7). Autologous bone grafts may be harvested from the ilium, tibia, or fibula (see Fig. 8). The overall results with this technique have been variable. Buckley et al. (6) reported the results of 20 hips in which either structural autografts or allografts were placed through the core decompression track (see Fig. 9). There was a suc-

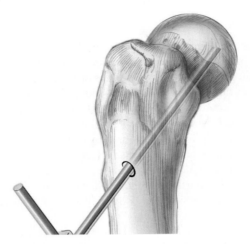

Figure 7. Diagram demonstrating a core decompression technique with a trephine for core biopsy and placement of a cortical strut graft.

cess rate of 90% in precollapse lesions at an average follow-up of 8 years (range, 2 to 19 years).

Bone Grafting through Articular Cartilage. Another method for debridement and grafting of an osteonecrotic lesion is through a "trapdoor" in the femoral head articular cartilage, which is lifted to expose the underlying lesion (see Fig. 10). Once the necrotic bone is removed, the cavity is filled with cancellous or cortical bone graft, or a combination of the two (see Fig. 11). The articular flap is then repaired with a bioabsorbable screw or absorbable sutures. Mont et al. (7) showed the early results using autogenous iliac cortical and cancellous bone graft combined with demineralized bone matrix and demonstrated good or excellent results in 22 of 30 procedures at a mean follow-up of 4.7 years. Meyers and Convery (8) also reported good results in 8 out of 9 postcollapse hips at a mean of 3 years.

Bone Grafting through the Femoral Head-neck Junction. Another bone-grafting technique that avoids entering the lesion through the articular cartilage is to create a cortical window at the base of the head (see Fig. 12). The necrotic area of bone is removed using a combination of burrs and curettes. Nonvascularized bone graft of choice is then placed into the defect. This technique has been referred to as the "lightbulb" procedure; good results have been reported at long-term follow-up for late precollapse and early postcollapse lesions (9).

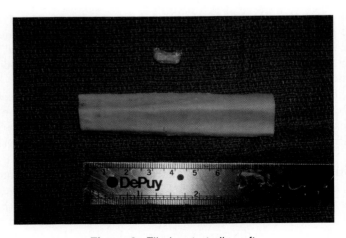

Figure 8. Fibular strut allograft.

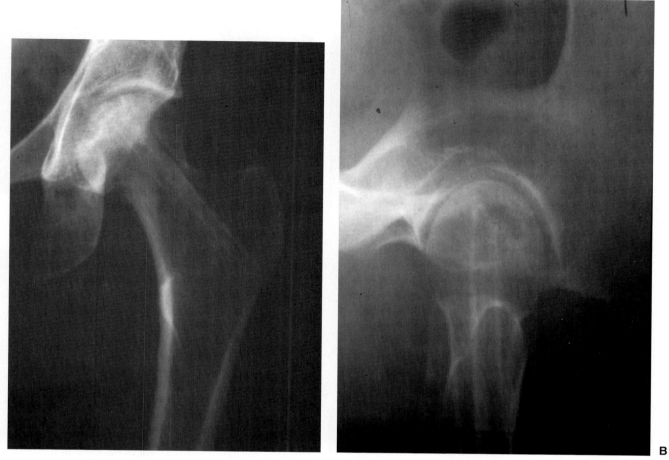

Figure 9. Anterior-posterior **(A)** and lateral **(B)** radiographs of a hip following cortical strut grafting.

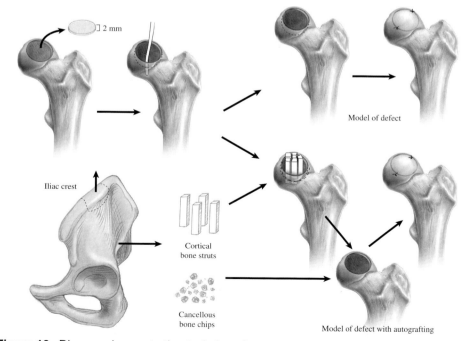

Figure 10. Diagram demonstrating technique for autogenous bone grafting through the femoral head cartilage.

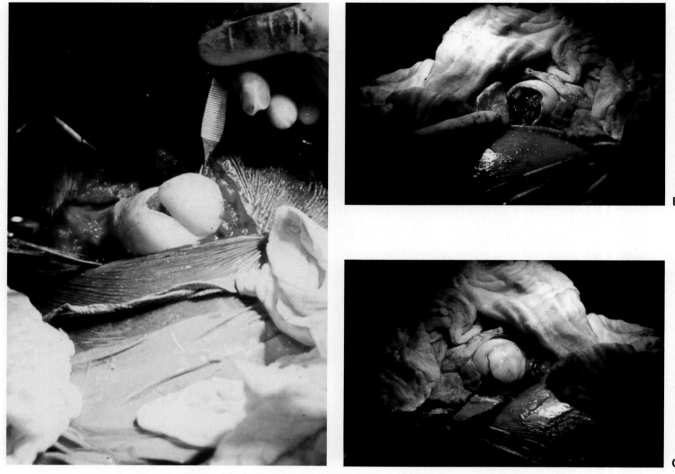

Figure 11. Intraoperative photographs of this bone-grafting technique through the femoral head.

Surgery

Patient Positioning. The patient is positioned laterally on the operating room table with the affected hip up and secured with a hip positioner. The underlying leg has a compression stocking and pneumatic pump applied and is then placed in flexion. All bony prominences are padded with special care to pad the area around the knee and fibular head. A compression stocking is placed on the operative leg. The affected leg is then prepped and draped free to allow full motion of the hip (see Fig. 13).

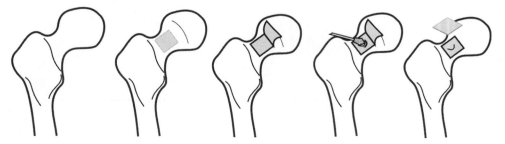

Figure 12. Diagrams of nonvascularized bone-grafting technique through a cortical window at the femoral head-neck junction.

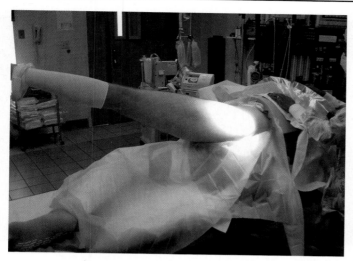

Figure 13. The patient is placed in a lateral position and secured with a hip positioner. The operative leg is prepped and draped free.

Surgical Technique. A straight lateral skin incision is made centered over the greater trochanter. The fascia lata is then exposed in an area slightly anterior to the greater trochanter. An incision is made in the fascia in a relatively amuscular plane and extended both proximally and distally with curved Mayo scissors. A blunt Hohmann retractor is placed directly posterior to the greater trochanter, and two right-angle Meyerding retractors are placed anteriorly and proximally to identify the abductor mass. Any overlying trochanteric bursa may be excised in order to clearly identify the abductor musculature. The anterior 40% of the gluteus medius muscle is elevated anteriorly with electrocautery proximally to its insertion on the trochanter. An adequate tissue sleeve must remain on the trochanter for subsequent repair. After this, the gluteus minimus is also elevated anteriorly off of the anterior capsule, and its tendinous insertion is dissected off the greater trochanter.

Hohmann retractors are placed anteriorly and superiorly around the femoral neck; a right-angle Meyerding retractor is placed anteriorly and cephalad to retract the anterior abductor mass and expose the anterior aspect of the acetabulum. A Cobb elevator is used to elevate the reflected head of the rectus femoris off of the anterior capsule. Once the entire anterior capsule is exposed, an anterior capsulectomy is performed with care to preserve the anterior labrum. The anterior femoral neck is then clearly exposed as well as the femoral head-neck junction. With careful longitudinal traction and rotation, most of the femoral head can be visually evaluated and directly palpated for evidence of chondral collapse. Please note that hip dislocation is not always necessary. However, in some cases, it may be required in order to fully evaluate the femoral head. When it is clear that there is no or minimal chondral collapse, an approximate 2 × 2 cm cortical window (trapdoor) at the femoral head-neck junction is outlined with electrocautery (see Fig. 14). Using a micro-oscillating sagittal saw, the window is cut in a beveled fashion. A quarter-inch osteotome is used to complete the corners and prevent propagation (see Fig. 15). The cortical window (trapdoor segment) is then elevated and preserved in normal saline-soaked gauze on the back table for later replacement. This window allows access to the necrotic bone, which is removed using a 6-mm mushroom-tipped burr and curettes (see Fig. 16). A fiber-optic, flexible light source or an arthroscope can be used to ensure adequate removal. The defect can be packed with a variety of bone grafts, including autogenous iliac crest bone graft. We have used bone morphogenetic protein-enriched allograft. A variety of other bone graft substitutes or autogenous bone graft may be utilized. Once the defect has been adequately packed, the cortical window is replaced and impacted. It is then held in place with three or four 2-mm Orthosorb absorbable

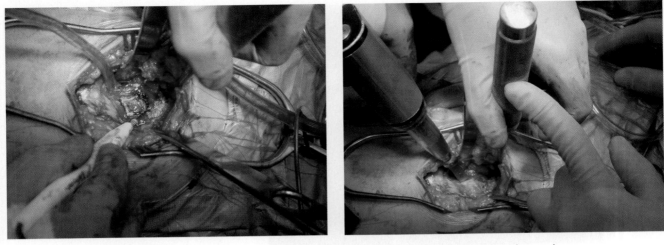

Figure 14. A 2 × 2 cm cortical window may be outlined at the head-neck junction and then cut using a microsagittal saw.

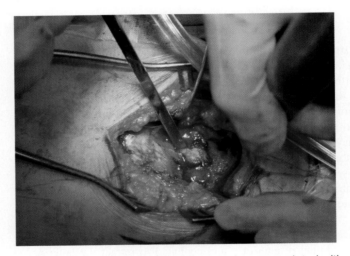

Figure 15. The corners of the cortical window (trapdoor) are completed with osteotomies.

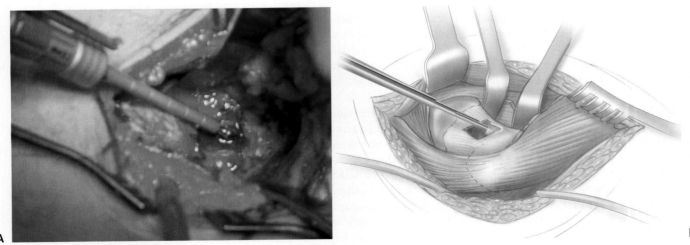

Figure 16. This window provides access to the necrotic bone in the femoral head, which is removed with an acorn burr and curettes. The defect is then packed with bone morphogenetic protein-enriched allograft.

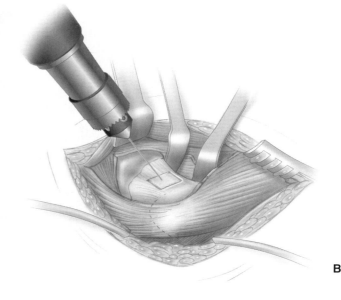

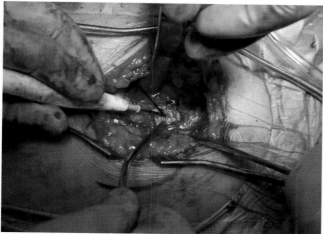

Figure 17. The cortical window (trapdoor) is replaced and secured with absorbable pins.

pins (Johnson & Johnson, New Brunswick, NJ) placed in diverging directions. The pin ends are cauterized in order to weld them in place (see Fig. 17).

A heavy 5-0 Ethibond suture is placed in the gluteus minimus with a Krackow stitch, and it is repaired back to the greater trochanter through drill holes (see Fig. 18). A drain is placed, and the gluteus medius is repaired back the remaining tissue sleeve on the greater trochanter with interrupted heavy absorbable suture. The fascia lata and wound are closed in a routine manner.

Alternatively, this procedure may be performed with femoral head dislocation for complete inspection of the femoral head cartilage (see Fig. 19).

Postoperative Management

The patient is transferred to a standard orthopaedic bed. Mobilization begins on the first postoperative day with toe-touch (20%) weight bearing. The drain is removed between 24 and 48 hours after surgery. The patient is typically discharged home 2 or 3 days following the surgery. Toe-touch weight bearing is maintained for 6 weeks following surgery with use of crutches or a walker. From 6 to 12 weeks, weight bearing is progressed to 50%, with interval radiographs to ensure no collapse. Full weight bearing may begin after 12 weeks, and physical therapy for abductor strengthening may be required. Impact loading of the hip is avoided for 1 year after surgery.

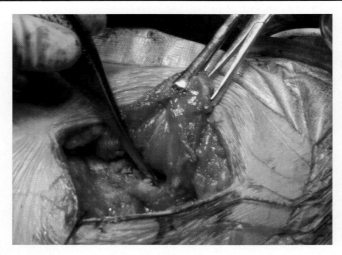

Figure 18. The minimus is repaired back to the trochanter with a Krackow stitch and through drill holes with heavy nonabsorbable sutures.

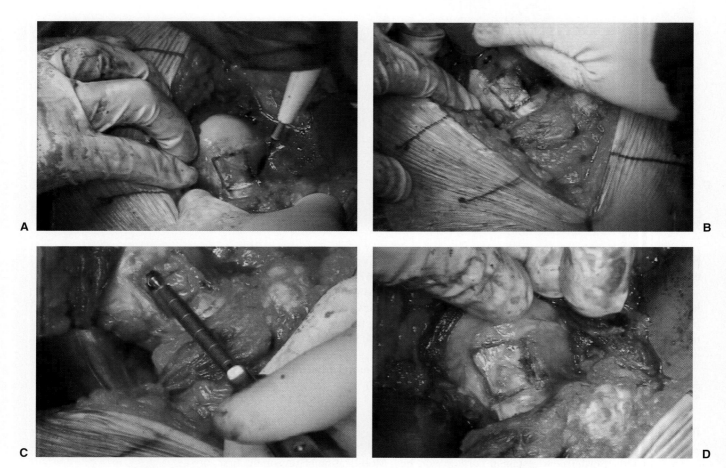

Figure 19. Alternatively, the femoral head can be dislocated, and the chondral surface can be inspected; after which, bone grafting through a cortical window in the head-neck junction can be performed in the manner previously described.

Results

Yamamoto et al. (10) reported on 38 hips at a mean follow-up of 9 years, of which 23 had good or excellent clinical results, using a combination of iliac crest cortical grafts and cancellous graft to fill the defects made after removal of the necrotic bone. Rosenwasser et al. (11) reported on the use of cancellous bone and found 13 of 14 hips to be symptom-free at a mean follow-up of 12 years. Mont et al. (9) also reported the results of bone grafting through a cortical window at the femoral head-neck junction in 21 hips at a mean follow-up of 48 months. In these hips, the necrotic bone was removed and replaced with bone graft substitute, combination of demineralized bone matrix, processed allograft bone, and a thermoplastic carrier. Eighteen of 21 hips (86%) were clinically successful at latest follow-up. Two of these patients had minimal roentgenographic progression with less than 2 mm of head collapse.

In summary, various bone-grafting techniques can be successfully used for precollapse lesions as well as postcollapse lesions, but all require that the femoral head articular cartilage be intact. This can be clearly ascertained at the time of surgery during open procedures. In some cases where the femoral head is not visualized directly, it might be useful to perform an arthroscopic procedure to delineate the status of the femoral head cartilage. If the femoral head cartilage is not intact or is found to be delaminated, these bone grafting procedures might not be successful. In these cases, other procedures such as limited femoral head resurfacing or total hip arthroplasty would be more appropriately indicated.

ARTHRODIASTASIS

Arthrodiastasis is a concept of joint distraction by means of an external fixator originally used to treat osteoarthritis of the hip (see Fig. 20). We have used this technique in young patients with osteonecrosis and collapse (see Fig. 21). The approach is very similar to that

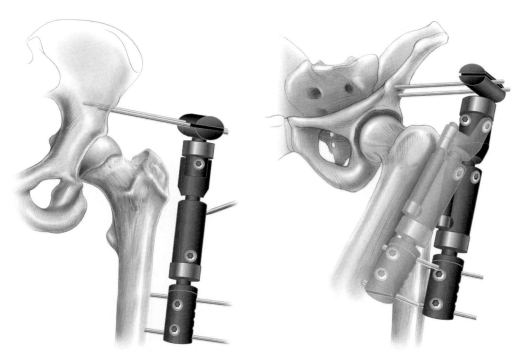

Figure 20. Schematic showing the external fixator spanning the ilium and femur and allowing for joint distraction.

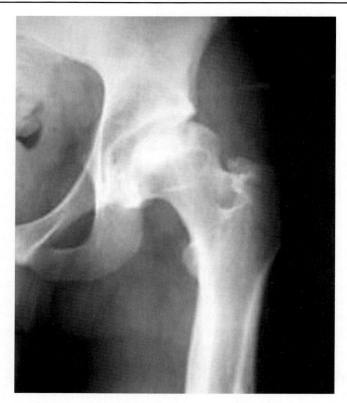

Figure 21. Preoperative anterior-posterior radiograph of the left hip in a patient undergoing nonvascularized bone grafting and arthrodiastasis.

of a standard bone-grafting procedure. If the articular cartilage is entirely delaminated, it is then repaired or reconstructed with periosteum from the ilium or graft tissue substitutes, such as Tissue Mend (Stryker Orthopaedics, Mahwah, NJ) or Graft Jacket (Wright Medical Technologies, Memphis, TN) (see Figs. 22–25). The bone-grafting procedure is performed either through a cortical window or through the cartilage lesion. The hip joint is then maintained in distraction for 3 to 4 months to allow the reconstruction to heal (Fig. 25).

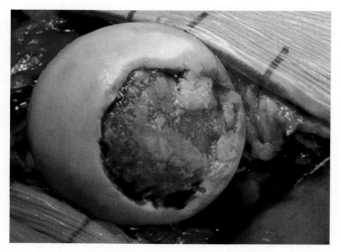

Figure 22. Intraoperative photographs demonstrating the degree of cartilage destruction.

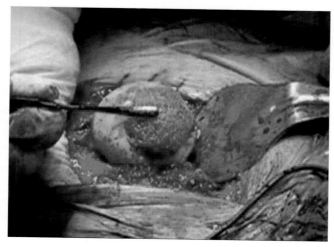

Figure 23. A combination of bone morphogenetic protein and corticocancellous allograft is applied.

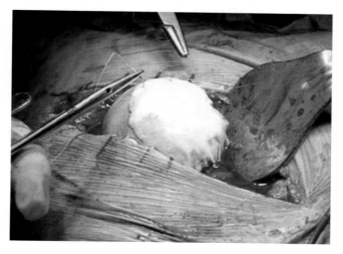

Figure 24. Reconstruction of the femoral head cartilage with graft substitute (Graft Jacket, Wright Medical Technologies, Memphis, TN).

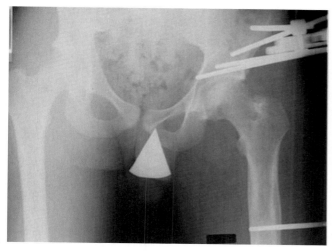
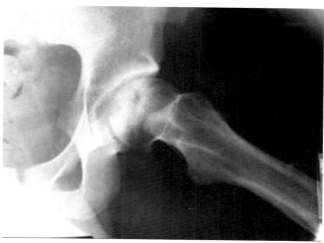

A

B

Figure 25. A: Postoperative anterior-posterior radiograph of the pelvis with the external fixator in place. **B:** Lateral radiograph of the hip 24 months following removal of the external fixator.

RECOMMENDED READING

1. Bozic KJ, Zurakowski D, Thornhill TS. Survivorship analysis of hips treated with core decompression for nontraumatic osteonecrosis of the femoral head. *J Bone Joint Surg Am* 81:200–209, 1999.

2. Fairbank AC, Bhatia D, Jinnah RH, Hungerford DS. Long-term results of core decompression for ischaemic necrosis of the femoral head. *J Bone Joint Surg Br* 77:42–49, 1995.

3. Mont MA, Carbone JJ, Fairbank AC. Core decompression versus nonoperative management for osteonecrosis of the hip. *Clin Orthop Relat Res* 324:169–178, 1996.

4. Kim SY, Kim DH, Park IH, et al. Multiple drilling compared with standard core decompression for the treatment of osteonecrosis of the femoral head. Presented at: Symposium of the Association Research Circulation Osseous; October 9–11, 2003; Jeju Island, Republic of Korea.

5. Mont MA, Ragland PS, Etienne G. Core decompression of the femoral head for osteonecrosis using percutaneous multiple small diameter drilling. *Clin Orthop Relat Res* 49:131–138, 2004.

6. Buckley PD, Gearen PF, Petty RW. Structural bone grafting for early atraumatic avascular necrosis of the femoral head. *J Bone Joint Surg Am* 73:1357–1364, 1991.

7. Mont MA, Einhorn TA, Sponseller PD, et al. The trapdoor procedure using autogenous cortical and cancellous bone grafts for osteonecrosis of the femoral head. *J Bone Joint Surg Br* 80:56–62, 1998.

8. Meyers MH, Convery FR. Grafting procedures in osteonecrosis of the hip. *Semin Arthroplasty* 2:189–197, 1991.

9. Mont MA, Etienne G, Ragland PS. Outcome of nonvascularized bone grafting for osteonecrosis of the femoral head. *Clin Orthop Relat Res* 417:84–92, 2003.

10. Yamamoto M, Itoman M, Sagamoto N, et al. Strut bone graft for aseptic necrosis of the femoral head: theory and surgical technique. *Orthop Surg* 34:902–908, 1983.

11. Rosenwasser MP, Garino JP, Kiernan HA, et al. Long term follow-up of thorough debridement and cancellous bone grafting of the femoral head for avascular necrosis. A comparison with osteoarthritis. *Clin Orthop* 306:17–27, 1994.

12. Camp JF, Colwell CW Jr. Core decompression of the femoral head for osteonecrosis. *J Bone Joint Surg Am* 68:1313–1319, 1986.

13. Ficat RP. Idiopathic bone necrosis of the femoral head: early diagnosis and treatment. *J Bone Joint Surg Br* 67:3–9, 1985.

14. Hungerford DS, Lennox DW. The importance of increased intraosseous pressure in the development of osteonecrosis of the femoral head: implications for treatment. *Orthop Clin North Am* 16:635–654, 1985.

15. Lieberman JR, Berry DJ, Mont MA, et al. Osteonecrosis of the hip: management in the 21st century. *Inst Course Lect* 52:337–355, 2003.

16. Mont MA, Pacheco I, Hungerford DS. Radiographic predictors of outcome of core decompression for hips with osteonecrosis stage III. *Clin Orthop Relat Res* 354:159–168, 1994.

PART V

Primary Total Hip Arthroplasty

13

Principles, Planning, and Decision Making

Robert L. Barrack and Shawn J. Nakamura

PREOPERATIVE PLANNING

Total hip arthroplasty (THA) is among the most successful interventions in all of medicine. The reported results are consistently excellent with a relatively low complication rate. This is, however, one of the most common surgical procedures performed, with the majority of the patients in the United States being in the Medicare population. There has been a substantial decline in reimbursements to surgeons and hospitals performing this procedure over the past several years, resulting in financial pressures in delivering this service efficiently. Fiscal restraints require that good results be consistently achieved with maximal efficiency in resource utilization. The resources that are under direct control of the surgeon include operating room time, the number of hospital days, rehabilitation services such as physical therapy and occupational therapy, and implants and instrumentation. The most significant factor in minimizing unnecessary resources is avoiding complications such as infection, dislocation, fracture, and neurovascular injury. The key to achieving optimal results and efficiency while minimizing complications is careful, consistent preoperative planning. This allows surgeons to shorten their learning curve on new techniques and implants, as well as anticipating and preparing for any potential problems that may occur during surgery.

Templating of adequate radiographs is a crucial step in the planning process. Preoperative planning, however, involves a number of steps prior to templating, which is the last in a series of steps involved in preoperative planning. Surgeons performing THA should have an organized, efficient process for planning each case that considers the individual patient and not just the hip joint. Planning for a THA can be approached by a logical sequence by first accurately determining the source of the patient's symptoms, confirming the specific diagnosis, determining if the patient is a reasonable surgical candidate, exploring nonsurgical and nonarthroplasty options, and determining the specific relevant findings on history and physical examination pertaining to THA. Following this, a standard set of radiographs should be carefully reviewed both for general assessment and finally for the purposes of templating and planning for specific technical details of implant selection and implantation.

Localization of Pathology

The most important first step in localizing the source of symptoms is the patient interview. It is most important to have the patient specifically identify the location of the symptoms. Many patients who are referred for hip pain and state that they have hip pain will point to the gluteal region or buttock as the actual location of their pain. Pain in the buttock is often of lumbar spine origin; however, pain in the groin is most specific for hip disease. It is important to distinguish between pain of lumbar spine versus pain of hip origin. This can be investigated further by having the patient describe the nature of the pain, such as whether it is radicular in nature and whether it is associated with any sensory deficit or muscle weakness. Physical examination findings such as a positive straight leg raise and diminished Achilles or patellar tendon reflex will also help distinguish lumbar pathology from pain emanating from the hip joint. Degenerative arthritis of the spine and hip frequently coexist and, on occasion, an epidural steroid injection may be administered if there are sufficient findings on physical examination and lumbar spine radiographs to support the diagnosis of lumbar pathology leading to the gluteal symptoms. If an epidural steroid injection completely relieves the symptoms, then it is reasonable to conclude that the symptoms are of lumbar spine origin, even in the presence of substantial radiographic changes of the hip.

Physical examination findings that support that the hip is the origin of the symptoms include the pain that is reproduced by resisted hip flexion (positive Stinchfield test) and pain and limitation of motion in internal rotation. Reproduction of the symptoms with hip rotation or axial load is a hallmark of hip pathology. Pain in the thigh or calf that is worse with prolonged activity is suggestive of vascular or neurogenic claudication, and careful evaluation of the patient's pedal pulses, as well as neurologic evaluation, should be performed.

Pain localized to the groin is commonly associated with hip pathology. Other extrinsic intrapelvic pathology can also present with groin pain, however, including inguinal hernia, retrocecal appendix, and ovarian cyst. Occasionally, hip pathology will present with knee pain in a patient that has normal knee radiographs and a normal knee exam, but abnormal hip radiographs. Referred pain from hip pathology is a distinct possibility. Once again, the symptoms are frequently reproduced with hip rotation, axial load, or assisted hip flexion and hip internal rotation. On occasion, it may be prudent to utilize intra-articular injection of the hip under fluoroscopy to confirm that knee pain is referred from the hip. Elimination of the knee pain with a hip injection helps confirm that diagnosis.

Once it has been determined that the hip is the source of symptoms, it is important to determine whether the pathology is intra-articular or extra-articular in origin. A number of entities can produce extra-articular hip pain, including trochanteric bursitis, piriformis syndrome, psoas bursitis or tendonitis, abductor strain or tendonitis, and ischiogluteal bursitis. Pain that is located directly over the trochanter that is worse with resisted hip abduction is the hallmark of trochanteric bursitis. Plain radiographs should be scrutinized for irregularity about the greater trochanter (see Fig. 1). A local injection into the area of maximal tenderness laterally over the trochanter will frequently alleviate the symptoms.

Specific Diagnosis

If the hip joint is determined to be the most likely source of symptoms, the next important step is to make a specific diagnosis. Although degenerative osteoarthritis is the most common cause for the need for THA, there are a number of other diagnoses that have extensive implications in the preoperative assessment. These include, in the approximate order of frequency: avascular necrosis (AVN), inflammatory arthritis, dysplasia, metastatic disease, occult infection, and occult trauma. In patients who have avascular necrosis, it is important to determine the etiology of the process. When an etiology can be determined, the most common are trauma, alcohol use, and steroid use. Patients with a history of heavy alcohol use may need treatment for this prior to undertaking a major elective procedure. Patients with hypercoagulable conditions often require anticoagulation or placement of a Greenfield filter prior to THA. Patients with sickle cell anemia often require preoperative transfusion. AVN is frequently bilateral. A patient with early stage AVN in the contralat-

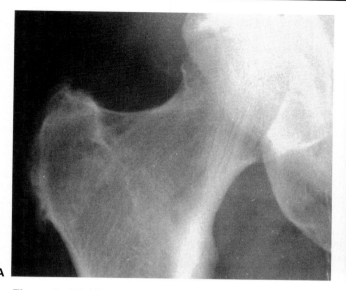
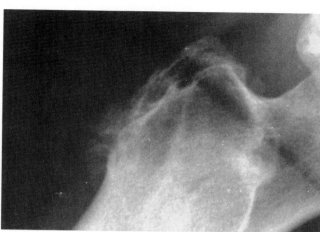

Figure 1. AP **(A)** and lateral **(B)** radiographs of the hip of a patient with localized trochanteric pain showing bony irregularity typical of trochanteric bursitis.

eral hip may be a candidate for core decompression or some other head-sparing procedure either prior to the contralateral hip replacement or concomitantly.

Patients with inflammatory arthritis have a number of relevant associated findings that impact preparation for hip replacement. Patients with rheumatoid arthritis frequently have involvement of the cervical spine and/or temporomandibular joint (TMJ). If the patient has headaches or neck pain, flexion/extension lateral radiographs to evaluate C1-2 instability should be considered. Patients with symptomatic C1-2 instability should have this assessed prior to hip replacement. Patients with TMJ involvement should be seen preoperatively for anesthesia consultation because of potential difficulty with intubation. These patients may require awake endoscopy-assisted intubation. Patients with rheumatoid arthritis are frequently on immunosuppressive agents such as corticosteroids. This may require a stress dose of steroids perioperatively to avoid Addisonian crisis. Rheumatoid patients may also be on other disease immunosuppressive agents such as methotrexate. It is prudent to discontinue these drugs for a period of time prior to elective surgery to minimize the risk of delayed wound healing or infection. Patients with gout, pseudo-gout, or other crystalline arthropathy may present with acute hip pain and chronic degenerative changes of the hip radiographically. If symptoms represent an acute flare of inflammatory disease, it is advisable to treat the flare appropriately before making further decisions about hip replacement. Occasionally, Paget disease presents with hip pain. It is important to assess the stage of the disease and to avoid elective surgery during the lytic phase of this disease. Serologic markers such as hydroxyproline can be utilized as measures of disease activity as can a technetium bone scan (1).

Other uncommon diagnoses to consider include occult infection, stress fracture, and occult hip fracture. The history and radiographs are crucial in considering these diagnoses. In an older patient with systemic symptoms, primary or metastatic disease should be considered. The most common primary malignancy involving bone is multiple myeloma, and it may present with anemia associated with hip pain. Myeloma lesions may involve the pelvis and can coexist with avascular necrosis from the disease or its treatment (see Fig. 2). Metastatic disease should also be considered in older patients with destructive lesions involving the periacetabular lesion or the intratrochanteric area. A bone scan in these cases may show multiple areas of skeletal involvement. Patients with a history of trauma may have an occult hip fracture while younger patients with a history of recent increase in activity may be at risk for stress fracture of the femoral neck, which can present with groin pain. Older patients may exhibit the insufficiency fractures of pubic ramus. Septic arthritis is an uncommon cause of debilitating groin pain, which on rare occasion can coexist with AVN, particularly in an immunocompromised patient. The index of suspicion should be

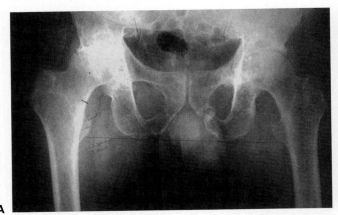
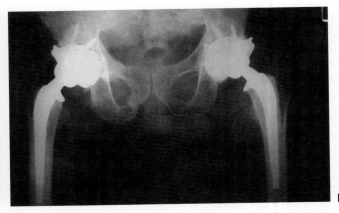

Figure 2. A: AP radiograph of patient with bilateral AVN associated with steroid treatment of myeloma. **B:** Because of the presence of tumor deposits in the pelvis and previous radiation, a protrusio ring was utilized on the acetabulum, and cemented stems were utilized on the femur.

raised when a patient with previous chronic symptoms develops a sudden increase in symptoms and intractable pain. In such cases, the sedimentation rate will be higher than expected, and radiographic appearance may be unusual with a more lytic appearance on both sides of the joint (see Fig. 3). Making a specific diagnosis helps ensure that conditions associated with the disease process are identified and appropriately treated prior to consideration of a major elective procedure such as total hip arthroplasty.

Is the Patient a Good Surgical Candidate?

After a specific diagnosis has been made and all associated conditions have been assessed and treated, the next step is to determine whether the patient is a good surgical candidate. The first criterion to satisfy is to determine whether there has been an adequate trial of non-

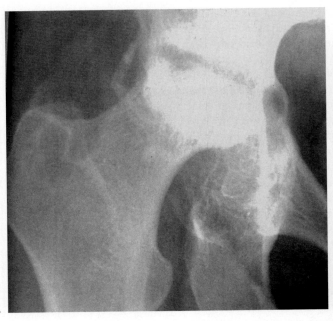
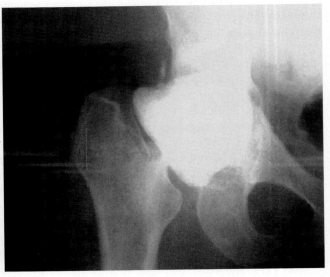

Figure 3. A: AP radiograph of an immunocompromised patient with severe exacerbation of hip pain with late stage AVN. **B:** Erythrocyte sedimentation rate (ESR) was markedly elevated, aspiration confirmed infection, and resection and antibiotic spacer was performed prior to THA.

operative measures, such as anti-inflammatory medication, activity modification, and weight loss if appropriate. Patients can obtain substantial relief by unloading the joint with the use of a cane or avoiding high-impact activities and losing weight. Obese patients should be counseled as to the increased risks associated with hip replacement in the presence of obesity and should be referred for counseling by a dietician with the aim of supervised weight loss. If appropriate nonoperative measures have failed, it is next prudent to determine whether the patient is realistic regarding the risks, benefits, and limitations associated with the procedure. It is important to determine what the patient's requirements are regarding his vocation and activities following surgery. A patient who is a laborer who is required to do heavy lifting and run and jump should be advised that these activities are not advisable following hip replacement. It is also important to determine whether the patient will be compliant with activities such as avoiding extreme positioning during the first several months to minimize the risk of dislocation and to avoid high-impact activities to lower the risk of early failure due to polyethylene wear, lysis, and loosening. There are certain patient characteristics that should be identified prior to major elective surgery. Patients who are seriously depressed should have this problem addressed prior to considering elective surgery. Counseling and medication may help address issues that are more important to the patient than their hip pain. In addition, patients who have significant psychosis or neurosis should be referred for evaluation and treatment to ensure that they are appropriately treated prior to considering hip replacement. Patients with pending worker's compensation claims have been associated with lower success rate. Other factors to consider are patients who are hostile or litigious. It is prudent to address these issues prior to proceeding with joint replacement.

It is crucial to determine if the patient is medically stable and optimal before a major elective procedure such as hip replacement. It is frequently advisable to have patients thoroughly evaluated by an internist to ensure that chronic conditions such as hypertension, diabetes, and pulmonary and cardiac disease are under maximal medical control prior to proceeding. It is also advisable to thoroughly screen patients for any potential source of hematogenous infection prior to hip replacement. The extremities should be assessed for cutaneous lesions such as venous stasis ulcers or infected toenails. These conditions should be treated prior to proceeding. Other potential sources of infection that should be addressed include urinary tract infection, prostatitis, periodontal disease, dental caries, and diverticulitis.

Nonarthroplasty Options

Once it has been determined that a patient is a good surgical candidate, the next step is to determine the most appropriate surgical intervention for each individual patient. Before proceeding with hip replacement, it is advisable to consider nonarthroplastic options. Patients with symptoms of a labral tear or loose body may be candidates for arthroscopy. In the presence of early degenerative changes with maintenance of articular cartilage and mechanical abnormalities, pelvic or femoral osteotomy may be an option. In the young active patient with unilateral hip disease and complete loss of articular cartilage, arthrodesis should be considered. A resection arthroplasty is rarely performed as a salvage procedure in patients who are poor ambulatory candidates.

Physical Examination

There are a number of details of physical examination that have a substantial impact on the preoperative plan for THA. The skin and soft tissue about the hip should be inspected, and previous incisions should be evaluated for the possibility of incorporation into the planned operative incision. Placement of a parallel incision anterior to a previous incision should be avoided since it is associated with increased risk of wound necrosis of the skin between the two incisions. The remainder of the extremity should also be evaluated to document both the neurovascular status and the presence of distal extremity infections. The patient's standing posture should be noted. Patients with excessive lumbar lordosis have a different orientation of the acetabulum in the erect posture. Hip surgery is frequently performed in the lateral decubitus position with the contralateral knee flexed; the lordosis is at least partially corrected. It may be advisable to place the acetabular component in more anteversion to compensate for the change in orientation of the acetabular component that will occur when the patient is upright. The iliac crest should be observed from behind for the presence of pelvic obliquity. This may result in an apparent limb length discrepancy. It is important to correlate the patient's own feeling about limb length with the measurements taken with blocks. The block test is generally considered the most accurate clinical measurement. In patients with fixed pelvic obliquity, the lumbar spine should be carefully evaluated for the presence of deformity that could be associated with pelvic obliquity. It is important to inform patients that apparent limb length discrepancy secondary to the lumbar spine may not be correctable at the time of hip replacement.

The surgeon should have an objective plan and strategy for the correction of limb length discrepancy. Following limb length assessment, the patient's gait should be observed for gait patterns, including antalgic, short limb, or Trendelenburg gait. The Trendelenburg test can also be performed as a clinical evaluation of abductor muscle weakness. This should be correlated with the observation of gait and manual muscle testing of abductor strength against resistance in the side-lying position. Patients with substantial muscle weakness should be evaluated for an underlying cause. Some degree of weakness can be secondary to pain; however, severe degrees of weakness and the inability to resist gravity in side-lying abduction are unusual, and an explanation should be sought. The presence of significant abductor weakness may be relevant in the operative plan. Strategies such as increasing lateral offset or lateralizing the trochanter may be advisable in the presence of significant laxity or weakness in the abductors. It also may be advisable to use a metal shell that can accommodate a constrained liner in the event that a patient with severely compromised abductors subsequently becomes a dislocator.

Rotational deformities may also be revealed on observation of gait. Patients with intoeing may also have increased femoral anteversion. This can also be determined by the presence of excessive passive internal rotation of the femur in combination with limited external rotation. This condition is usually bilateral, and patients should be advised that limb rotation may be somewhat asymmetric postoperatively.

After gait observation, active and passive range of motion of the hip should be recorded. Patients with severe flexion or adduction contractures present substantial problems. Preoperative physical therapy might be advisable in order to lessen the degree of contracture. Patients with flexion and adduction contractures may benefit from a transgluteal surgical approach to minimize the risk of dislocation. A posterior approach may place such a patient at an increased risk of postoperative dislocation. In patients with a severe degree of adduction contracture, percutaneous adductor tenotomy may be considered prior to beginning the case.

Physical exam of the contralateral hip and other joints also significantly impacts the preoperative plan. If the patient has severe bilateral hip involvement that would preclude ambulation postoperatively, bilateral hip replacement should be considered. The status of other joints is particularly relevant in patients with rheumatoid arthritis, who frequently have other joints involved. If the upper extremities are involved to the extent that it would prevent postoperative ambulation with assistive devices, typically the upper extremity should be addressed first. Likewise, a plantigrade foot is essential for effective ambulation. If foot or ankle pathology does not allow normal plantigrade gait, then corrective foot or ankle surgery prior to hip replacement should be considered. When both the ipsilateral hip and knee joints are markedly symptomatic, hip replacement is generally performed prior to knee replacement; however, there are exceptions. In patients with severe flexion contractures of the knees that will prevent ambulation, consideration should be given to performing knee arthroplasty prior to hip replacement.

Radiographic Evaluation

It is prudent to defer review of radiographs until after the history and physical examination are performed so as not to bias the examiner. The first step in preoperative radiographic analysis involves obtaining consistent, appropriate radiographs for review. A minimum of two views is required, one in the anteroposterior (AP) projection and one lateral view. In practice, three views are preferable. An AP view of the pelvis is necessary to estimate relative limb length. A more accurate assessment of the dimensions of the proximal femur is obtained from an AP view centered over the hip. The standard distance from the x-ray tube to the tabletop is 40 inches. If a grid cassette is placed directly beneath the hip, magnification of the bones of approximately 10% is seen in an average size patient. Placing a cassette directly beneath the extremity is common in the operating room, but in most radiology departments a Bucky tray is placed in a compartment approximately 2 inches below the tabletop, resulting in magnification of 15% to 20% (2). The degree of magnification is directly related to the distance from the bone to the cassette. In an obese patient, therefore, the magnification can be over 25%, whereas in a thin patient it, can be less than 15%. In patients who are substantially larger or smaller than average, a magnification maker can be utilized to quantify the degree of magnification.

The AP pelvis and hip radiograph should be obtained with the patient lying flat on the table and the lower extremities internally rotated 15° to 20°. If a flexion contracture is present as noted on physical examination, the radiographic technique should be modified. If a standard AP radiograph is obtained in the presence of a flexion contracture, typically the femur will be off of the tabletop with the patient supine, or there will be increased lumbar lordosis. If the hip is flexed for an AP radiograph, it will result in a greater degree of magnification, foreshortening the image, and often rotation of the femur as well. These inaccuracies can be minimized by obtaining the AP radiographs in a semisitting position (see Fig. 4). It is also desirable to obtain the AP radiographs in 15 to 20 degrees of internal rotation to bring

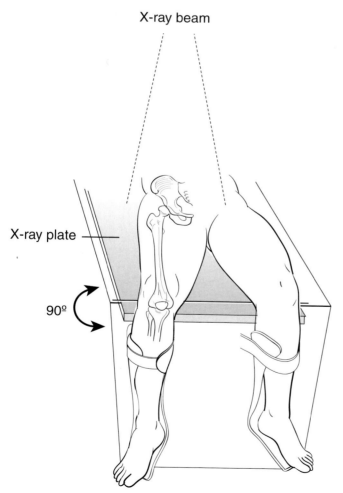

X-ray beam

X-ray plate

90°

Figure 4. Positioning of the patient with flexion contracture of the hip and/or knee. (After Engh C, Bobyn LD, eds. *Biological Fixation in Total Hip Arthroplasty*. Thorofare, N. J.: Slack; 1985:47.)

the femoral neck into a parallel orientation relative to the cassette and thus perpendicular to the x-ray tube in the average patient. This gives a more accurate depiction of the proximal femoral geometry and true femoral offset. Patients tend to naturally assume a posture of external rotation of the hips when lying supine. In addition, patients with degenerative disease tend to lose internal rotation early and later develop external rotation contractures, accentuating the tendency for AP radiographs to be taken with the hip externally rotated. Radiographs in external rotation make the intertrochanteric area appear more narrow, the femoral offset less, and the lesser trochanter more prominent. Internal rotation has the opposite effect: increasing the offset, making the intertrochanteric area larger, and making the lesser trochanter much less prominent (see Fig. 5). Rotation of the femur has a significant effect on the measurement of both the neck-shaft angle and femoral offset. As a result of all of these factors, preoperative planning based on malrotated radiographs is inaccurate and will provide suboptimal information for the preoperative plan. If the pathologic hip cannot be internally rotated 15 degrees, templating can be done on the contralateral normal or less involved side (see Fig. 6). This assumes that the internal geometry of the contralateral hip is an accu-

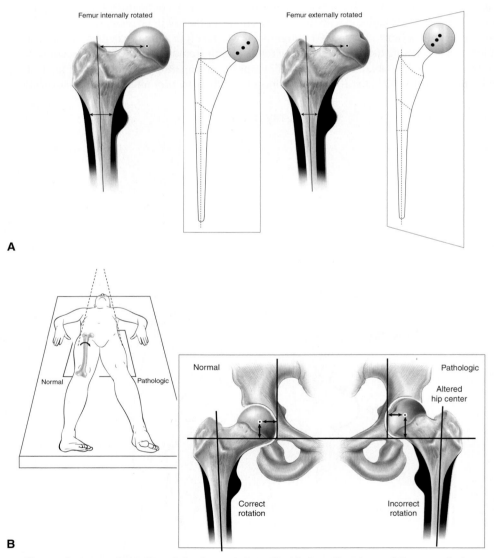

Figure 5. Internal rotation of the femur brings the hip into the plane of the acetabulum, which changes the apparent offset, metaphyseal dimensions, and neck-shaft angle **(A)** and makes the lesser trochanter less prominent **(B)**. (After Engh CA. Recent advances in cementless total hip arthroplasty using the AML prosthesis. *Tech Orthop* 6(3):60–61, 1991.)

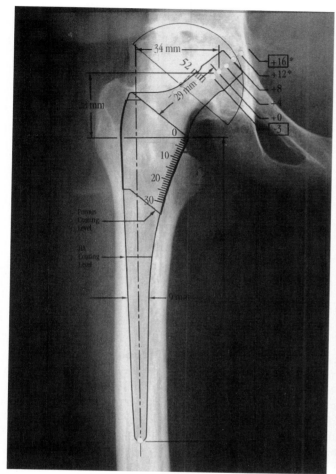

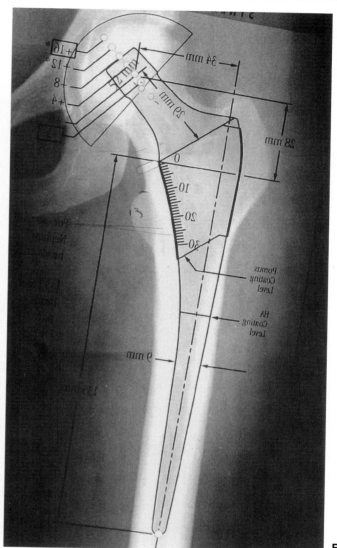

A

B

Figure 6. A: AP radiograph of affected hip with external rotation contracture as evidenced by prominent lesser trochanter, diminished intertrochanteric area, and decreased offset. **B:** Templating of contralateral hip in this case is much more accurate.

rate representation of that of the pathologic hip, a supposition that has been supported by a number of authors (3,4). In many cases, however, both hips have external rotation contractures. In such cases, a posteroanterior radiograph can be obtained with the patient placed prone, with the affected limb in 15 to 20 degrees of external rotation and the hip directly against the tabletop (see Fig. 7).

If there has been a previous fracture or osteotomy, long films of the entire femur are advisable. A standing film that includes the hip, knee, and ankle will give a more accurate assessment of the effect of the angular deformity on the overall limb alignment. Previous internal fixation devices may require special equipment for removal as well as special components to compensate for bone loss from component removal (see Fig. 8).

The preferred lateral projection of the hip advocated by most authors for preoperative planning is a modification of the frog leg lateral: the table-down or Löwenstein lateral x-ray. This is obtained with the patient supine and the hip externally rotated such that the hip, knee, and ankle are contacting the tabletop (see Fig. 9A). The femur is usually closer to the table in this position than in the standard AP radiograph, because the distance to

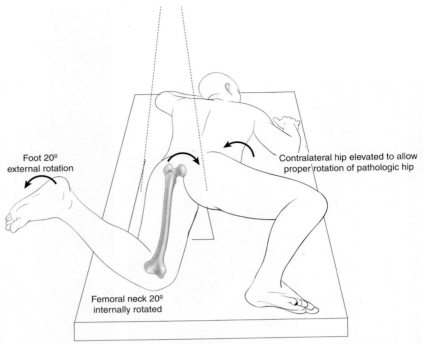

Foot 20°
external rotation

Contralateral hip elevated to allow
proper rotation of pathologic hip

Femoral neck 20°
internally rotated

Figure 7. Positioning of the patient with external rotation contracture of both hips. (After Engh CA. Recent advances in cementless total hip arthroplasty using the AML prosthesis. *Tech Orthop* 6(3):62, 1991.)

the femur is less and results in less magnification. This projection is best for determining the maximum bow of the femur and estimating the true degree of anteversion of the femoral neck. To obtain an orthogonal view to the AP projection with the limb internally rotated, the knee can be lifted at an angle of 15 to 20 degrees from the tabletop (Fig. 9B).

General Radiographic Review. Once standard radiographic views are obtained, it is appropriate to review the films in a general way to confirm the original or working diagnosis prior to embarking on preoperative planning. If the trabecular pattern is coarsened and irregular, for instance, Paget disease should be considered. Laboratory values from serum and urine may be appropriate to determine if the patient is in the active, lytic phase of the disease, in which case medical treatment with deferral of surgery may be appropriate. This would also alert the surgeon to carefully review long films of the femur in the AP and lateral projections for bowing, which could make stem insertion difficult. It may be difficult to distinguish bone pain from Paget disease from the accompanying degenerative joint disease. Intra-articular injection of a local anesthetic has been suggested as a method of making this distinction (1).

Other relevant systemic diseases may be discovered by general radiographic review. If the patient is a male with hypertrophic osteoarthritis and prominent syndesmophytes are visible in the lower lumbar spine on the AP pelvis view, the diagnosis of diffuse idiopathic skeletal hyperostosis (DISH) should be entertained. Perioperative radiation or indomethacin may be elected in such cases for prophylaxis of heterotopic ossification. In patients with sickle cell disease, the intertrochanteric region should be examined for evidence of bone infarcts or obliteration of the intramedullary canal (see Fig. 10A). The bone can be very sclerotic and require awls or drills to penetrate and reestablish the canal (Figs. 10B and 10C) prior to placement of a small cementless stem (Fig. 10D). There is a high risk of perforation in such cases, and fluoroscopy may even be advisable to lower the risk. Similar concerns exist in osteoporosis and Paget disease. Patients with severe osteoporosis may be candidates for preoperative medical treatment to increase bone mass. These patients are also at increased risk of intraoperative fracture, and the surgeon should be alerted to this.

Figure 8. A: Preoperative radiograph demonstrating multiple pins embedded in bone. **B:** A long cementless stem was elected to bypass the femoral window necessary to remove the pins.

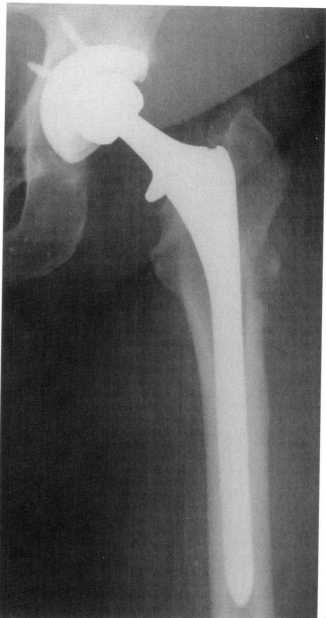

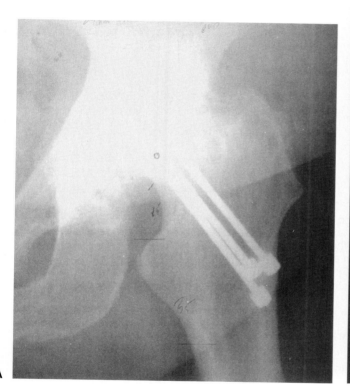

A

B

After confirming the diagnosis, radiographs should be examined for bone quality. This is an important factor for prosthesis selection for many surgeons (3). In the past, the Singh index was commonly utilized (6), and it has been modified for purposes of classifying bone density for preoperative component selection. More recently, Dossick et al. (7) described a method of classifying proximal femoral geometry based on the calcar-to-canal ratio. The outer diameter of the femur at the midportion of the lesser trochanter is divided by the diameter at a point 10 cm distal. A ratio of less than 0.5 is classified as type A, between 0.5 and 0.75 is type B, and more than 0.75 is type C. Type A bone has also been described qualitatively as demonstrating thick cortices on both the AP and lateral radiographs, while type B bone has thinning of the posterior cortex on the lateral view and type C has thinning of cortices on both views, typical of a "stovepipe" femur (7). Type A bone is generally believed to be most amenable to an uncemented femoral component. Type C bone favors the use of a cemented stem, and type B bone is intermediate.

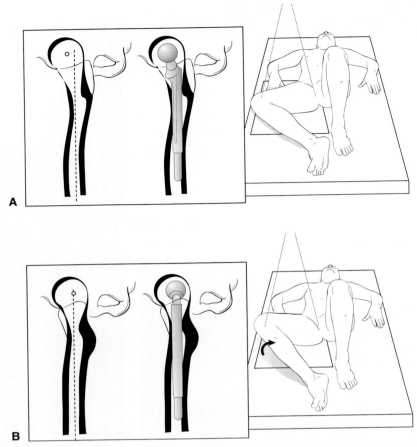

Figure 9. Patient positioning for modified frog leg lateral (Lowenstein lateral). With the knee flat on the table, the maximum anterior bow of the femur is visualized **(A)**; with the knee 20 degrees elevated, the view is rotated 90 degrees (orthogonal) from the AP view **(B)**. (After Engh CA. Recent advances in cementless total hip arthroplasty using the AML prosthesis. *Tech Orthop* 6(3):63, 1991.)

Radiographic Landmarks. Prior to actual templating, it is useful to mark anatomic landmarks and record certain measurements. In the past, the ilioischial line (Kohler's line) has been used to estimate the degree of protrusio acetabuli radiographically. Kohler's line is actually posterior to the medial wall of the pelvis and only overlies it on a true AP view. The acetabular teardrop is an anatomic landmark present in the inferomedial aspect of the acetabulum just superior and lateral to the obturator foramen. Its lateral lip represents the exterior of the acetabular wall, and the medial lip represents the interior margin of the wall. These relationships do not vary as much with rotation as does Kohler's line, and the teardrop represents an actual anatomic landmark of the inferomedial acetabulum rather than a radiographic image. The teardrop has become a pivotal landmark for preoperative planning as well as postoperative measurement of component migration (8). A horizontal line can be constructed connecting the inferior margins of both teardrops on the AP pelvis radiograph. Vertical lines are constructed bisecting the teardrops extending superiorly. The centers of the femoral heads are located, and the horizontal and vertical distances from the teardrop to the center of the head can be determined (see Fig. 11). The horizontal and vertical coordinates give an accurate recording of the center of rotation of the normal and pathologic hip. Average coordinates reported in normal adults are 14 mm vertical and 37 mm horizontal from the acetabular teardrop.

Another important radiographic measurement is that of limb length. This is commonly estimated by drawing a horizontal line along the inferior margin of both ischial tuberosities (interischial line). The vertical distance from this line to either the top or the bottom of the lesser trochanter of each hip is measured. The difference between the two is recorded as the radiographic limb length discrepancy (see Fig. 12). This should be correlated with clinical measurements, and any significant difference should be evaluated and resolved prior to surgery. The presence of a flexion contracture may result in a clinical measurement of shortening, whereas adduction contracture may give the appearance of lengthening. The amount of desired lengthening should be well established preoperatively and incorporated into the plan. If the operative limb appears long preoperatively, the patient should be advised that it may well remain long postoperatively, because shortening may increase the risk of instability. Change in limb length is a major cause of litigation in total hip replacement, the most common problem being lengthening of the operative limb. This risk can be minimized by careful preoperative planning, and if lengthening appears to be a potential problem, this should be emphasized in preoperative counseling and informed consent.

The neck-shaft angle, defined as the angle between the central axis of the femur and the axis of the femoral neck, is a useful measurement. There is wide variation of this angle, with a reported mean of 124.7 ± 7.4 (9). If the neck-shaft angle of the component utilized varies significantly from the anatomic angle, the level of the neck resection will be affected.

The femoral offset is defined as the perpendicular distance from the neutral long axis of the femur and the center of rotation of the hip. Restoring the normal degree of offset is a

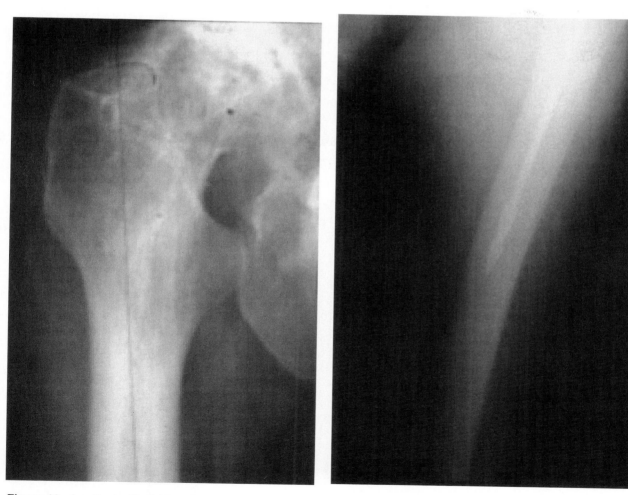

A

B

Figure 10. A patient with sickle cell anemia and subtle calcification and density changes in the intertrochanteric area **(A)**. A pointed awl was necessary to reestablish the canal as confirmed on AP and lateral intraoperative radiographs (*continues*)

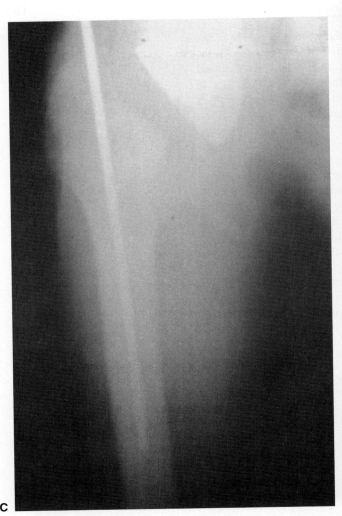

C

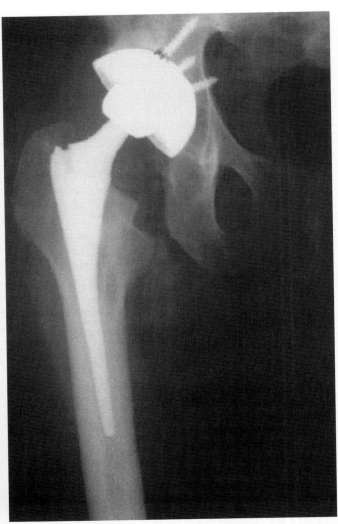

D

Figure 10. *(continued)* **(B,C)** prior to insertion of a small cementless femoral stem **(D)**.

Figure 11. A: AP radiograph demonstrating horizontal and vertical coordinates from teardrop to the center of hip rotation of the left, normal hip as determined from the acetabular teardrop. **B:** Placement of the acetabular component adjacent to the teardrop on the left side restored the center of rotation to within 2 mm.

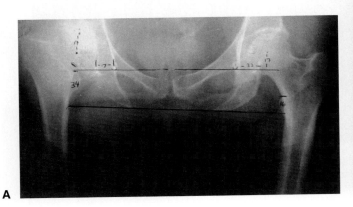

A

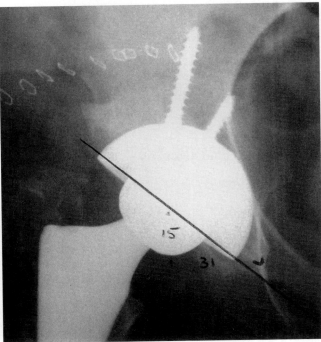

B

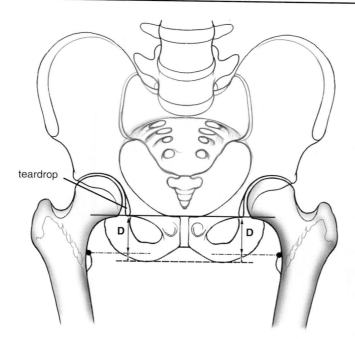

Figure 12. Preoperative measurements include interischial line *AB* and interteardrop line.

primary goal of hip replacement, thus making this measurement valuable. Because the amount of offset is affected by the degenerative process, it is useful to measure the offset on the contralateral normal hip.

TEMPLATING

Restoring proper hip biomechanics was a primary objective of total hip replacement as described by Charnley (10). This can best be accomplished by careful preoperative templating of appropriate radiographs. The general goals are to restore as nearly as possible the anatomic or premorbid center of rotation and femoral offset, while equalizing limb length.

Acetabular Side

Templating appropriately begins with the acetabular side because this is the sequence that is followed in surgery. The acetabular template is placed just lateral to the lateral edge of the teardrop at a 45-degree angle. Ideally, the cup should be completely covered by bone and should span the distance between the teardrop and the superolateral margin of the acetabulum. The component size that best accomplishes this with minimal removal of subchondral bone is selected. For cemented sockets a uniform 2- to 3-mm space must be left for cement. This is often indicated on templates by a dashed line. The center of rotation is marked through the template. If the component's medial edge is just lateral to the teardrop, the horizontal and vertical distances from the teardrop should closely approximate those of the contralateral normal hip.

Protrusio Acetabuli Cases. Protrusio acetabuli is present in a number of primary hip replacements, particularly in cases of rheumatoid arthritis, ankylosing spondylitis, Paget disease, and any metabolic bone disease that weakens the subchondral bone. Leaving the hip center in the medialized location is not advisable, because there is often not optimal structural support for the component in that position and the opportunity to restore medial bone should be utilized. The femoral head can be morselized and used as a medial graft to lateralize the component to a more normal anatomic position. It should be noted that a large

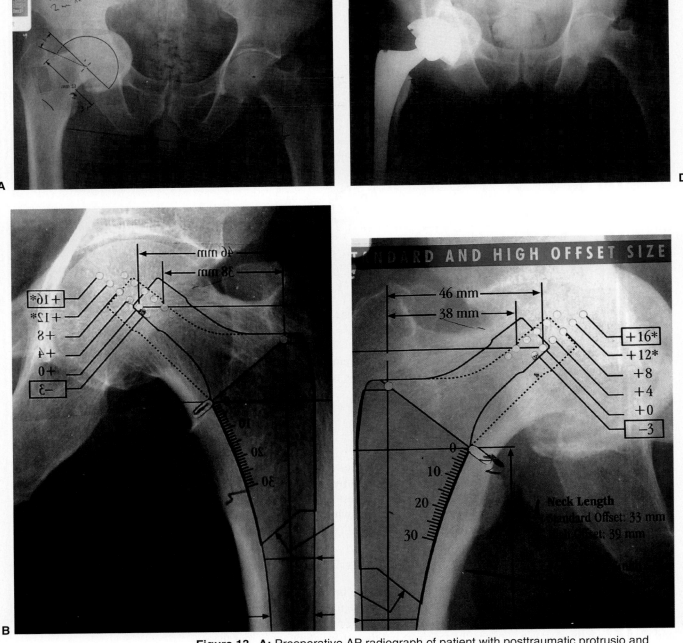

Figure 13. A: Preoperative AP radiograph of patient with posttraumatic protrusio and minimal shortening. **B:** The center of rotation is moved proximally by the amount of lengthening planned, and a high-offset component is predicted to be necessary. **C:** Templating of the contralateral hip also predicts a high offset and low neck cut. **D:** A low neck cut avoided overlengthening, and 60 cc of allograft in addition to the morselized autograft from the head was required.

volume of morselized bone may be necessary to achieve component lateralization, and it may be necessary to use additional allograft material in addition to the autograft from the femoral head (see Figs. 13A and 13B).

Lateralizing the component in cases of protrusio acetabuli has the additional advantage of increasing femoral offset and decreasing the tendency for impingement. Because the cup is contacting bone graft medially rather than structurally supportive subchondral bone, a large component is needed to achieve peripheral rim contact. Failure to achieve initial stability through a tight rim fit risks fracture of the medial wall during insertion or medial migration and recurrence of protrusio over time.

Significant shortening can occur through the acetabulum in cases of protrusio acetabuli. Therefore, it is common to lengthen the involved extremity during reconstruction. This is often desirable, since the limb is often short in these cases. Protrusio acetabuli is often bilateral, and the patient should be advised that there may be a significant degree of lengthening of the first hip but that there will be the opportunity to equalize the limb length when the other hip replacement is performed.

In cases of long-standing protrusio acetabuli, there is often ankylosis of the hip with contracture of the capsule and surrounding soft tissue. When lengthening occurs through lateralizing the socket, the amount of lengthening that can reasonably be obtained may be limited. As a result, a lower neck cut and shorter modular head may be utilized in these cases (Figs. 13C and 13D).

In cases where protrusio acetabuli is associated with severe osteoporosis, as in juvenile rheumatoid arthritis, it is occasionally prudent to consider a protrusio ring or cage. Insertion of an uncemented press-fit component in such cases can risk acetabular or pelvic fracture.

Lateralized Acetabulum. In many cases of degenerative osteoarthritis, the presence of hypertrophic osteophytes in the acetabulum causes lateralization of the hip's center of rotation. This occurs most often in men with hypertrophic osteoarthritis. This becomes apparent during templating when 1 or 2 cm of reaming is noted to be necessary to place the component in the vicinity of the teardrop. Failure to recognize this will result in placement of the acetabular component in a lateralized position with incomplete bony coverage and suboptimal stability, particularly when a press-fit cementless acetabular component is implanted without screws. Complete peripheral rim contact is desirable to obtain immediate stability with press-fit acetabular components. Complete bony coverage is also desirable for cemented sockets. Higher degrees of cemented acetabular component coverage have been associated with lower loosening rates (11). An increased horizontal distance from the teardrop (lack of adequate medialization of a lateralized acetabulum) has been shown to be a significant factor predictive of an unfavorable radiographic appearance of a cemented acetabular component (12).

Identifying the anatomic location of the hip joint in such cases can be difficult. The most reliable structural landmark is the transverse acetabular ligament that marks the inferior border of the true acetabulum and the location of the teardrop (8). Often, the cotyloid notch is completely overgrown with cartilage and not visually discernible. If reaming is initiated above the transverse acetabular ligament in a straight medial direction for several millimeters, the location of the notch becomes apparent; it can be curetted of bone, cartilage, and soft tissue, and the unicortical inner plate of the acetabulum which corresponds to the teardrop can be visualized at its base. Straight medial reaming to within a few millimeters of the planned depth of reaming is advisable to avoid superior placement of the component. If reaming is initiated at the 45-degree angle from the outset in such a scenario, the reamers will cut a path that is equally superior and medial, resulting in higher cup placement. This can be avoided by straight medial reaming with smaller reamers to close to the desired depth initially, followed by progressively larger reamers to enlarge the periphery in the optimal orientation (see Fig. 14).

Superolateral Migration. In addition to medial and lateral displacement, many degenerative hips migrate in a superolateral direction. This is most common in women with some degree of dysplasia. Because of the shallowness of the acetabulum and the incomplete coverage of the femoral head, forces are concentrated on the superolateral joint margin, which initially becomes flattened and eventually erodes away with subsequent superior migration of the hip and shortening of the extremity (see Fig. 15). This becomes apparent when the template is placed adjacent to the teardrop and a significant portion of the lateral margin remains uncovered (Fig. 15A).

When the template is placed adjacent to the teardrop and the lateral margin is uncovered, a number of options exist. Medial reaming to the subchondral plate and use of a low-profile cup will minimize the degree to which the femoral head is uncovered. A 10% to

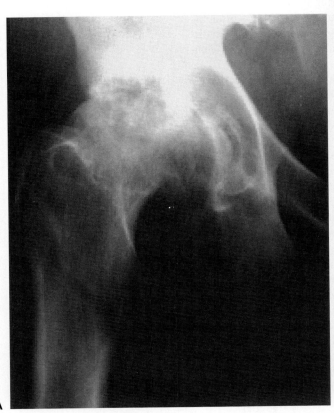
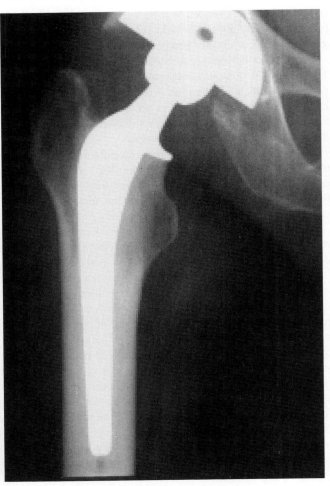

A

B

Figure 14. A: Lateralized acetabulum with extensive medial osteophyte. **B:** Medial reaming allowed complete coverage and placement of component at level of teardrop.

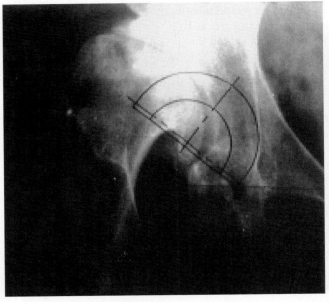
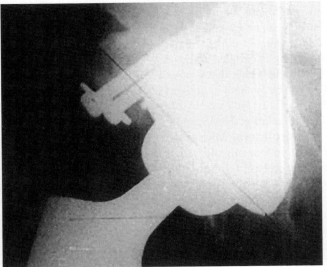

A

B

Figure 15. A: Significant superior deficit remains with cup placed in anatomic position.
B: Structural graft allows complete coverage and restoration of normal center of rotation.

20% uncovered femoral head can be accepted, and screws can be used to augment fixation of cementless components, because there will not be circumferential peripheral contact. In cemented components, cement augmentation of the superolateral deficiency has been described without deleterious effects on component fixation in the 5- to 10-year time frame. The acetabular component can be positioned somewhat vertically, and an elevated rim liner can be placed in the superior position to compensate for this. If the cup remains more than 10% to 20% uncovered in spite of all of these maneuvers, a structural graft fixed to the pelvis can be considered (Fig. 15B). This possibility should be recognized during templating, because a significant amount of additional equipment may be required. Surgical techniques for implanting cementless components with structural femoral head autograft have been described (13).

When structural grafting is performed, significant lengthening will occur through the acetabular component. This may necessitate a lower neck cut and shorter prosthetic neck length to avoid overlengthening. In cases in which significant length changes are anticipated, it is particularly appropriate to use one of a number of intraoperative devices to measure length.

The presence of hip dysplasia should also alert the surgeon to the possibility of excessive femoral anteversion, which is a common coexisting condition. If a cemented stem is selected, a smaller, straighter stem, such as a congenital hip dysplasia (CDH) stem, may be necessary. The stem can simply be rotated within the cement column to compensate for the excessive anteversion. In these cases, however, the greater trochanter is often posteriorly rotated; during trial reduction the direction of pull of the abductors should be observed, and the hip should be carefully checked for impingement of the trochanter in extension and external rotation. It may be necessary to osteotomize the trochanter and reattach it further anteriorly, laterally, and distally.

If an uncemented, press-fit stem is selected, excessive anteversion presents a challenge for which there are a number of potential solutions. A modular stem can be used, with a metaphyseal portion oriented to the degree of anteversion of the patient's anatomy. The stem can then be rotated within the metaphyseal segment in a variety of positions until maximal stability is achieved. If an off-the-shelf cementless stem is utilized, there are at least two options. If the stem is straight and parallel-sided and the neck is anteverted 10 degrees, implanting a left stem in a right hip (or vice versa) will provide relative retroversion of 20 degrees, which may be adequate for mild or moderate degrees of excessive anteversion.

Because of all of the surgical implications of increased femoral anteversion, it is important to recognize this entity preoperatively. With careful attention to the details of the physical examination and radiographic review, this should not be difficult in the majority of cases.

Identifying the Center of Rotation. The ideal position for the acetabular template (and component) is achieved by placing the inferomedial edge adjacent to the lateral margin of the teardrop. In most patients, this will restore the center of rotation very close to an anatomic and desirable location. This can be checked by measuring the horizontal and vertical distance from the teardrop to the templated center of rotation, compared to the coordinates from the teardrop to the center of the normal or unaffected contralateral hip. If the distances are equal and there is no difference in limb length, then this point can be utilized as the point about which the reconstruction can be planned. If a limb length discrepancy is present with the affected side short, which is most often the case, the center of rotation planning point is moved superiorly above the templating point the number of millimeters of the planned correction, and this point is utilized for subsequent templating. Generally, correction of two thirds to three fourths of the shortening is a prudent goal.

Femoral Templating

After the planned center of rotation of the reconstruction is marked on the radiograph, the femur is templated, referencing from this point. The goals and emphasis of femoral templating vary depending on whether a cementless proximally coated, cementless extensively coated, or cemented stem is planned. Although in practice most surgeons have a strong tendency to implant the same type of stem for most of their cases, it is prudent to template for both a cemented and cementless stem, particularly in cases where any anatomic abnormality is identified.

Component size is judged from the AP radiograph of the hip. For proximally coated components, proximal fit and fill are generally emphasized. For extensively coated cementless stems, fixation is obtained distally, so a tight fit in the isthmus is sought. Contact of the stem medially and laterally with the endosteal sidewalls over several centimeters is recommended (2). For cemented stems, it is important to leave adequate room for a cement mantle. A 2- to 3-mm circumferential cement mantle is optimal. It is crucial to perform femoral templating on radiographs with the correct degree of rotation (15 to 20 degrees of internal rotation) to most accurately predict stem size, neck length, offset, and neck resection level. If the affected side has an external rotation contracture and the contralateral side is normal, then templating begins with acetabular templating on the affected side. The center of rotation is marked on the x-ray, and the horizontal and vertical distances from the teardrops are measured. These coordinates are used to transpose the center of rotation to the unaffected side, where femoral templating can be performed (2).

The femoral template is moved vertically until the center of the femoral head template is at the same vertical height as the planned acetabular center of rotation. Regardless of the stem type utilized, the templates should be kept centered along the neutral axis of the femur, rather than in any varus or valgus inclination. Ideally, femoral bone stock should be maintained, and neck cuts should be planned between 1 and 2 cm above the lesser trochanter. If the center of rotation of the femur overlies the planned center of rotation of the hip, then length and offset will be restored. The neck resection level is marked through the template, and the distance above the lesser trochanter can be measured with a ruler with the appropriate level of magnification, so the correct neck resection level can be reproduced during surgery. If the center of the femoral head template lies medial to the planned center of hip rotation when the template is at the appropriate height, stem insertion to this level will increase femoral offset, which is generally an advantage, particularly if it is a matter of a few millimeters. Excessive increase in offset may cause prominence of the trochanter with a tendency toward bursitis, adductor tightness, and restricted rotation, and should be avoided.

If the center of the femoral head template lies *lateral* to the planned center of hip rotation, then the reconstruction will decrease femoral offset, and this is particularly to be avoided. Charnley (10) was among the first to emphasize restoring normal hip biomechanics as a goal of hip replacement, and one of the cornerstones of this philosophy was restoring or increasing the abductor moment arm. He accomplished this by utilizing a component of appropriate offset, making the neck cut at the appropriate level, and lateralizing the trochanter. Now that trochanteric osteotomy is rarely performed in primary THA, the major tool at the disposal of the surgeon for increasing the abductor moment arm is restoring or increasing the femoral offset (14).

Decreasing offset has a number of negative effects that have been associated with decreased strength, increased limp, increased polyethylene wear, and instability. A study from McGrory et al. (15) showed less strength in isokinetic testing in hips with lesser offset. Another study by Rothman et al. (16) showed a higher incidence of limp when femoral offset was decreased. Decreasing the abductor moment arm increases joint reaction forces, which could lead either to higher rates of acetabular loosening or to increased rates of polyethylene wear. Robinson et al. (17) were able to demonstrate a correlation between low offset and higher rate of polyethylene wear. Finally, decreasing offset leads to laxity in the abductor musculature, which could lead to a higher incidence of instability. Increasing evidence of the advantage of restoring offset has led to a resurgence of interest in this concept (14).

A number of options exist to avoid performing a reconstruction that decreases offset. Seating the femoral component lower, using a low neck cut, and utilizing a longer head will compensate for small decreases in offset (see Fig. 16). This sacrifices bone, however, and changes the fit of the proximal femoral component, which is a particular concern in proxi-

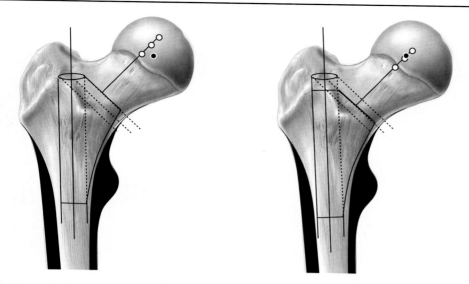

Figure 16. Seating the femoral component lower and using longer neck affects offset as well as proximal fill. (After Engh CA. Recent advances in cementless total hip arthroplasty using the AML prosthesis. *Tech Orthop* 6(3):67, 1991.)

mally coated cementless stems. A larger-sized component may be considered if going to the next size increases the base offset. The anatomy of the femur may preclude this, however. If a cemented stem is utilized, adequate room for the cement mantle must be assured if a large stem is considered. This might entail drilling of the femur to ensure a 2-mm mantle. Another option is switching to a different stem design that has a higher base offset. There are a number of component design strategies for increasing offset, including changing the neck-shaft angle, changing the proximal geometry, and medializing the takeoff point of the neck from the stem. Because of the complexity of going from one stem to another, it is important to plan the strategy for restoring offset preoperatively. In recent years, a popular solution has been the dual offset total hip. This allows the same stem and same neck resection level to be utilized with two different base offsets (see Fig. 17).

The neck resection should be planned so as to utilize a neck length without a "skirt," or thickened extension of the head, as this tends to impinge at extremes of motion. Such impingement will result in restricted motion, polyethylene wear, and/or instability. Most implant systems offer four or five head choices, of which the first three or four do not have a skirt or extension. Generally, reconstructions are planned around a short neck length (high neck cut), since calcar planers are often utilized, the broach can always be countersunk, and further planing can be done. Alternatively, the neck can be recut. This is preferable to too low a resection level, resulting in the necessity of utilizing a long or extralong neck, which typically comes with a skirt.

The AP radiograph is also useful for planning an entry point for the femoral stem. By drawing a line along the lateral margin of the femur and extending it proximally, the appropriate entry point can be located. This is more crucial in a cementless stem. Typically, this involves a lateral entry site near the pyriformis fossa and requires removal of any remnants of the lateral aspect of the femoral neck to avoid varus stem placement.

The planned component size and distal canal diameter should be measured on the AP radiograph and used as a reference during surgery. If difficulty is encountered seating reamers and broaches below the planned size, often the entry point is incorrect, usually medial, and reaming and broaching are often being done in a varus orientation. If difficulties persist, an intraoperative x-ray with a broach in place will often confirm the problem (see Fig. 18). If reaming of the femur is proceeding *above* the planned size, it may also be prudent to obtain an intraoperative radiograph with a reamer or broach in place. Reamers can ream away cortical bone, particularly in osteoporotic patients, leading to potential compli-

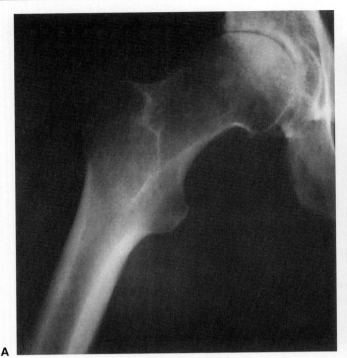
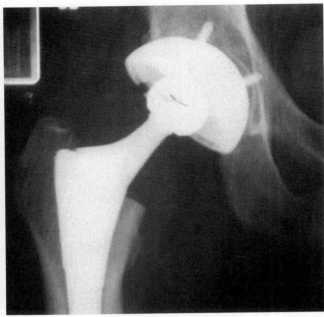

Figure 17. A: Preoperative radiograph of a patient with a high-offset hip; requires the extra offset option to reproduce the patient's anatomic offset. **B:** A high-offset component restored the anatomic offset.

cations. If cortical bone is being reamed without significant resistance, the choice of a cementless stem should probably be reconsidered.

Neck-shaft Angle

If the neck-shaft angle is measured preoperatively, it can be compared with the neck-shaft angle of the implant to be utilized. If there is a difference of more than a few degrees, a predictable pattern of intraoperative adjustments can be made. The average neck-shaft angle is approximately 125 degrees, whereas most implant systems have a neck-shaft angle of 130 to 135 degrees. Values significantly lower than this represent coxa vara, while values above this represent coxa valga.

Coxa Vara. Patients with coxa vara frequently have higher than usual femoral offset. This can be compensated for by utilizing a stem with a lower neck-shaft angle or by making a lower neck cut and utilizing a longer neck. Making a standard length neck cut can significantly lengthen the leg without restoring offset. The use of high-offset components or components with a lower neck-shaft angle helps preserve bone by minimizing the necessity of the low neck cut (see Fig. 19A).

Coxa Valga. The opposite situation exists when the patient's neck-shaft angle significantly exceeds that of the prosthesis. There is relatively low offset and more length. To compensate for this with a component with less valgus, it is necessary to make a higher neck cut and use a shorter neck to maintain length and offset. Coxa valga is frequently associated with low offset and a narrow intertrochanteric area, which may necessitate a CDH stem design. Making a standard neck cut in a valgus hip is a serious error from which recovery is difficult (Fig. 19B).

Coxa Breva. When avascular necrosis of the capital femoral epiphysis occurs early in life, as in Perthes disease, a short femoral neck (coxa breva) can result. In these cases, length and offset are usually increased when using a standard acetabular component. If a standard neck cut and neck length are employed, overlengthening may occur. Often, a low

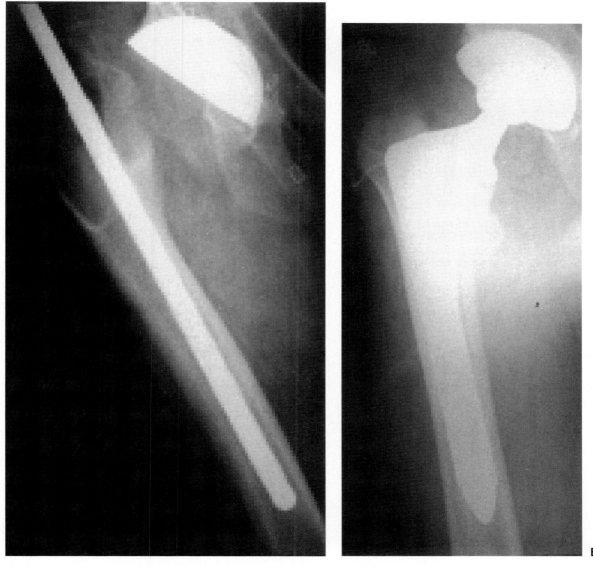

Figure 18. A: Intraoperative radiograph with a reamer and broach well below the templated size showing relative varus and medial entry point. **B:** A more lateral entry point allowed implantation of a larger stem in accordance with the preoperative plan.

neck cut and short head may be necessary to avoid this (see Fig. 20). Perthes disease may also be associated with coxa plana and trochanteric impingement.

High Offset. Large-stature patients may have increased femoral offset with a normal neck-shaft angle. These patients in particular benefit from a stem with a high-offset option.

CHOICE OF OPERATIVE APPROACH

On the basis of the patient's history and physical examination, a plan for the operative approach should be formulated. Most surgeons will utilize the same operative approach to the hip based on their training and experience. There are cases, however, in which modification of the surgeon's operative approach may be advisable. As previously mentioned, a previous surgical scar may require modification of the operative approach. Longitudinal incisions should be incorporated whenever possible. A longitudinal incision anterior and

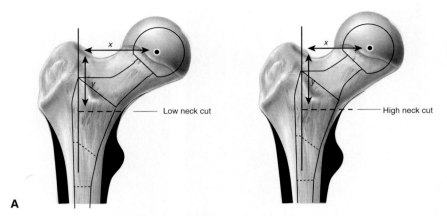

A

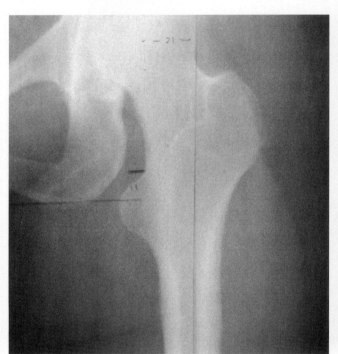

B

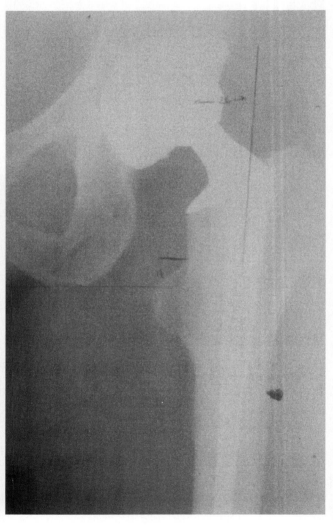

C

Figure 19. A: Coxa vara generally requires high-offset components and a low neck cut while coxa valga calls for a low-offset component, a high neck, and a high neck cut. **B:** Clinical example of preoperative coxa valga. **C:** Postoperative radiograph showing the high neck cut and low-offset component required to maintain equal limb length and restore biomechanics. (**A** after Engh CA. Recent advances in cementless total hip arthroplasty using the AML prosthesis. *Tech Orthop* 6(3):71, 1991.)

parallel to a previous incision has the highest risk for necrosis. In this case, it may be necessary to use the same incision with proximal and distal extensions.

In obese patients, longer incisions are necessary to adequately visualize the underlying structures. It may be necessary to have longer, self-retaining retractors that reach the depth of the wound. In extremely large patients, it is advisable to have a second assistant available. Patients with neuromuscular problems (a history of polio, cerebral palsy, previous stroke, or Parkinson disease) are at an increased risk for dislocation. In these cases, the surgeon may want to avoid the posterior approach in favor of a transgluteal approach (4).

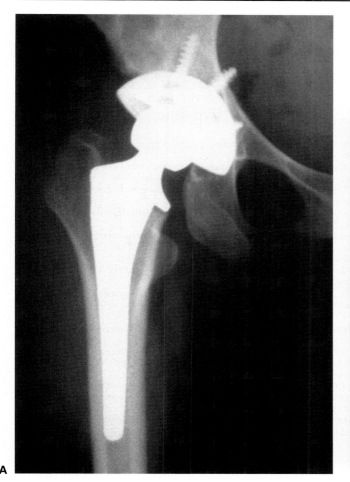
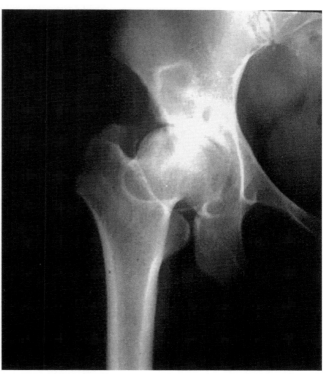

A   B

Figure 20. A: Preoperative radiograph demonstrating coxa breva secondary to Perthes disease. **B:** Postoperatively: A standard cup resulted in lengthening, which restored equal lengths, but a low neck cut and short neck were necessary to avoid overlengthening.

The presence of a stiff or ankylosed hip will influence the operative approach. If the posterior approach is utilized, it may be necessary to do further releases to mobilize the femur for adequate exposure. The entire quadratus femoris and gluteal sling can be released from the femur. Also, the reflected head of the rectus femoris and the anterior capsule can be released in order to mobilize the femur to access the acetabulum. A trochanteric osteotomy or slide or can be considered for exposure. However, if perioperative radiation therapy is being considered for heterotopic ossification, trochanteric osteotomy is less attractive because of the risk of nonunion.

Protrusio acetabuli should be considered when planning the operative approach. In most cases, the femoral head can be cut in situ allowing the use of a standard operative approach. Significant force should be avoided in dislocating the hip. This could lead to fracture of the femur, acetabulum, or pelvis. A trochanteric osteotomy can aid significantly with exposure. If a trochanteric osteotomy is planned, it is best to avoid the direct lateral approach.

The need for access to a particular anatomic region is important for planning the operative approach. If a posterior column plate is present from a previous acetabular fracture, a posterior approach may be necessary to remove the plate for access to the acetabulum. The sciatic nerve may be encased in scar tissue adherent to the nerve. In these cases, it is prudent to localize the nerve in an area away from the plate prior to dissection. Somatosensory evoked potentials (SSEP) monitoring may be considered to warn of potential nerve damage. If an anterior acetabular deficiency is present, an anterior or anterolateral approach may be necessary for access to this area.

RECOMMENDED READING

1. Kaplan FS, Singer FR. Paget's disease of bone: pathophysiology, diagnosis, and management. *J Am Acad Orthop Surg* 3(6):336–344, 1995.
2. Engh CA. Recent advances in cementless total hip arthroplasty using the AML prosthesis. *Tech Orthop* 6(3):59–72, 1991.
3. D'Antonio JA. Preoperative templating and choosing the implant for primary THA in the young patient. *Instr Course Lect* 43:339–346, 1994.
4. Dore DD, Rubash H. Primary total hip arthroplasty in the older patient: optimizing the results. *Instr Course Lect* 43:347–357, 1994.
5. Carter LW, Stovall DO, Young TR. Determination of accuracy of preoperative templating of noncemented femoral prostheses. *J Arthroplasty* 10(4):507–513, 1995.
6. Singh M, Nagrath AR, Maini PS. Changes in trabecular pattern of the upper end of the femur as an index of osteoporosis. *J Bone Joint Surg Am* 52(3):457–467, 1970.
7. Dossick PH, Dorr LD, Gruen T, Saberi MT. Techniques for preoperative planning and postoperative evaluation of noncemented hip arthroplasty. *Tech Orthop* 6(3):1–6, 1991.
8. Goodman SB, Adler SJ, Fyhrie DP, Schurman DJ. The acetabular teardrop and its relevance to acetabular migration. *Clin Orthop Relat Res* (236):199–204, 1988.
9. Noble PC, Alexander JW, Lindahl LJ, et al. The anatomic basis of femoral component design. *Clin Orthop Relat Res* 235:148–164, 1988.
10. Charnley J. *Low Friction Arthroplasty of the Hip.* New York: Springer-Verlag; 1979.
11. Sarmiento A, Ebramzadeh E, Gogan WJ, McKellop H. Cup containment and orientation in cemented total hip arthroplasties. *J Bone Joint Surg Br* 72:996–1002, 1990.
12. Karachalios T, Hartofilakidis G, Zacharakis N, Tsekoura M. A 12 to 18 year radiographic follow-up study of Charnley low-friction arthroplasty. The role of the center of rotation. *Clin Orthop Relat Res* 296:140–147, 1993.
13. Barrack RL, Newland CC. Uncemented total hip arthroplasty with superior acetabular deficiency. *J Arthroplasty* 5(2):159–167, 1990.
14. Steinberg B, Harris WH. The "offset" problem in total hip arthroplasty. *Contemp Orthop* 24:556–562, 1922.
15. McGrory BJ, Morrey BF, Cahalan TD, et al. Effect of femoral offset on range of motion and abductor muscle strength after total hip arthroplasty. *J Bone Joint Surg Br* 77(6):865–869, 1995.
16. Rothman RH, Hearn SL, Eng KO, Hozack WJ. The effect of varying femoral offset on component fixation in cemented total hip arthroplasty. Presented at: 60th Annual Meeting of the American Academy of Orthopaedic Surgeons; February, 1993; San Francisco, Calif.
17. Robinson EJ, Devane PA, Bourne RB, et al. Effect of implant position on polyethylene wear in total hip arthroplasty. Presented at: 62nd Annual Meeting of the American Academy of Orthopaedic Surgeons; February, 1995; Orlando, Fla.

14

The Cemented Stem

John J. Callaghan, Steve S. Liu, David A. Vittetoe, and Lucian C. Warth

INDICATIONS/CONTRAINDICATIONS

Total hip replacement is indicated for any cause of end-stage arthritis of the hip. Cemented femoral fixation was the only form of fixation used by surgeons on the femoral side of the total hip arthroplasty construct, except for a few pioneers who used cementless fixation, until the early to middle 1980s. Femoral cementing techniques evolved during the 1970s from hand-packing the cement into the femoral canal to plugging the distal canal with a cement or plastic plug and filling the canal with cement in a retrograde fashion with a cement gun delivery system. Pressurization techniques for introducing the cement into the femoral canal were also developed.

Durable results were obtained with these techniques in the vast majority of patients with end-stage hip arthritis. However, cemented fixation was found to be less durable in younger, active patients and in heavier patients. Although some surgeons continue to use cemented femoral fixation in all patients, most surgeons today use only cemented fixation in the smaller, less active, elderly patient, especially when the femoral canal is capacious and osteopenic. Cemented femoral fixation is also utilized in cases of previous sepsis because antibiotics can be added to the cement. Most surgeons agree that cemented femoral fixation should not be utilized in heavy, young, active patients, especially if they have excellent femoral bone stock. In our hands, that would include patients younger than 65 or 70 years who are active, especially if they weigh more than 175 pounds, since they may not be ideal candidates for cemented fixation on the femoral side of the total hip arthroplasty construct.

PREOPERATIVE PLANNING

Preoperative planning of the total hip arthroplasty procedure has been discussed previously. If a cemented femoral component is to be utilized, the surgeon must plan to use a component size that allows for at least 2 to 3 mm of cement mantle around the entire prosthesis. If the patient has a large osteopenic canal, up to three or four packs of cement may be needed to adequately fill and pressurize the canal with cement. Especially for the case of previous sepsis and cases with a higher risk of infection (i.e., diabetes mellitus, rheumatoid arthritis, and patients on chronic steroid therapy), antibiotic-impregnated cement should be available and utilized.

SURGICAL TECHNIQUE

Any surgical approach can be used to insert a femoral component with cement. As with all total hip arthroplasty procedures, adequate exposure must be obtained for the surgeon to be able to adequately prepare the femoral canal, introduce the cement with a cement gun delivery system, and introduce and seat the femoral component without the introduction of blood and debris around the component and without excessive toggle of the component.

After the hip is exposed and the femoral neck osteotomy has been performed (Fig. 1) at the level determined to provide appropriate leg length at the time of preoperative planning, the femoral canal is prepared. Use a box-cutting chisel to resect the lateral femoral neck bone, as well as the bone in the greater trochanter. This allows neutral placement of the stem and adequate lateral cement mantles (Fig. 2). Alternatively, a high-speed burr can be used to take out this bone. Use a canal-finding reamer to open the femoral canal and to direct future broaching (Fig. 3). Remember to direct this reamer and subsequent broaching from superolateral to inferomedial to avoid varus positioning of the component.

Although in the mid-1980s some surgeons used reamers to prepare the femoral canal, it was found that removal of bone to the cortex did not allow adequate cement penetration into the reamed bone. Hence, use only broaches to prepare the femoral canal. Start with a broach that is smaller than the size for the prosthesis that has been preoperatively templated (Fig. 4). Progress to the broach that fills the femoral canal (Fig. 5). Always err on the side of caution by using a smaller broach rather than a large one that may become incarcerated in the canal or fracture the femur. Remember, the goal is to place a component with a 2- to 3-mm circumferential cement mantle around it.

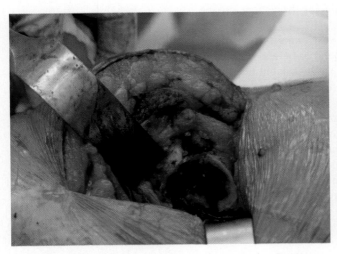

Figure 1. Femoral exposure after femoral neck osteotomy to allow femoral canal preparation.

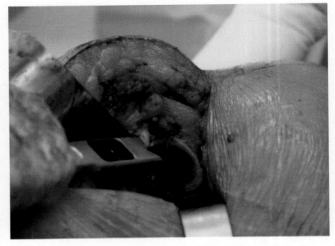

Figure 2. Box chisel used to resect lateral femoral neck and medial greater trochanteric bone.

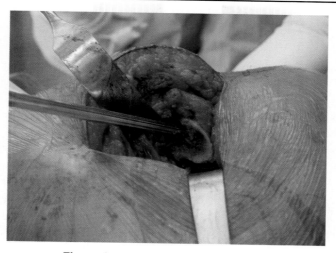

Figure 3. Use of canal-finding reamer.

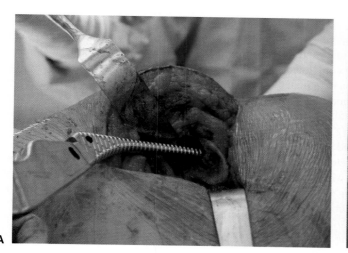

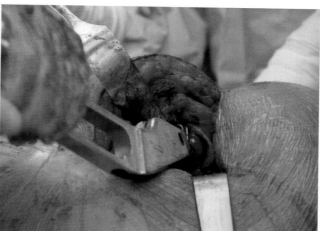

A

B

Figure 4. Use of small broach for initial canal preparation.

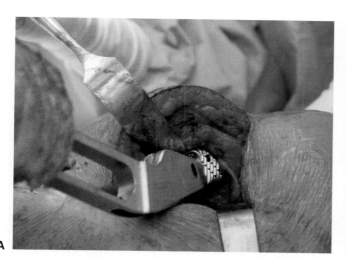

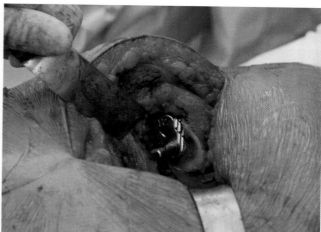

A

B

Figure 5. Use of optimally sized broach for final implant.

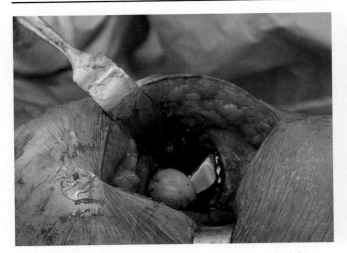

Figure 6. Placement of appropriate femoral head trial to determine leg length and hip stability.

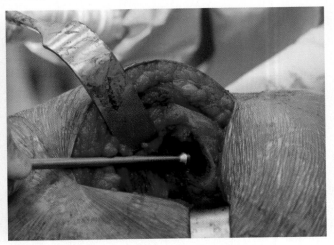

Figure 7. Final canal preparation with remaining 2 or 3 mm of firm cancellous bone.

Usually, the broach is anteverted in 15 degrees of anteversion, but when a cemented stem is used, this can easily be modified to a position that provides optimal stability in combination with the acetabular component. Use the broach and trial component to check leg length and stability (Fig. 6). (We match the distance from the center of the femoral head to the top of the lesser trochanter before our femoral neck osteotomy, using the appropriate modular head length to obtain this distance.) On trial reduction, we try to maintain hip stability in full extension with external rotation to 45 degrees and flexion to 100 degrees, with adduction to 20 degrees and internal rotation to 60 degrees.

Anterior femoral neck osteophytes should be resected to avoid anterior impingement on the acetabular component, which can lead to posterior instability. Remove loose cancellous bone in the proximal femur with a curette, leaving only the strong cancellous bone, which is within 2 to 3 mm of the cortex (Fig. 7). Remove loose distal canal cancellous bone with a stiff brush (Fig. 8).

Place a cement restricting plug 1 to 2 cm distal to the end of the prosthesis and any centralizer (Fig. 9). Use a restrictor large enough to fit into the canal and to avoid plug dislodgement during cement introduction. If the distal canal is larger than 25 mm, we use a cement plug. Clean the femoral canal with jet lavage and pack the canal with an epinephrine-soaked sponge (Figs. 10 and 11).

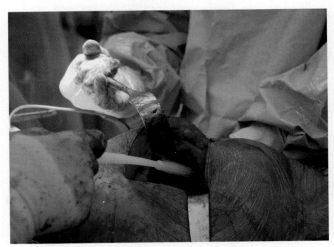

Figure 8. Use of brush to remove loose distal cancellous bone.

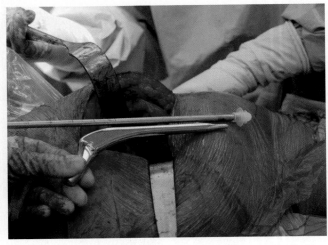

Figure 9. Determination of distance from the prosthetic tip to seat the distal cement plug.

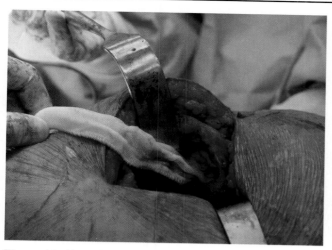

Figure 10. Use of epinephrine-soaked sponge to provide hemostasis in the femoral canal.

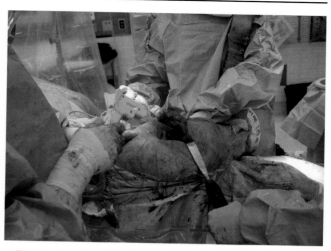

Figure 11. Use of jet lavage to clean the femoral canal.

Use vacuum mixing or centrifugation for porosity reduction and introduce the cement in a doughy state (Fig. 12). Pressurize the cement with a thumb or proximal seal. Introduce the stem in a neutral (valgus–varus) position and at 15 degrees of anteversion when the cement is in the middle to late doughy stage (Fig. 13). Be sure to have the assistant who is holding the leg apply counter-resistance. We impact the modular head before stem introduction, but if one is concerned about stability, it can be done after cement curing so that trial reduction can be performed. Either way, place the femoral head on a clean taper (Fig. 14) and close the wound.

POSTOPERATIVE MANAGEMENT AND REHABILITATION

Patients begin full weight-bearing walking with crutches and advance to a cane when it is tolerated. They perform muscle-strengthening exercises with the hip and lower extremity. They leave the hospital when they can independently transfer themselves into and out of bed, go to and from the bathroom, negotiate stairs, and understand hip dislocation precautions.

Most patients can perform their exercises and walk at home without the aid of a therapist. By 2 to 3 months, they are usually walking without aids and without a limp unless they have other musculoskeletal problems.

A
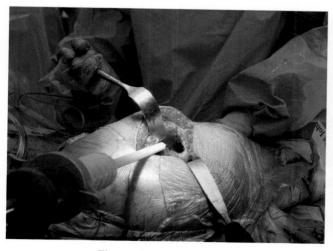

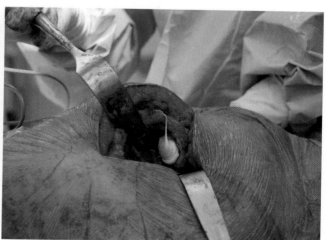
B

Figure 12. Introduction of cement in the doughy phase.

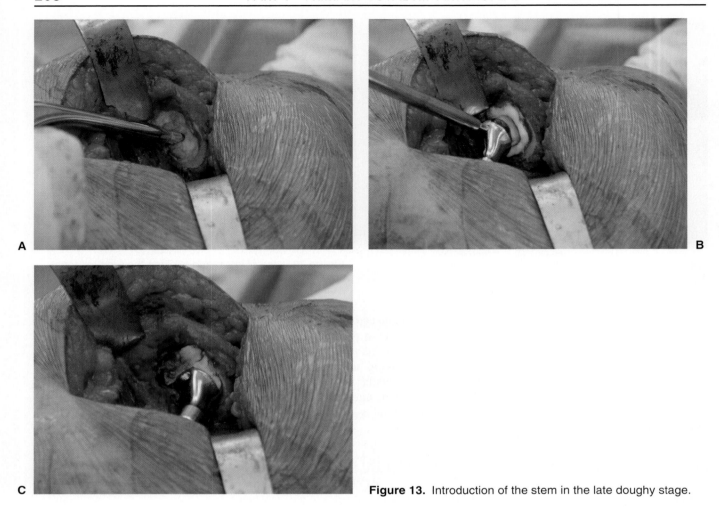

Figure 13. Introduction of the stem in the late doughy stage.

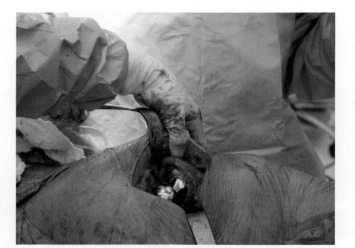

Figure 14. Application of the femoral head on a clean trunnion.

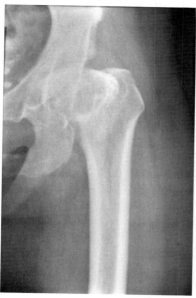
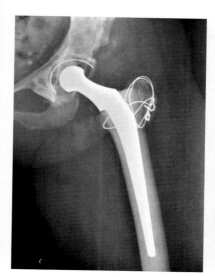
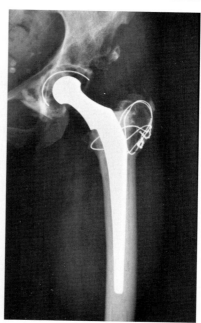

A,B

C

Figure 15. Preoperative **(A)**, postoperative **(B)**, and 25-year follow-up **(C)** using a Charnley femoral component, a distal plug, and cement delivery gun cementing technique.

RESULTS

Our results with polished cemented femoral components have demonstrated excellent durability, with less than 5% revision of the femoral component for loosening in 20- to 30-year follow-up studies (Fig. 15). Results have been durable in younger patients, but most of these patients were in their late thirties or forties. Although most surgeons who use cemented femoral stems in young patients prefer stems with a polished surface finish, the optimal surface finish of the component remains somewhat controversial.

COMPLICATIONS

The complications specifically related to cemented femoral stems include femoral fracture resulting from too large a broach or too large and stiff a cement restrictor, inadequate cement mantles and bone-cement radiolucencies resulting from aggressive reaming of the femoral canal, too little cement or inadequate pressurization of the cement, and insertion of the component before the cement is allowed to reach the doughy phase. The final complication is the inability to seat the prosthesis because the cement has hardened during the time the surgeon has been introducing the prosthesis into the femoral canal.

RECOMMENDED READING

1. Callaghan JJ, Templeton JE, Liu SS, et al. Results of Charnley total hip arthroplasty at a minimum of thirty years. *J Bone Joint Surg Am* 86-A(4):690–695, 2004.
2. Collis DK, Mohler CG. Comparison of clinical outcomes in total hip arthroplasty using rough and polished cemented stems with essentially the same geometry. *J Bone Joint Surg Am* 84-A(4):586–592, 2002.
3. Crowninshield RD, Jennings JD, Laurent ML, Maloney WJ. Cemented femoral component surface finish mechanics. *Clin Orthop Relat Res* Oct(355):90–102, 1998.
4. Klapach AS, Callaghan JJ, Goetz DD, et al. Charnley total hip arthroplasty with use of improved cementing techniques: a minimum twenty-year follow-up study. *J Bone Joint Surg Am* 83-A(12):1840–1848, 2001.
5. Keener JD, Callaghan JJ, Goetz DD, et al. Twenty-five-year results after Charnley total hip arthroplasty in patients less than fifty years old. *J Bone Joint Surg Am* 85-A(6):1066–1072, 2003.

15

Extensively Porous Coated Femoral Components

Andrew H. Glassman

Extensively porous coated stems are defined as those in which the ingrowth surface extends into the femoral isthmus. The first such stem approved for use without cement in the United States was the anatomic medullary locking (AML) prosthesis (see Fig. 1). The clinical and radiographic results using this stem were characterized in a number of seminal studies conducted by its chief proponent, Charles A. Engh, MD, and coworkers (1–4). The immeasurable value of this body of work is in large part attributable to the implantation of the same basic stem design in a large series of consecutive patients, regardless of age, gender, diagnosis, or bone quality. As a consequence of these works, extensively porous coated stems are the most thoroughly studied and longest followed cementless stems still currently in widespread use. Moreover, the studies alluded to have provided valuable insight into the biology of cementless stems in general, including the requirements for bone ingrowth (1,2), the radiographic features of cementless stem fixation (2,3,5), and the patterns of adaptive remodeling of bone following cementless stem implantation (2,3,5,6). Understandably, the common perception of an extensively porous coated implant is that of a straight, distally cylindrical monobloc design, fabricated of cobalt chromium alloy coated with two to three layers of sintered cobalt beads. In actuality, contemporary extensively porous coated stems comprise a significantly more diverse variety of designs—including both modular and monobloc stems fabricated of cobalt chromium, titanium, or even composites—and have a variety of different surface treatments, including sintered beads, plasma spray, titanium fiber metal, corundumization, or calcium-phosphate bioceramics (see Fig. 2).

INDICATIONS/CONTRAINDICATIONS

Extensively porous coated femoral components can be used in most primary cases and with excellent outcomes in terms of fixation and clinical results (2–4). Currently, other designs of cemented or cementless implants are often preferred in primary interventions because of the perceived drawbacks of extensively porous coated stems, namely stress shielding and the difficulty of their removal (2,6–10). In the author's view, there are

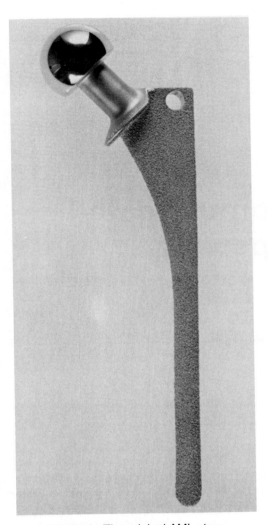

Figure 1. The original AML stem.

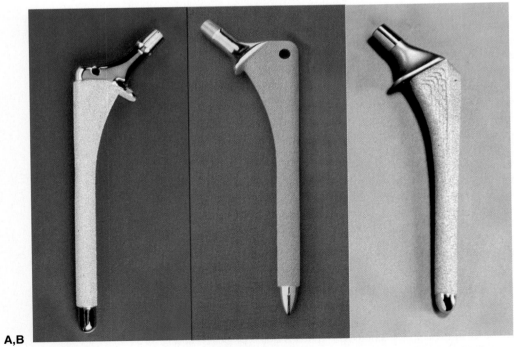

Figure 2. Various contemporary designs of extensively porous coated stems. **A,B:** Cast cobalt chromium stems with porous surfaces of sintered beads. **C:** Cast cobalt chromium stem with a plasma-sprayed porous surface.

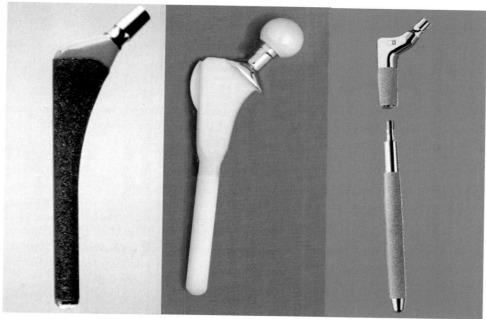

D,E   **F**

Figure 2. *(continued)* **D:** The Epoch composite stem. **E:** An extensively hydroxyapatite-coated stem. **F:** An extensively coated modular titanium stem.

several situations in which an extensively porous coated stem is preferable to other designs (see Table 1).

PREOPERATIVE PLANNING

A minimum of three high-quality radiographic views is required for proper templating and planning of the actual surgical procedure. These include an anteroposterior (AP) view of the entire pelvis with the beam centered on the symphysis pubis, a long AP view of the involved femur, and a Lauenstein lateral projection of the femur. The latter two films should include the hip joint and extend distally to the isthmus. Several technical details are important. Specific measures are taken to minimize and control for magnification. The tube-film distance should be a known constant. A general estimate of the magnification can be obtained using several techniques. A marker with two points separated by a known dis-

Table 1. *Indications for the Use of Extensively Porous Coated Stems in Primary Total Hip Replacement*

Indication*
1. To restore hip biomechanics
2. Champagne flute canal
3. DDH
4. Prior surgery
a. With bone deficit
i. Traumatic bone loss
ii. Defect from removal of internal fixation devices
b. Deformity
i. Prior osteotomy
ii. Malunion
5. MIS: two-incision
6. Osteoporosis (stovepipe canal)

*DDH, developmental dysplasia of the hip; MIS, minimally invasive surgery.

tance can be taped to the thigh at the level of the femur. The distance between the markers is then measured on the radiograph, and the magnification factor is calculated using the following formula:

$$\frac{(\text{measured distance} - \text{actual distance})}{\text{actual distance}} \times 100 = \% \text{ magnification}$$

This percentage can be used as a guide in selecting the appropriately magnified templates for most average-sized patients, bearing in mind that the magnification error will vary among individuals depending upon their soft tissue mass. For extremely thin or obese patients, a radiographic marker should always be used.

Because the femur is normally held in slight external rotation, the lower extremity should be internally rotated 15 to 20 degrees when the AP view of the femur is obtained (see Fig. 3). Osteoarthritis and various other conditions frequently cause a fixed external rotation contracture of the hip, and a standard AP roentgenogram will underestimate the medial to lateral dimension of the metaphysis. Therefore, a posteroanterior view of the femur is obtained by first placing the patient prone and then elevating the normal side of the pelvis to an angle equivalent to the contracture (see Fig. 4). This internally rotates the affected thigh and places the coronal plane of the femur parallel to that of the film cassette.

In most cases, leg length discrepancy can be measured radiographically by comparing the distances between the superior aspects of the lesser trochanters and a line drawn across the ischial tuberosities or the radiographic teardrops. If the physical examination suggests fixed pelvic obliquity, standing roentgenograms of the lumbosacral spine are obtained, including bending films. When planning total hip replacement (THR) for posttraumatic arthritis following acetabular fractures, bony deficiencies, or malunions, nonunions about the acetabulum should be identified with internal and external pelvic oblique (Judet) views, plain tomography, or computed tomographic scanning.

The goals of templating for cementless total hip arthroplasty are twofold: selecting the appropriate-sized components to ensure initial implant stability (intraosseous considerations) and planning the placement of the implants so as to reestablish proper hip mechanics (extraosseous considerations).

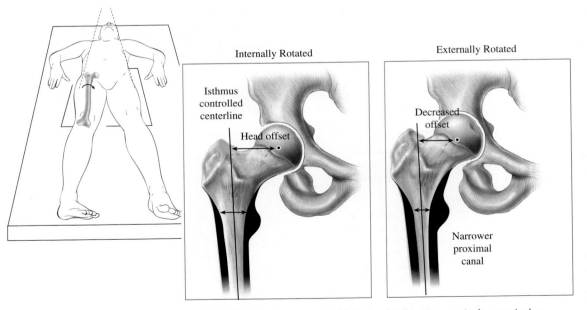

Figure 3. Internally rotating the femur allows one to obtain a true anterior-posterior projection of the proximal femur. (After Glassman AH. Preoperative planning for primary total hip arthroplasty. *Oper Tech Orthop* 5:296–305, 1995.)

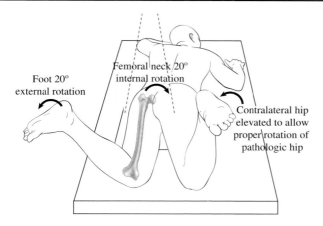

Figure 4. In the presence of a fixed external rotation contracture, a posterior-anterior view of the femur is obtained with the contralateral aspect of the pelvis elevated to a degree equal to the contracture. (After Glassman AH. Preoperative planning for primary total hip arthroplasty. *Oper Tech Orthop* 5:296–305, 1995.)

Templating is begun on the acetabular side, using the AP pelvic roentgenogram. This establishes the center of rotation of the prosthetic joint. The center of the prosthetic acetabular component should mirror that of the contralateral hip, assuming that it is normal. The center of the contralateral, normal hip is located using a series of concentric circles. A coordinate system is then established using a horizontal line through either the teardrops or across the bottom of the ischial tuberosities. Vertical axes are established bilaterally, usually through the teardrops. The coordinates of the center of the normal joint are then transposed to the diseased side, as a guide to the ideal position of the prosthetic acetabular component. Templating of the diseased acetabulum is then performed. The template is positioned to approximate the subchondral plate superiorly and the lateral aspect of the teardrop inferomedially. Ideally, it should be inclined 40 to 50 degrees from the horizontal, as referenced from the interteardrop line, and it should be completely contained within the acetabular cavity. The center of the templated acetabular component is marked, and any deviation of that mark from the transposed location of the normal acetabular center is noted, as compensation for the discrepancy may be made on the femoral side. The templated size of the acetabular component actually defines a range of potential sizes that may be required. Patient malposition on the x-ray table, magnification errors, and variability in bone quality may dictate the need for a component one or two sizes larger or smaller than that templated.

In cases of acetabular dysplasia, several choices exist. In mild cases, the socket may be adequately contained in the anatomic position with some lack of superolateral coverage. Coverage may be improved by deliberate medialization of the component. In more severe cases in which a false acetabulum is present, the cup can be placed in the high position, 1 to 2 cm above the anatomic position without undue compromise of hip biomechanics, as long as the component is not lateralized. In more severe cases, this may not be possible, and one can then plan femoral head autografting or even distal femoral allografting of the defect, with placement of the prosthetic component in the anatomic position. It is sometimes impossible to know which of the above options is optimal until the time of surgery. Acetabular arthroplasty for developmental dysplasia therefore requires the availability of a much broader than usual range of implant sizes.

On the femoral side, provisional templating for intraosseous fit is begun on the AP roentgenogram of the femur. The longitudinal axis of the component is aligned with that of the femur. The template is then lowered to the estimated level of the femoral neck resection, which is generally about 1 cm above the superior border of the lesser trochanter. Fit is then critically assessed. When templating for the distal dimension of an extensively porous coated stem, one should select a size that will provide for contact in the isthmus both medially and laterally over a distance of 4 to 5 cm. Because significant disproportion may exist between the dimensions of the metaphysis and the isthmus, it may be difficult to simultaneously achieve ideal component fit and fill in both areas. Most contemporary extensively porous coated stems are now available with multiple proximal sizes for each distal diameter of stem to reconcile such discrepancies. Nonetheless, when templating reveals extreme mismatches, one may anticipate the need to adjust one's surgical technique to optimize stem fit. For example, in the case of a "champagne flute" femur, one may need to ream the isthmus aggressively and use the largest metaphyseal size available for a relatively small distal stem diameter. One should avoid implanting an extensively porous coated stem that is press fitted distally and grossly undersized proximally. Distally ingrown stems lacking proximal support—in particular, ones smaller than 13.5 mm—are susceptible to late fatigue fracture from cantilever bending (6,10). Conversely, in the case of a "stovepipe" femoral canal, the metaphysis may need to be sculpted with a burr to accommodate the smallest metaphyseal size available for a large-distal-diameter stem.

Once satisfied with the size and orientation of the AP template, its proximal-distal position is marked in reference to an anatomic landmark such as the tip of the greater trochanter. That position is then transferred to the lateral femoral radiograph, and lateral templating is begun. Straight-stemmed implants generally achieve point contact with the femoral endosteum at predictable points on the lateral x-ray. These include the posterior femoral neck, the anterior cortex just below the lesser trochanter, and the posterior cortex at midstem (see Fig. 5). In short-stature patients or those with an exaggerated anterior femoral bow, a fourth point of contact may occur between the stem tip and the anterior femoral cortex. Anterior cortical impingement or perforation should be avoided. If templating suggests that this may be a risk, then one has several choices, including the use of a different stem or attempting to rotate the stem (proximal stem anterior, distal tip posterior) by biasing the pilot hole used for reaming anteriorly and milling the posterior femoral cortex at midstem with a high-speed burr.

Once the component sizes have been determined in terms of intraosseous fit, the surgeon should focus upon reestablishing appropriate leg length, offset, and component version, in other words, the extraosseous relationships. These are important determinants of hip mechanics, together influencing abductor function and, therefore, gait, stability against dislocation, joint reactive force, and implant loading. In most instances, the position of the prosthetic acetabular component is dictated by the individual patient's anatomy. It is on the femoral side of the arthroplasty that the surgeon has the most latitude in adjusting extraosseous relationships. Thankfully, many contemporary systems of cementless implants offer a choice of different extraosseous designs for any given implant size, including extended offset and low-head-center options. These allow one to optimize the stem selection on the basis of both intraosseous and extraosseous considerations without compromising either. With any given implant, one can further adjust extraosseous relations by altering the level of neck resection, the level of implant seating, and the choice of head and neck length. Such alterations will, however, to some extent influence the intraosseous fit of the femoral

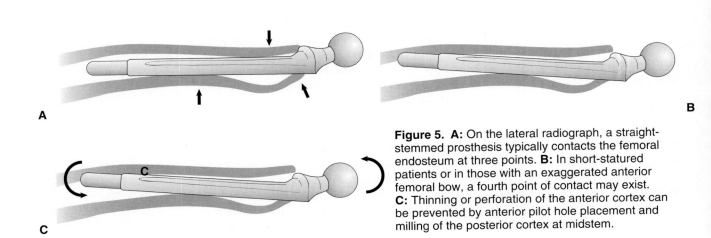

A

B

C

Figure 5. A: On the lateral radiograph, a straight-stemmed prosthesis typically contacts the femoral endosteum at three points. **B:** In short-statured patients or in those with an exaggerated anterior femoral bow, a fourth point of contact may exist. **C:** Thinning or perforation of the anterior cortex can be prevented by anterior pilot hole placement and milling of the posterior cortex at midstem.

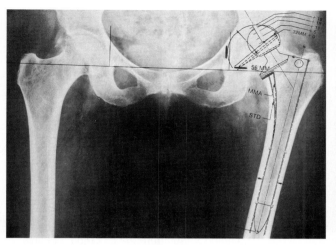
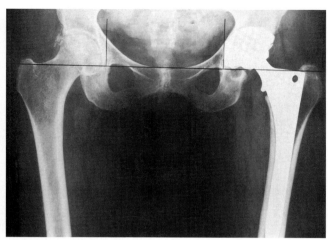

Figure 6. A: Preoperative film showing superior and cephalad migration of the femoral head in osteoarthritis with templating of the acetabular and femoral head centers. **B:** Postoperative film showing an increase in leg length and a decrease in offset corresponding to the vertical and horizontal distances between the templated head centers.

component. Specifically, a higher neck resection may dictate the need for a larger metaphyseal segment. Conversely, a low neck resection may require the use of a smaller metaphyseal segment.

The recommended sequence for templating to optimize extraosseous relationships is as follows. After the appropriate femoral implant is selected during intraosseous templating, the level of neck resection for that implant is marked, as is the planned center of the prosthetic femoral head. If the disease process has resulted in distortion of anatomic relationships, this center of the femoral head will not correspond with the center of the templated acetabular component. Assuming that the acetabular component is placed at the normal anatomic hip center, the effect of a particular femoral component size and position on leg length and offset can be assessed by measuring the vertical and horizontal distances between the templated component centers. For example, in a typical case of osteoarthritis, the femoral head center may be displaced cephalad and laterally with resultant limb shortening and increased offset. After appropriate templating, the center of the prosthetic femoral head will occupy a position cephalad and lateral to the center of the prosthetic acetabulum. After reduction of the hip, the leg will be lengthened by an amount equal to the vertical distance between the templated head centers, and the offset will be reduced by an amount equal to the horizontal distance (see Fig. 6). The amount of leg lengthening predicted by this technique must be compared with the preoperative leg length discrepancy measured clinically and radiographically.

The discussion thus far has assumed that the acetabular component can be placed at or near the anatomic position. Distortions of acetabular anatomy in cases of posttraumatic arthritis, tumor reconstruction, and developmental dysplasia may render this impossible. Recreating the proper relationship of the femur to the pelvis is then accomplished as follows: The acetabular component is placed at the abnormal location as dictated by the anatomy, and this position is measured using the coordinate system. This nonanatomic center is then transposed onto the normal side (see Fig. 7). The femur on the normal side is then templated to optimize fit and fill, while placing the center of the prosthetic femoral head as near as possible to the mark for the transposed acetabular center. The level of the femoral neck resection is marked, and the required head-neck length is noted. Implantation of the templated femoral component at that level on the diseased side, combined with the appropriate length head-neck segment, will restore the normal spatial relationship of the femur to the pelvis despite the nonanatomic location of the acetabular component (1).

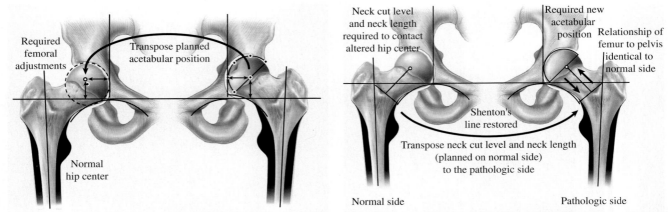

A

B

Figure 7. The Engh technique for templating in the face of a markedly abnormal acetabulum. **A:** The abnormal (left) acetabulum is templated for the appropriate component size and position as dictated by the disease-altered anatomy. The coordinates of the planned cup center are transposed onto the normal (right) side. **B:** The right femur is then templated to determine the stem size and neck length necessary to place the prosthetic femoral head center exactly at the transposed acetabular component center. The required level of neck resection is marked. The neck resection level marked on the right is transposed to the abnormal left femur. Placement of the templated femoral component at this level will restore the normal spatial relationship between the pelvis and the femur. (After Engh CA. Recent advances in cementless total hip arthroplasty using the AML prosthesis. *Tech Orthop* 6:59–72, 1991.)

Anteversion is an important determinant of range of motion, stability against dislocation, and torsional loading of the femoral component. Anteversion is assessed preoperatively on the lateral radiograph by measuring the angle between the axes of the femoral neck and shaft (see Fig. 8). Normally, it ranges between 10 and 20 degrees. Extreme deviation must be noted. Excessive anteversion is far more common than relative retroversion, the classic example being developmental dysplasia, where anteversion may exceed 45 degrees. There are five basic designs of extensively porous coated stems currently available with regard to anteversion. The first type is axisymmetric: no anteversion, in which the same stem can be used for either a left or a right femur, and the neck axis is in the same plane as the remaining implant. These implants allow for some intraoperative adjustment of anteversion by adjusting the orientation of proximal femoral broaching and sometimes using an implant with a smaller metaphyseal segment. The second type of implant is axisymmetric and anteverted. The body of these stems is identical for both right and left stems, but the neck is anteverted. A left stem can be implanted into a right femur to reduce the inherent anteversion.

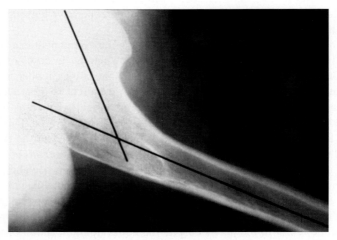

Figure 8. Femoral anteversion is assessed on a true lateral femoral radiograph.

The third type of stem is nonaxisymmetric (anatomic) and anteverted. The geometry of such stems closely approximates that of the proximal femur, and most such stems actually have antetorsion of their metaphyseal portion, in addition to anteversion of the neck. Such stems are available as dedicated right and left implants: A left stem cannot be implanted into a right femur and vice versa. Because of their complex geometry and having greater metaphyseal filling than the other designs mentioned, there is limited ability to adjust the anteversion dictated by the patient's anatomy. The fourth stem type is the modular design, which has adjustable anteversion. The fifth and final category is that of custom stems, which can be fabricated with whatever degree of anteversion that is desired. Each of these designs has different capabilities in terms of ability to adjust anteversion. This should be borne in mind when selecting the optimum stem.

SURGERY

Standard Technique for Routine Primary Total Hip Replacement

For routine primary total hip arthroplasty, extensively porous coated femoral components can be implanted using virtually any standard surgical approach. Special circumstances (developmental dysplasia, prior trauma, retained hardware, etc.) may require alternative, more extensile approaches. Various aspects of the techniques to be described will vary, depending upon the particular design of extensively porous coated stem to be utilized, and the reader is encouraged to carefully study the surgical technique recommended by the stem's manufacturer. Certain principles to be presented have general applicability regardless of the implant design utilized. Femoral preparation is composed of two major steps: reaming of the femoral isthmus and broaching or otherwise machining the metaphysis (1).

Reaming. Achieving initial mechanical implant stability is a fundamental requirement for successful bone ingrowth fixation of cementless components (2). For straight-stemmed extensively porous coated femoral components, immediate axial and rotational stability requires 4 to 5 cm of press fit in the femoral isthmus. This is accomplished by incremental reaming with appropriately designed, fully fluted, rigid reamers in serial fashion, followed by impaction of a stem that is slightly oversized in relation to the prepared isthmus.

Most contemporary extensively porous coated stems designed for primary THR have a straight stem distally. Accurate reaming for such stems is facilitated by first creating a pilot hole. Optimum pilot hole location generally corresponds to the insertion site of the piriformis tendon within the trochanteric fossa. The pilot hole can be created with either a reamer specifically designed for that purpose or a high-speed burr (see Fig. 9). Pilot hole placement can be checked by passing either a tapered "canal finder" or the smallest avail-

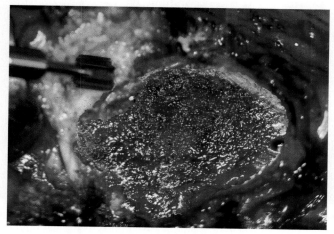

Figure 9. The pilot hole is created in the piriformis fossa using a high-speed burr or specially designed reamer.

able cylindrical reamer down the intramedullary canal by hand (see Fig. 10). The reamer should pass easily and should remain centered within the pilot hole without abutting its walls (see Fig. 11). The position of the reamer should be dictated by its fit within the femoral isthmus. Eccentric pilot hole placement can bias subsequent reaming into varus, valgus, or anterior or posterior malalignment. If the smallest reamer cannot be passed a depth corresponding to the length of the implant for which the case has been templated, one must suspect an error in pilot hole placement or an unrecognized deformity of the femur. The pilot hole should be cautiously enlarged, and the reamer should be reoriented. If it still cannot be passed to the appropriate depth, intraoperative anterior-posterior and lateral radiographs are obtained. After successful passage of the initial reamer, serial hand reaming proceeds in 1-mm increments. One should be able to continue hand reaming to the appropriate depth with progressively larger reamers to within 2 mm of the templated stem diameter. If one is deliberately expanding the isthmus, as one might in a case with a pronounced "champagne flute" canal or femoral stenosis, hand reaming may only be possible to within 3 or 4 mm of the templated stem diameter. Upon completion of hand reaming, one then proceeds with power reaming in 0.5-mm increments. Copious irrigation during power reaming speeds the process through fluid lubrication and the flushing away of reaming debris. As an added benefit, the cooling effect helps to minimize thermal necrosis of bone.

It is critical to obtain the appropriate tolerance between the final reamer and the distal, cylindrical portion of an extensively porous coated stem. One must achieve an adequate press fit to assure initial stability without incurring femoral fracture. This requires familiarity with the implant and the instrumentation. Manufacturers commonly recommend underreaming of the isthmus by 0.5 mm relative to the stem size. Femoral implant size most commonly refers to the stem diameter in its distal, cylindrical portion. However, the true dimension of the stem can vary from its nominal size. A "15-mm" stem may in actuality be 14.9 or 15.1 mm, depending on the manufacturer. Likewise, the true size of a cylindrical reamer may differ from its stated size. Frequent sharpening of the reamers eventually results in diminution of their size. This is most likely when well-used "loaner" instrument sets are utilized. The variability in sizing of implants and reamers may be additive and predispose to fracture unless specific precautions are taken. As an example, the surgeon templates for a size 15-mm stem and, in accordance with the manufacturer's recommendation, elects to underream the femoral canal by 0.5 mm (to 14.5 mm). If the reamer is

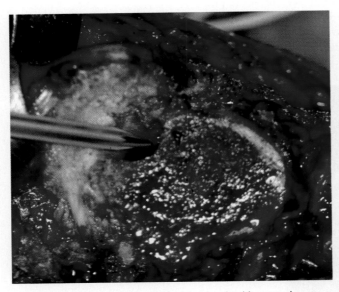

Figure 10. Pilot hole placement is checked by passing an awl or starter reamer down the intramedullary canal.

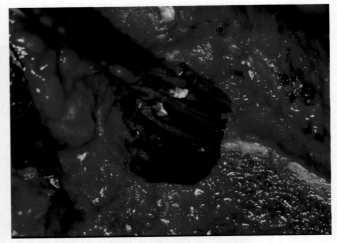

Figure 11. The reamer should remain centered in the pilot hole as it enters the isthmus. Here, the reamer abuts the posterior edge of the pilot hole, indicating the need to enlarge the pilot hole in that direction.

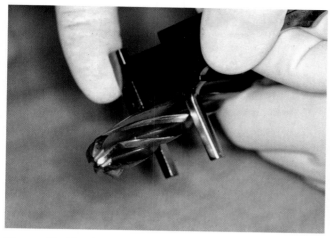
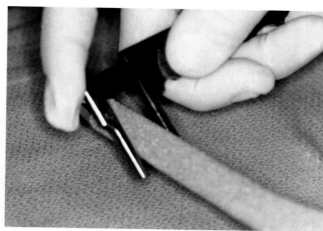

Figure 12. Vernier calipers are used to measure the reamer **(A)** and stem **(B)**.

actually 14.4 mm and the stem is 15.1 mm, a press fit of 0.7 mm is created, and fracture is possible. As such, it is recommended that the final reamer and the actual femoral implant be measured either with Vernier calipers, a dial micrometer, or hole gauges (see Fig. 12).

After reaming is completed, metaphyseal broaching is performed to accommodate the implant's proximal geometry. It is recommended that one begin with a broach two to three sizes smaller than the size corresponding to the last reamer used. To help reconcile mismatches in proximal-distal geometry, most currently available stems are available with at least two metaphyseal sizes for each distal stem diameter. These vary only in their medial-to-lateral dimension. Broaching is begun with the smallest-metaphyseal-sized broaches and continues up to the size corresponding to the distal reaming. If considerable metaphyseal bone then remains medial to the broach, one can consider repeating the broaching process with the larger metaphyseal broaches. Before making this decision, it is strongly recommended that one first perform a trial reduction with the smaller metaphyseal broach in place to ensure that it is seated at the appropriate level. If a high initial neck cut was made, the smaller broach may reside more proximally than ideal, in the broader portion of the metaphysis, lending the impression that it is undersized. In this case, one will find that it is difficult or impossible to perform a trial reduction, even with the shortest neck length. Recutting the femoral neck and seating the broach more deeply may reveal that the smaller metaphyseal size is appropriate. At this juncture, one must also consider whether it might be preferable to deliberately seat the broach and hence the implant at a low position and use a longer neck length in order to increase femoral offset. On the other hand, one may find that the smallest-metaphyseal-sized broach cannot be adequately seated, even after removal of all proximal-medial cancellous bone. Broaches or rasps are ineffective and risk fracture if used in an attempt to remove endosteal cortical bone. In this situation, one must sculpt the proximal-medial endosteum with a high-speed burr in order to allow full broach seating (see Fig. 13).

Once the surgeon is satisfied with the size and depth of broach seating, a trial reduction is performed, and leg length, offset, and stability against dislocation are assessed. As stated, some implant systems offer a choice of neck configurations in terms of offset and/or neck shaft angle, and when using such systems, it is at this juncture that the most appropriate geometry is selected.

The extent of anterior-posterior metaphyseal filling varies among different designs of extensively porous coated stems (see Fig. 14). Some offer very little fill in this dimension and rely largely upon medial-to-lateral fill for proximal implant stability. These stems are more forgiving in terms of allowing the surgeon to implant the actual stem in slightly more or less anteversion than that achieved during broaching without incurring a fracture. Other stems fill the metaphysis in the anterior-posterior dimension and require that the stem be inserted in exactly the same orientation as the broach. When using these implant systems,

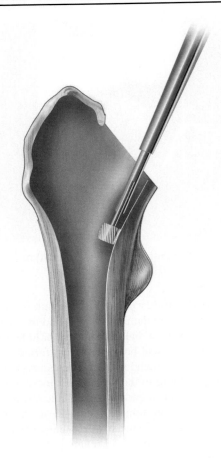

Figure 13. A high-speed burr should be used when removal of proximal-medial endosteal cortical bone is necessary.

the rotational alignment of the fully seated final broach should be carefully marked on the medial aspect of the femoral neck. Some broaches for metaphyseal filling stems feature a centerline scored on the medial aspect of the broach for this specific purpose (see Fig. 15).

Stem Impaction. The stem is first placed down the intramedullary canal in the appropriate rotational alignment as far as is possible by hand. Many stem designs have impaction handles or guides to control rotational alignment, while others do not. For the latter, either the surgeon or the assistant carefully controls stem anteversion, while the other impacts the stem. The stem will begin to achieve rotational stability as its distal cylindrical portion enters the isthmus. Stem rotation can be adjusted during initial impaction, guiding the proximal portion of the stem to match the prepared envelope of the femur and achieve the desired anteversion. Some manufacturers provide a rotational alignment guide that is affixed to the stem and has a stylus that is aligned to a centering mark on the cut femoral neck created with the broach in place (see Fig. 16).

The stem is impacted with repetitive blows of the mallet. The impaction force should be firm but not violent. The stem should be observed to advance within the femoral canal by 2 to 3 mm per blow. Using appropriate reaming tolerance and broach preparation, in combination with proper instrumentation, one should be able to achieve full implant seating with most contemporary designs of extensively porous coated stems. The impaction process provides visual, auditory, and tactile feedback as to when the stem will no longer advance without risk of fracture. Unfortunately, the ability to accurately interpret these signals is acquired only through experience with these stems. As maximum seating is approached, stem advancement visually slows to as little as 1 mm with each blow.

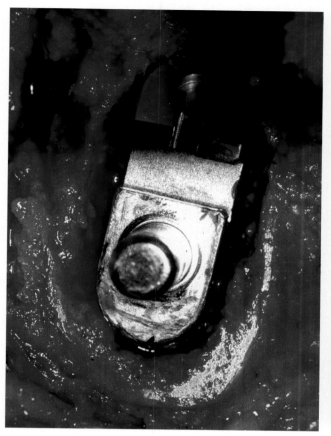
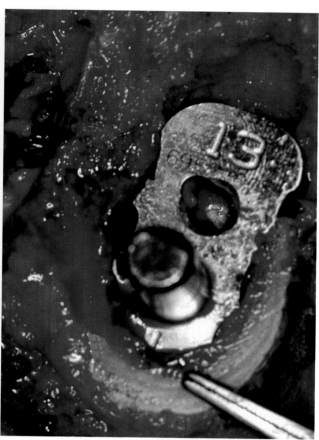

Figure 14. A: The broach corresponding to an extensively porous coated stem with flat anterior and posterior sides fills the metaphysis medially to laterally but leaves gaps anteriorly and posteriorly. **B:** The broach for a stem with divergent anterior and posterior sides results in greater metaphyseal filling.

Increasing resistance to impaction is felt. The sound produced changes from hollow to a sharper, higher-pitched tone. At this point, one should resist the temptation to increase the force of impaction. If progress is halted far short of complete seating (e.g., 4 cm or more), one should consider removing the stem, remeasuring both the reamer and the stem, and perhaps reaming line-to-line. Under no circumstances should one overream when preparing to implant a straight-stemmed extensively porous coated implant that depends upon a press fit in the isthmus for initial mechanical stability. If the stem system being used employs broaches that are undersized in their metaphyseal portion relative to the actual implant, countersinking the broach by 2 to 3 mm relative to the neck cut is considered. Despite these measures, the inability to completely seat an extensively porous coated stem can and does occur. For this reason, it is recommended that the femur be prepared in such a fashion that appropriate leg length, offset, and stability against dislocation can be achieved during trial reduction using a trial head at least one length longer than the shortest head available. If this is done and the actual stem cannot subsequently be fully seated, one can then resort to the use of a shorter head to compensate.

Extensively Porous Coated Stems for Restoration of Hip Biomechanics

Extensively porous coated stems achieve initial mechanical stability and subsequent biologic fixation in the isthmus as well as in the metaphysis and generally do not fill the metaphysis completely. As a result, these stems can be seated at various levels within the

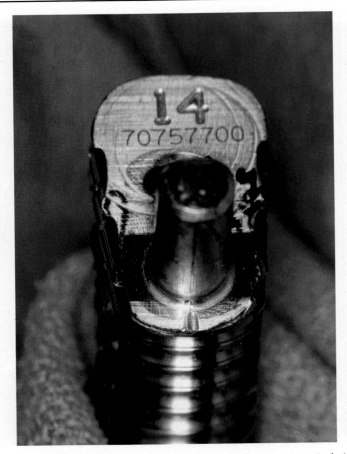

Figure 15. This broach for a metaphyseal filling extensively porous coated stem is scored along the medial centerline.

femur in order to adjust both leg length and offset, without compromising initial or late stability. For example, in cases of marked coxa vara, an extensively porous coated stem can be seated lower within the proximal femur and combined with a relatively long neck length in order to achieve the amount of offset required. Likewise, in cases of coxa valga, the neck can be resected at a higher level, and a shorter neck length is used (see Fig. 17).

Establishing correct leg length and offset requires careful preoperative templating and intraoperative measurement. *Femoral* offset and head height can be measured intraoperatively after dislocation and prior to the provisional neck resection. These values are then compared to the same measurements made with the trial femoral component and trial head in place. Exact reproduction of femoral head height and offset does not, however, assure restoration of overall offset and leg length because of variability in acetabular component placement. In cases with unusually large offset or extreme coxa valga, a measuring stylus can be affixed to the iliac wing and used to measure overall offset and leg length prior to dislocation and at the completion of the arthroplasty (see Fig. 18).

The preparation of the femur in these situations is substantially similar to the technique described above for routine arthroplasty. Seating of the femoral component deeper within the femoral canal in order to use a longer head and thereby enhance offset entails some special consideration. First, when using an implant system offering different metaphyseal sizes, the smallest size available is selected. After appropriate distal reaming, the broach corresponding to that implant is seated to the maximum depth. The neck resection is revised as needed, and a trial reduction is performed. If measurements indicate the need to further countersink the broach, bone should be removed from the medial neck and calcar area. Use of a rasp to remove hard endosteal bone in this area is ineffective and risks fracture. A high-speed burr should be used instead.

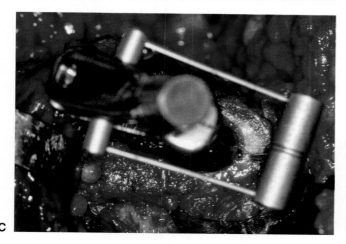

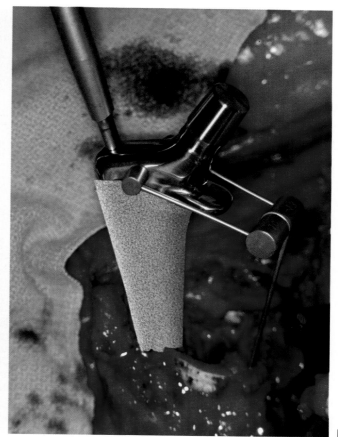

A

B

C

Figure 16. The technique for assuring proper rotational alignment of the stem. **A:** After seating the broach the cut surface of the medial femoral neck is scored to mark rotational alignment. **B:** A stylus is affixed to the stem. The femoral impactor is keyed into the stem and used to control rotation as the stem is advanced. **C:** The stylus is kept centered over the score mark made on the medial femoral neck.

Champagne Flute Canals and Femoral Stenosis

The femoral canal may present an exaggerated metaphyseal flare in combination with a very narrow isthmus. Extreme isthmic narrowing is termed femoral stenosis. It may be difficult if not impossible to reconcile extreme proximal-distal mismatch with standard monobloc proximally porous coated femoral components. A stem small enough to seat within the isthmus is generally undersized in the metaphysis, resulting in poor rotational stability and limited contact between the porous coated portion of the stem and the endosteum. While cemented fixation is an option, the distal canal may not be large enough to accommodate an adequate cement mantle. The remaining options include custom or modular implants, or an extensively porous coated stem (see Fig. 19).

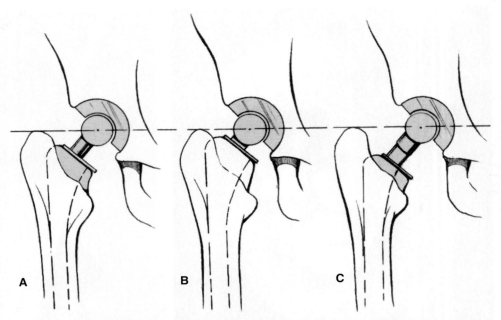

Figure 17. Offset can be adjusted without altering leg length by selection of the level of neck resection, the metaphyseal size of the prosthesis, and head length. **A:** Normal anatomy. A standard neck cut is combined with a standard-metaphyseal-sized implant and a standard length head. **B:** Coxa valga. A high neck resection is combined with a larger-metaphyseal-sized implant and a short neck length. **C:** Coxa vara. A low neck cut is combined with a smaller-metaphyseal-sized stem and a long neck length.

Preparation of such femora for the implantation of an extensively porous coated stem involves expansion of the intramedullary canal. Proportionally more endosteal cortical bone must be sacrificed than is customary. Thankfully, in the majority of these cases the cortices are thick and remain sufficiently strong even after aggressive reaming. Initially, it can be impossible to pass either a canal finder or the smallest rigid reamer down the intramedullary canal. Flexible intramedullary reamers with diameters as small as 5.0 mm are therefore used for initial reaming. Power reaming is required and proceeds in 0.5-mm increments. Copious irrigation is imperative. As of this writing, the smallest known

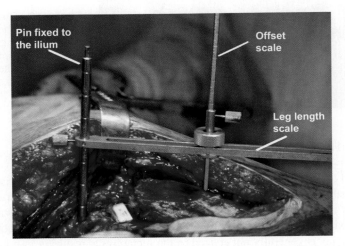

Figure 18. Offset/leg length gauge for complex cases requiring significant change in leg length and/or offset. The device is fixed to the ilium. The stylus is set to a reference point on the femur prior to dislocation. The leg length and offset can be read from the scales on the device. The gauge is then removed, leaving the pin fixed in the ilium. During trial reduction, the device is reapplied, and changes in both leg length and offset can be measured.

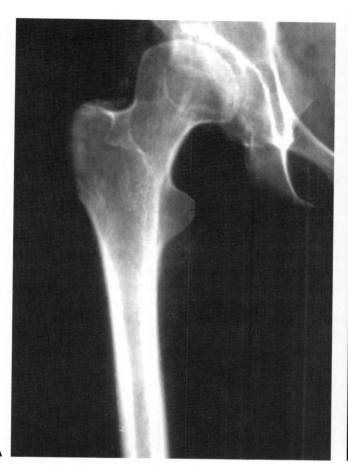
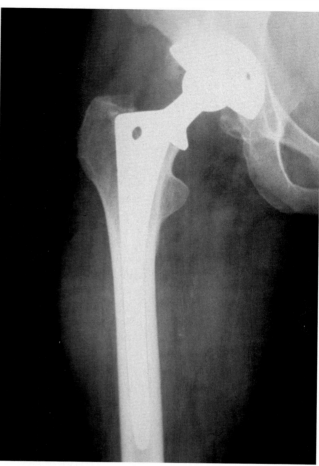

A   B

Figure 19. Champagne flute morphology and moderate femoral stenosis treated with an extensively porous coated stem. **A:** Preoperative film. **B:** Postoperative film.

standard size extensively porous coated stem is 9.0 mm in diameter. As such, flexible reaming is continued up to 8.0 mm. Further reaming is performed with rigid, fully fluted reamers, beginning at 8.5 mm, and is again continued in 0.5-mm increments. Because of proximal-distal disproportion, there is a tendency for the proximal aspect of the stem to be undersized relative to the metaphysis, and the largest proximal body size available should be used. If possible, the femoral isthmus should be reamed up to a size that will allow the implantation of a stem that provides some endosteal contact proximally and hence some metaphyseal support of the implant. Extensively coated stems that are "potted" distally, with no proximal support, are at risk of fatigue failure through cantilever bending (6,10). This is particularly so for smaller-diameter stems, which are often needed in these cases. If some proximal filling and therefore implant support cannot be achieved, an alternative stem design such as a modular or custom stem should be considered.

Developmental Dysplasia

The spectrum of anatomic defects possible in developmental dysplasia of the hip is well known (11). More severe cases, particularly Crowe type IV (11), are particularly challenging in that the femoral head is displaced proximally, while ideal socket placement is in the true acetabulum. The limb is usually considerably shortened, yet a femoral prosthesis placed at the anatomic level is often impossible to relocate into an acetabular component placed in the true acetabulum because of soft tissue contractures and the risk of stretch injury to surrounding neurovascular structures (11–13). In addition, there may be excessive femoral neck anteversion and metaphyseal antetorsion, as well as some degree of isthmic stenosis. An effective solution is a shortening, derotational, subtrochanteric osteotomy, as summarized in Figure 20. This procedure allows for correction of anteversion and relief of soft tissue tension. The challenges with this technique are establishing rotational stability of the stem within both the proximal, metaphyseal segment, and the (often narrow) distal, diaphyseal segment, while avoiding distraction at the osteotomy site. An extensively porous coated straight-stemmed prosthesis is particularly effective in meeting these challenges and, in effect, functions like an intramedullary rod (13).

The recommended surgical approach is posterolateral. The acetabulum may be prepared either before or following initial femoral preparation. Preliminary femoral preparation, including the initial subtrochanteric osteotomy, greatly facilitates exposure for complex acetabular reconstruction and will be described. After dislocation of the hip, the pilot hole is placed. Reaming and broaching are performed in routine fashion. The final broach is aligned over the femur (see Fig. 21). The vastus lateralis muscle is elevated from the anterior and lateral aspects of the femoral shaft and held there with a Bennett retractor. The osteotomy is planned at the level corresponding to the junction of the proximal metaphyseal and distal cylindrical portions of the broach (see Fig. 22). The osteotomy is performed with an oscillating saw and may be transverse, oblique, or step-cut, according to the surgeon's preference. A transverse osteotomy facilitates derotation of the femur to correct excessive anteversion but provides little inherent rotational stability. After completion of the osteotomy, the proximal segment can be retracted anteriorly and cephalad, affording the

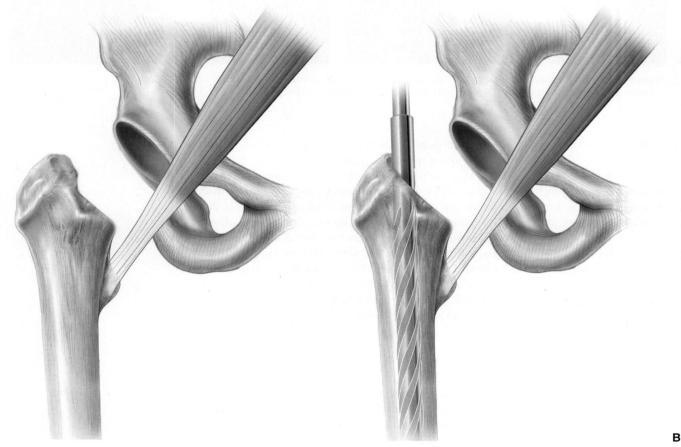

A

B

Figure 20. Steps in the management of developmental dysplasia with a shortening, derotational, subtrochanteric osteotomy. **A:** Neck resection. **B:** Reaming in standard fashion.

(continues)

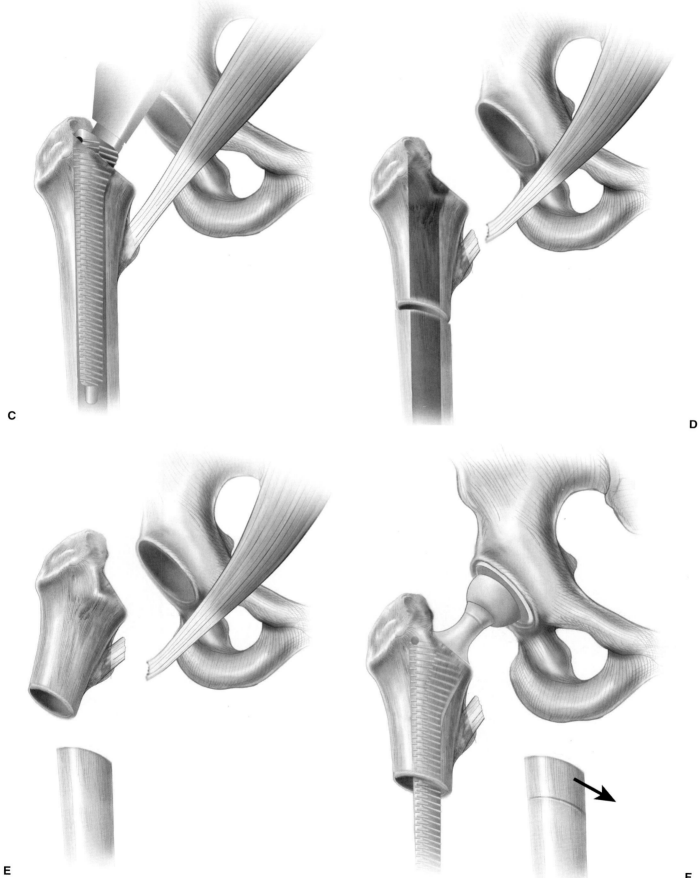

C

D

E

F

Figure 20. *(continued)* **C:** Broaching. **D:** Oblique subtrochanteric osteotomy and release of the iliopsoas tendon. **E:** Retraction of the proximal segment anteriorly and cephalad. **F:** A second, shortening osteotomy. *(continues)*

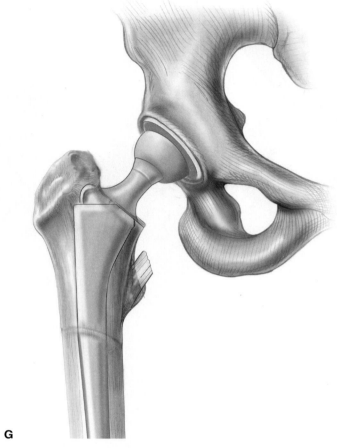

G

Figure 20. *(continued)* **G:** Stem implantation.

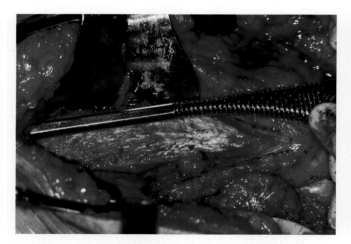

Figure 21. Locating the appropriate level for the initial osteotomy at the junction of the proximal, metaphyseal segment of the broach with the distal, cylindrical segment.

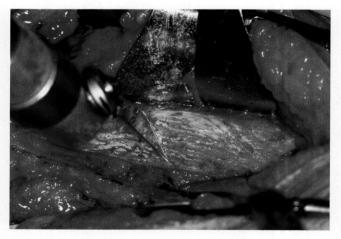

Figure 22. Creation of an oblique osteotomy with the oscillating saw.

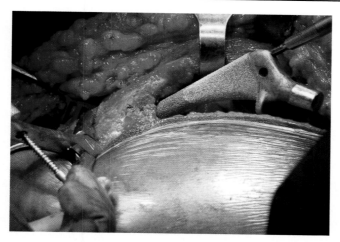

Figure 23. Impacting the stem while holding the osteotomy reduced with bone-holding forceps.

surgeon outstanding exposure of and access to the acetabulum. Mobilization of the proximal segment is enhanced by release of the iliopsoas tendon. Acetabular preparation and component implantation are performed. Structural allografting of the acetabulum may be required and is facilitated by the wide exposure provided by displacement of the proximal femur. The broach is then reinserted into the proximal but not the distal segment of the femur. A trial head is placed on the broach and reduced into the acetabulum. The distal segment of the femur is allowed to lie beside the proximal segment in "bayonet" fashion. Gentle longitudinal traction is applied to the leg. The point of overlap of the proximal and distal femur is marked on the distal fragment. A second osteotomy, parallel to the first, is performed at the level marked, thereby shortening the distal fragment. The osteotomy site is then reduced and provisionally held in place with bone-holding forceps. Derotation of the osteotomy to correct excessive anteversion is performed at this point. It is important to realize that after shortening the femur, the depth of reaming into the distal segment will be inadequate. Therefore, a critical technical point is that the shortened femur must be rereamed to the appropriate depth. After reaming, broaching is also repeated, and a trial reduction is performed. Leg length, offset, and stability are assessed. Final adjustments in anteversion are made. The osteotomy is held firmly reduced. Our preference is to use a six-hole dynamic compression plate temporarily affixed with plate-holding clamps. The trial components are removed, and the femoral component is impacted (see Fig. 23). Care is taken to avoid distraction at the osteotomy site. Axial counterpressure applied at the knee by an assistant is helpful in this regard. After stem impaction is complete, the stability of the osteotomy is assessed. One may choose to fix the osteotomy with plates or cerclage, although in general, we have not found this to be necessary (see Fig. 24).

Prior Surgery

The residua of prior, nonarthroplasty procedures about the hip such as internal fixation of fractures and corrective osteotomies include bone defects, angular deformities, proximal-distal axial misalignment, and retained hardware that must be removed, creating stress risers in the proximal femur. Metaphyseal distortion may obviate primary mechanical stability with a stem designed for proximal fit and fill. Angular or bayonet deformities in the coronal or sagittal plane may require corrective osteotomy. An extended trochanteric osteotomy may be required to access and remove broken screws or other retained hardware (see Fig. 25). Plates used for osteotomy fixation decades earlier may occupy an intracortical position, and their removal can result in the creation of mechanically significant bony defects. Most of these situations can be addressed using an extensively porous coated stem

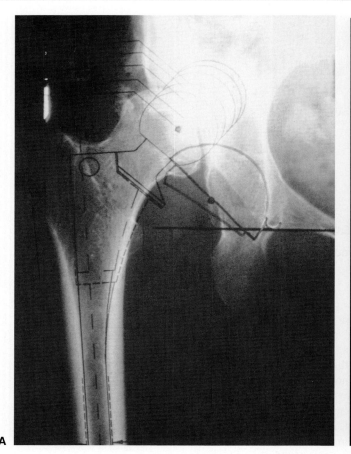
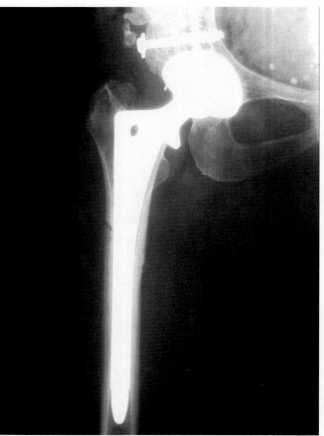

Figure 24. Crowe IV developmental dysplasia managed with a subtrochanteric osteotomy. **A:** Preoperative radiograph. **B:** Postoperative radiograph.

that achieves initial mechanical stability and subsequent biologic fixation in the femoral isthmus (see Fig. 26).

Two-incision Minimally Invasive Total Hip Replacement

In recent years, there has been growing interest in surgical techniques that minimize soft tissue dissection. One method that has gained considerable attention is the two-incision approach. This technique involves preparation of the femoral canal under fluoroscopic guidance. Reaming of the femoral isthmus with a rigid, fully fluted reamer in this manner is similar to the technique for closed intramedullary nailing and is particularly well suited for the implantation of an extensively porous coated stem (see Fig. 27). The surgical technique is covered in detail elsewhere in this text.

Osteoporosis

The use of a cementless stem for the management of patients with osteoporotic "stovepipe" canals requires a larger stem to achieve canal filling and initial implant stability. In the past, a larger stem equated with a stiffer stem and was associated with a higher incidence and severity of stress shielding. This was particularly so when an extensively porous coated stem was used. Cemented stems are therefore often recommended. The drawbacks of cemented stem fixation include difficulty in adequately pressurizing cement to achieve an ideal cement mantle in a large femoral canal and the risk of embolic

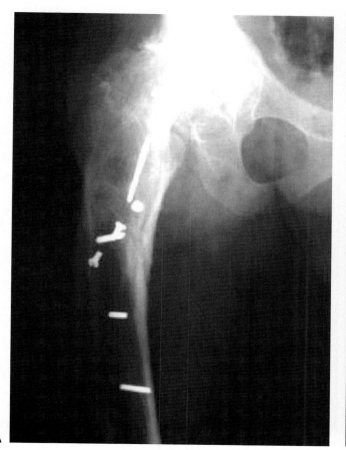
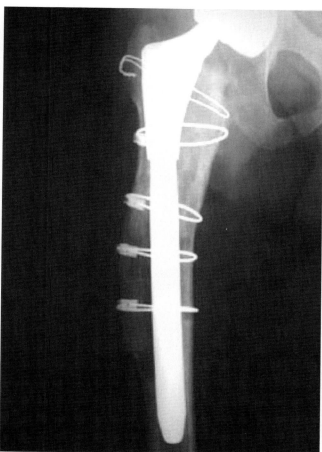

A   **B**

Figure 25. A: Preoperative radiograph of a patient with osteoarthritis, status post internal fixation of a femoral fracture, with several retained broken screws and an apex lateral subtrochanteric angular deformity. **B:** Postoperative radiograph following THR with an extensively coated modular stem. The hip was approached with an extended trochanteric osteotomy.

phenomenon associated with the large volume of cement required (14,15). An alternative is the use of a low-modulus, composite, extensively porous coated stem. Initial studies of one such stem demonstrate predictable fixation, favorable clinical results, and a significant increase in the retention of bone mineral density as compared to similarly shaped solid metal cementless stems (16,17) (see Fig. 28).

Currently, the only extensively porous coated low-modulus femoral component available is the Epoch stem (Zimmer Inc., Warsaw, Indiana) (see Fig. 2D). This stem features a solid cobalt chromium core surrounded by the thermoplastic adhesive polymer polyaryletherketone (PAEK). The entire intraosseous portion of the implant is then "jacketed" in commercially pure titanium fiber metal mesh (see Fig. 29). The stem has a unique geometry, an understanding of which is essential to the surgical technique. The distal aspect is cylindrical and is available in 1-mm increments from 14.0 to 19.0 mm in diameter. Only one proximal metaphyseal size is available for each distal stem diameter. The proximal segment is anatomically shaped and metaphyseal filling and, therefore, it comes in right and left designs. The femoral neck segment is anteverted.

As with other extensively porous coated stems, preparation of the femur involves distal reaming and proximal broaching. Reaming of the isthmus is performed in routine fashion with the exception that reaming to the exact diameter of the distal stem size is recommended rather than underreaming by 0.5 mm. This allows slight rotational "self-adjustment" of the implant as the large metaphyseal segment seats in the proximal femur.

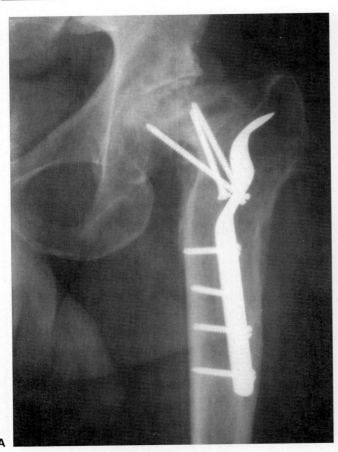
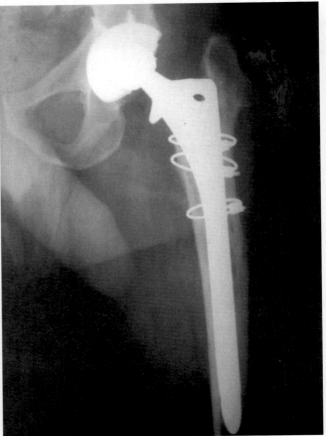

Figure 26. A: Preoperative radiograph of a patient status post valgus osteotomy with re-tained fixation plate. **B:** Postoperative radiograph after THR with an extensively porous coated stem. This case also employed an extended trochanteric osteotomy. (From Della Valle CJ, Berger RA, Rosenberg AG, et al. Extended trochanteric osteotomy in complex primary total hip arthroplasty. *J Bone Joint Surg Am* 85:2385–2390, 2003.)

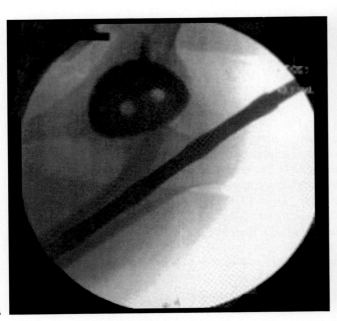
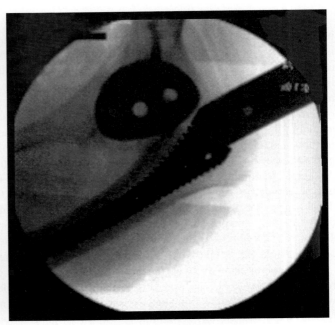

Figure 27. Two-incision minimally invasive total hip replacement. **A:** Fluoroscopic image of intramedullary reaming during two-incision THR. **B:** Broaching under fluoroscopic guidance.

(continues)

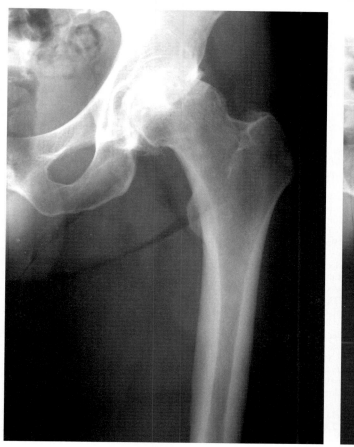

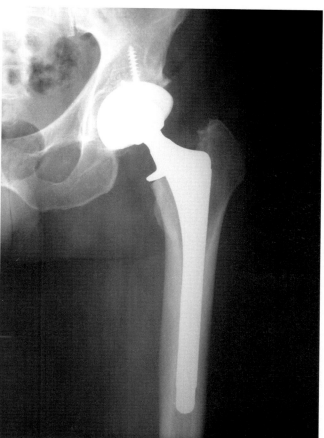

Figure 27. *(continued)* **C:** Preoperative radiograph. **D:** Postoperative radiograph.

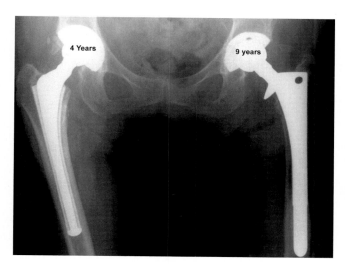

Figure 28. Bilateral THRs with a low-modulus Epoch composite stem on the right and an extensively porous coated solid cobalt chromium stem on the left. Significantly greater bone is retained about the composite stem.

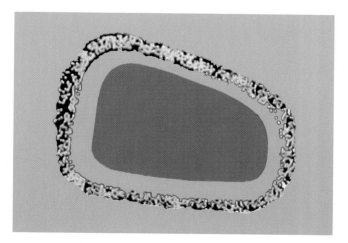

Figure 29. Cross section of the Epoch composite stem demonstrating the cobalt chromium core (*gray*), surrounded by the thermoplastic polyaryletherketone (*green*), with an outer layer of commercially pure titanium fiber-metal mesh.

RECOMMENDED READING

1. Engh CA. Recent advances in cementless total hip arthroplasty using the AML prosthesis. *Tech Orthop* 6:59–72, 1991.
2. Engh CA, Bobyn JD, Glassman AH. Porous-coated hip replacement. factors governing bone ingrowth, stress shielding, and clinical results. *J Bone Joint Surg Br* 69:45–55, 1987.
3. Engh CA Jr, Culpepper WJ II, Engh CA. Long-term results of the anatomic medullary locking prosthesis in total hip arthroplasty. *J Bone Joint Surg Am* 79:177–184, 1977.
4. McAuley JP, Moore KD, Culpepper WJ, et al. Total hip arthroplasty with porous-coated prostheses fixed without cement inpatients who are sixty-five years of age or older. *J Bone Joint Surg Am* 80:1648–1655, 1998.
5. Engh CA, Massin P, Suthers KE. Roentgenographic assessment of biological fixation of porous-surfaced femoral components. *Clin Orthop* 257:107–128, 1990.
6. Engh CA. Mechanical consequences of bone ingrowth in a hip prosthesis inserted without cement [Letter]. *J Bone Joint Surg Am* 78:312, 1996.
7. Bobyn JD, Glassman AH, Goto H, et al. The effect of stem stiffness on femoral bone resorption after canine porous-coated total hip arthroplasty. *Clin Orthop Relat Res* 261:196–213, 1990.
8. Engh CA, Glassman AH, Bobyn JD. Surgical principles in cementless total hip arthroplasty. *Tech Orthop* 1:35–53, 1986.
9. Glassman AH, Engh CA, Bobyn JD. The removal of porous-coated femoral hip stems. *Clin Orthop* 285:164–180, 1992.
10. Keaveny TM, Bartel DL. Mechanical consequences of bone ingrowth in a hip prosthesis inserted without cement. *J Bone Joint Surg Am* 77:911, 1995.
11. Crowe JF, Mani VJ, Ranawat CS. Total hip replacement in congenital dysplasia and dislocation of the hip. *J Bone Joint Surg Am* 61:15–23, 1979.
12. Dunn HK, Hess WE. Total hip reconstruction in chronically dislocated hips. *J Bone Joint Surg Am* 58:838–845, 1976.
13. Yasgur DJ, Stuchin SA, Adler EM, DiCesare PE. Subtrochanteric femoral shortening osteotomy in total hip arthroplasty for high-riding developmental dislocation of the hip. *J Arthroplasty* 12:880–888.
14. Christie J, Burnett R, Potts HR, et al. Echocardiography of transatrial embolism during cemented and uncemented hemiarthroplasty of the hip. *J Bone Joint Surg Br* 76:409–412, 1994.
15. Ries MD, Lynch F, Rauscher LA, et al. Pulmonary function during and after total hip replacement. Findings in patients who have insertion of a femoral component with and without cement. *J Bone Joint Surg Am* 75:581–587, 1993.
16. Glassman AH, Crowninshield RD, Herberts P, Schenck R. Early results of a low-modulus composite hip stem. *Clin Orthop* 393:128–136, 2001.
17. Karrholm J, Anderberg C, Snorrason F, et al. Evaluation of a femoral stem with reduced stiffness. *J Bone Joint Surg Am* 84:1651, 2002.

16

The Tapered Stem

Peter F. Sharkey and Frazer A. Wade

Hip replacement is arguably the most effective health care intervention introduced in the last four decades. The gold standard for hip arthroplasty in the elderly, osteoarthritic patient remains the cemented Charnley hip replacement. It has proven to be both reliable and durable in the hands of a number of skilled surgeons. Durability limits the results of cemented hip arthroplasty in young and active adults with osteoarthritis. Increasing life span coupled with large numbers of these high-demand patients prompts a search for an alternative to cemented femoral fixation.

Currently in the United States, 85% of hip arthroplasties are performed by surgeons who undertake 10 procedures or less per annum. An ideal hip replacement must give reliable and dependable performance among hip surgeons of all levels of experience and not simply in the hands of the originator or within large tertiary referral centers.

Cemented total hip arthroplasty has yielded variable results depending on surgical technique, implant, and patient population. Results with tapered stems appear reproducible and require fewer surgical steps (1). We feel this surgical simplicity produces predictable results. Ten-year results in a number of patient groups seem to indicate that the technique is more versatile than cemented stem fixation (1–5).

Initial experiences with uncemented fixation yielded results that were marred by a number of problems such as femoral fracture, subsidence, thigh pain, osteolysis, and stress shielding. We believe that many of the problems associated with early uncemented femoral components have been addressed by the latest generation of components (6,7). We also believe that uncemented femoral fixation with a well-designed prosthesis is a straightforward and reliable alternative to more technically demanding cemented femoral fixation.

INDICATIONS/CONTRAINDICATIONS

The tapered stem is ideally suited to provide fixation in femora with a broad spectrum of bone stock, bone quality, and underlying patient biology. Dorr type A and B femora ensure that stable initial fixation vital for bone ingrowth takes place. Initially, uncemented fixation was thought unsuitable for the patients with rheumatoid arthritis and osteoporotic Dorr type C proximal femora. The Dorr type C femur occurs in markedly osteoporotic femora and results in an increased risk of intraoperative femoral fracture. Additionally, a larger implant is required to produce primary stability. This unfortunately results in the use of a stiffer implant, and greater stress shielding or thigh pain have been found in this situation when tapered cobalt chrome implants are utilized. Experience and published results have shown this not to be the case with a tapered titanium implant (5). We caution against the use of cementless fixation where there is any concern about the stability of initial fixation.

PREOPERATIVE PLANNING

Precise preoperative planning is obligatory for any arthroplasty surgery. It enables the element of surprise to be removed from any operating room and ensures that the highest standard of surgery can be undertaken.

Good-quality anteroposterior and lateral radiographs allow planning to accommodate abnormalities such as increased femoral anteversion, femoral bowing, or deformity. These conditions may require alteration of the femoral canal entry point, osteotomy, or a change in prosthetic choice. In particular, where a proximal femoral osteotomy will be required, a fully coated and distally fixed prosthesis might be a more appropriate choice.

Preoperative templating should determine the appropriate center of rotation of the hip and femoral neck resection level (see Fig. 1). Varus femoral necks are radiographically identified, and often it can be predicted that a high-offset (varus-angled) prosthesis is required to restore stability without leg lengthening.

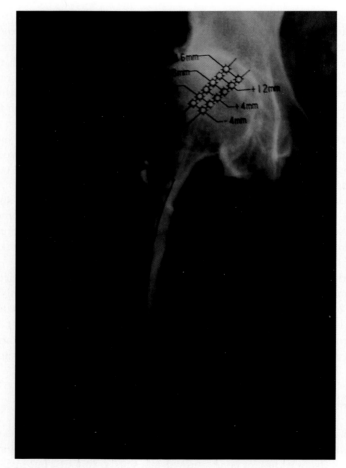

Figure 1. Careful templating offers a guide to femoral sizing, but it should never be viewed as absolute. Templating may be influenced by radiological magnification, and the definitive size is a complex three-dimensional interaction between fit and fill in both sagittal and coronal planes.

The ability to template and plan component size allows the surgeon to recognize problems intraoperatively. A discrepancy between templated and actual size should alert the surgeon to an undersized femur or a femoral fracture. Final component sizing should ultimately be determined by intraoperative trials using broaches.

Templating inaccuracies are compounded by radiographic projection and magnification. Standardized films or digital templating systems assist in compensating for these variables. In contrast to standard arthroplasty, the three-point fixation in the diaphyseal region seen on the lateral film may be equally as important as the metaphyseal fill seen on the antero-posterior (AP) radiograph in determining size of implant.

The eventual size is therefore determined by a complex interaction between the three-dimensional anatomy of the proximal femur and operative variables such as entry point, neck resection, and component orientation.

Design Rationale

We believe that the double-tapered design is ideally suited to permit fixation within the proximal femur and to provide immediate axial and rotational stability. Cadaver studies by Sharkey et al. have demonstrated that initial axial and rotational stability following implantation of a tapered stem (Taperloc®) was comparable to that of a cemented prosthesis (8). Should initial stability be insufficient for bone ingrowth, the component will subside. Unlike some alternative designs, subsidence of a tapered stem may reestablish the hoop stresses within the proximal femur, providing again the environment for bony ingrowth. The disadvantage is that the restoration of leg length and stability might be compromised. Hence, only small amounts of subsidence can be tolerated.

The wide variation in proximal femoral anatomy and concerns about creating an excessively stiff prosthesis are a further endorsement of the tapered stem. A tapered titanium stem provides a progressive transition from bulky and relatively inflexible proximal segment to the narrower and more flexible distal section. This, in turn, permits the loading of the proximal femur and theoretically protects against the effects of stress shielding.

A collared prosthesis has the theoretical benefits of providing absolute axial stability and loading the calcar, thus preventing stress shielding. This has not proven to be true when reviewing clinical data. We feel that a collar also has several potential drawbacks. First, if there is failure of initial rotational stability, then subsidence will be prevented, and stability will not be restored. Slight undersizing of the component or a high neck cut might create this scenario. Second, if component removal is required for any reason, then direct access to the bone prosthesis interface can be obscured by the collar. Third, for a collar to function with a stable component, there must be a very precise relationship between neck resection level, component design, and the complex three-dimensional anatomy of the proximal femur. Finally, the collar may prevent full "seating," creating an unstable prosthesis with axial stability yet unsatisfactory rotational stability.

We have opted for a circumferential proximal porous coating on the tapered stems we utilize. This permits bone ingrowth on the proximal femur and also promotes loading of the metaphyseal bone. Should the prosthesis require removal, a more extensive femoral osteotomy would not be required. Perhaps the greatest benefit from a complete proximal coating is that it creates a seal separating any debris generated by the bearing surface from gaining access to the bone prosthesis interface and inducing femoral osteolysis.

Metallurgical advances have developed stronger and yet more flexible titanium alloys (see Fig. 2). The reduced modulus of elasticity, although still several times that of bone, has a beneficial effect on the incidence of thigh pain and stress shielding. There is good evidence that thigh pain in earlier uncemented hips was associated with the larger and hence more rigid components (9,10). Titanium permits bone ongrowth more readily than cobalt chrome. Early titanium implants in orthopaedics displayed significant notch sensitivity. This tendency for imperfections to propagate under loading has been reduced with the newer alloys such as TZMF® (Ti-12Mo-6Zr-2Fe).

The majority of currently available components permit a degree of modularity in terms of neck length (see Fig. 3). Additionally, it is desirable to have lateral offset components to permit soft tissue tensioning and yet prevent the dissatisfaction and legal repercussions associated with limb lengthening.

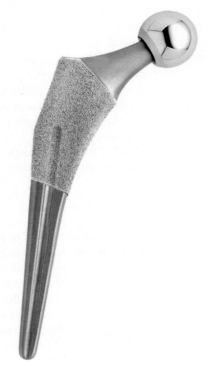

Figure 2. The titanium alloy tapered stem with circumferential proximal coating and trapezoidal neck. (Courtesy of Stryker Orthopaedics.)

SURGERY

Patient Positioning

Patients are placed in the supine position with a firm support raising the pelvis and keeping it level. The buttock and gluteal mass should be unsupported, preventing them from being forced up into the wound and occluding satisfactory visualization. Supine positioning in this manner permits more accurate assessment of leg length intraoperatively as the

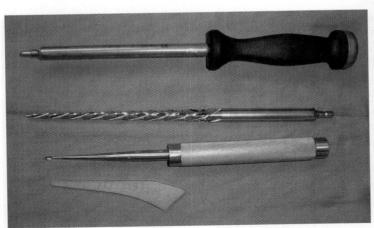

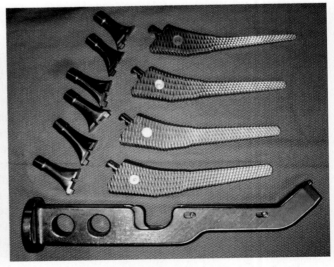

A   B

Figure 3. Femoral preparation requires a relatively limited set of instruments. Modularity of the broaches allows trialing of standard (132-degree) and lateral offset (127-degree) implants.

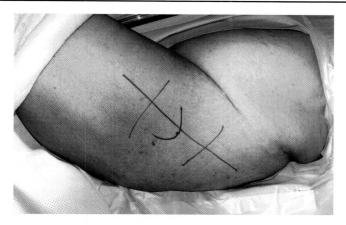

Figure 4. The patient is positioned supine and on a bolster.

confounder of pelvic obliquity is removed. We employ the direct lateral approach for all routine primary hip replacements (see Fig. 4). Trochanteric osteotomy is reserved for a small group of individuals in whom the exposure is unlikely to be satisfactory with the modified Hardinge approach. We employ the trochanteric osteotomy with decreasing frequency within the setting of primary hip replacement but would have no hesitation in recommending it for those with morbid obesity (particularly young males) and individuals with abnormal proximal femoral anatomy.

Surgical Technique

The practical points of the modified Hardinge approach are extensively covered elsewhere in this text. Variations important to the technique of uncemented tapered stem insertion are addressed here.

Following approach and dislocation, the level of neck resection can be determined by referring to the preoperative film and referenced from the tip of the greater trochanter (see Fig. 5). Contralateral leg length and hip pathology should be taken into account.

Following acetabular preparation and insertion, attention is returned to the femur. The proximal extent of the incision must permit satisfactory access to the femoral canal without

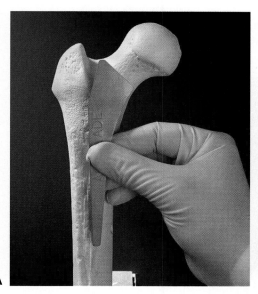
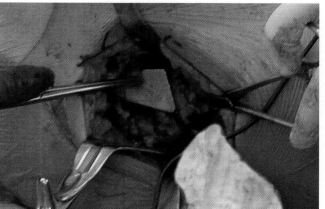

A   B

Figure 5. With the assistance of a template, the neck resection is marked with diathermy.

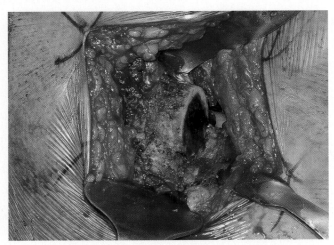

Figure 6. The femoral neck cut should be checked employing the templated relationships to the piriform fossa and lesser and greater trochanters.

compromising the procedure or traumatizing the wound margins. The neck cut should be checked and revised if required (see Fig. 6). Poor exposure can result in an improperly rotated stem.

The entry point of initial reaming is carefully determined with reference to the preoperative radiographs. Pitfalls that should be avoided are the medial and anterior entry points. These result in both a posterior trajectory and a varus stem. This should be guarded against by ensuring that the femur is appropriately projected up into the wound with retraction. When necessary, there should be no hesitation about extending the wound proximally. Employing large, angled rongeurs/nibblers, the entry point is appropriately lateralized (see Fig. 7). Often, there will be a small amount of bone to resect at the base of the piriform fossa that might otherwise have diverted the path of the reaming and subsequently forced the stem into varus.

The canal is opened first with a blunt-ended curette (see Fig. 8). Take great care not to perforate the shaft, particularly in patients with obesity, osteoporosis, or femoral deformity. A powered reamer is then employed to open the canal (see Fig. 9). The trajectory is toward the center of the knee joint in both sagittal and coronal planes (see Fig. 10). To guard against malalignment or perforation, the reamer should be advanced without marked force.

Broaches are employed to contour the femur in both mediolateral (ML) and AP dimensions. The broaches follow the same trajectory as the initial reaming (see Fig. 11). Fewer repeated blows with the mallet and frequent backstrokes with occasional rest help to prevent femoral fracture by permitting stress relaxation of the bone. Anteversion should be

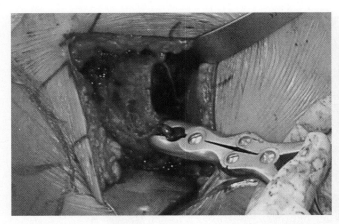

Figure 7. The entry point of initial reaming is lateralized with large, angled rongeurs or nibblers.

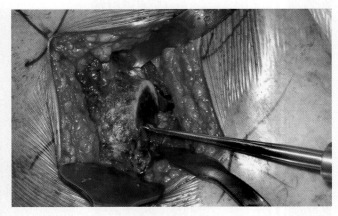

Figure 8. A blunt-ended curette is used to open the canal initially.

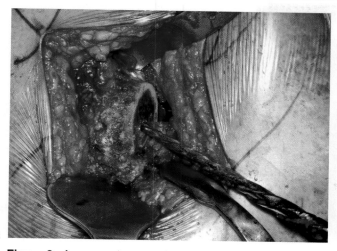
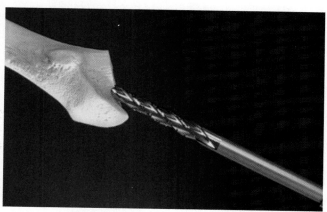

Figure 9. A powered reamer is then used to gently further open the canal. Great care must be taken to avoid femoral perforation.

kept constant and carefully controlled throughout femoral preparation. Altering anteversion after femoral broaching might compromise rotational stability of the definitive implant.

The surgeon should be vigilant to the change in pitch that signifies that the broach is fully seated. At that point, it should be backed out before any attempt is made to advance it further. Backing out the broach has the effect of removing the debris from the interface. Lavage of the broach and canal can both reduce systemic embolism and assist in advancing the broach.

A standard head/neck combination is first employed unless preoperative templating determines otherwise (see Fig. 12).

Trial reduction with the broach and a standard neck segment allows the assessment of stability. Rotational stability is assessed in both flexion and extension. Longitudinal traction with the knee flexed, and hence the hamstrings relaxed, allows the assessment of "shucking" (see Fig. 13). If this is greater than a few millimeters, then abductor tension can be modified by increasing the offset or length. With reference to the preoperative radio-

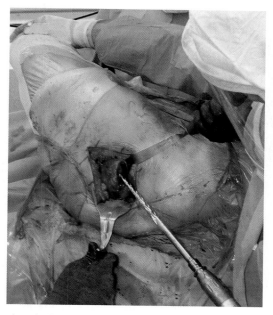

Figure 10. Firmly gripping the flexed knee assists in aiming the power reamer.

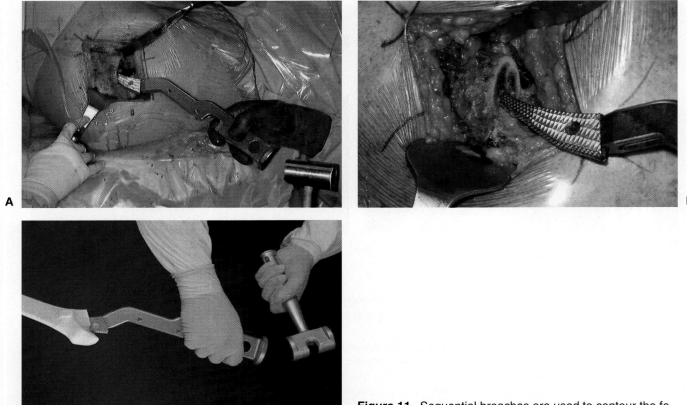

Figure 11. Sequential broaches are used to contour the femur in both ML and AP dimensions.

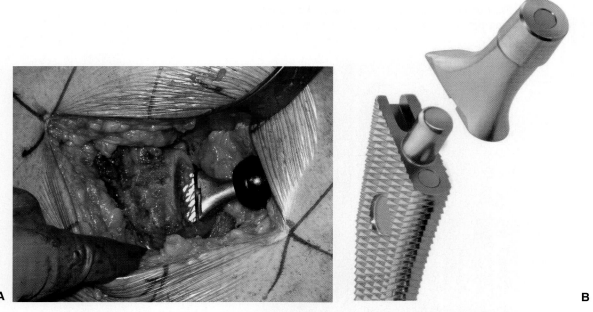

Figure 12. A. The modular broach is left within the femur, and **(B)** a standard head/neck combination is used in most cases for the first trial reduction (**B**, Courtesy of Stryker Orthopaedics.)

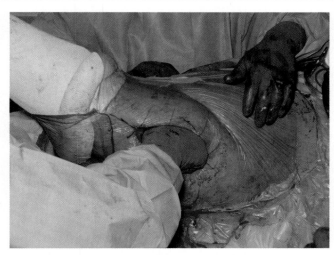

Figure 13. With the knee flexed and hamstrings relaxed, an assessment of offset can be made.

graphs and intraoperative assessment, it can be determined whether offset or length is required to produce satisfactory soft tissue tension and stability.

Definitive component insertion should be preceded by lavage of the canal (see Fig. 14). Lavage reduces embolic load and prevents insertion being halted by debris. Once again, short repeated taps, occasional rests, and listening for a change in pitch are employed. If the prosthesis fails to advance, it should be removed, and the canal should be lavaged and rebroached. Incomplete broaching with the next larger size trial may open the canal slightly and allow complete seating of the true implant.

Following definitive prosthesis insertion with a trial head in place (see Fig. 15), a further assessment of leg length and stability is made. Following lavage, the interior of the acetabulum should be carefully inspected for debris. The trunion is carefully cleaned and dried. The definitive head is applied, and reduction is undertaken (see Fig. 16).

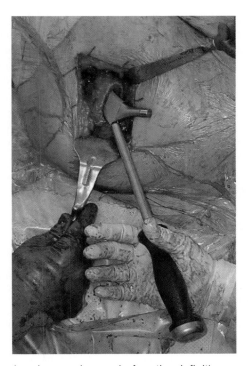

Figure 14. The canal undergoes lavage before the definitive component is inserted.

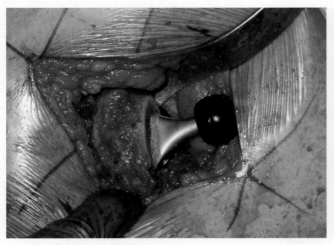

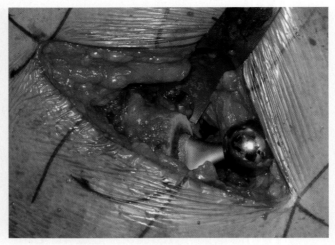

Figure 15. The definitive prosthesis has been inserted, and a final trial is undertaken.

Figure 16. Finally, the definitive head is applied, and reduction is undertaken.

POSTOPERATIVE MANAGEMENT

We permit all patients to fully weight bear immediately following their operation; however, we advise the use of crutches or a cane for 6 weeks to guard against falls (11). The typical postoperative management regimen is covered extensively elsewhere.

COMPLICATIONS

A three-tiered approach should be employed involving prevention, recognition, and management of intraoperative femoral failure. Prevention requires recognition of those at risk with osteoporotic, deformed, or "tight" femora. Reaming should be careful and controlled in both force and direction. The surgeon should also be aware of the change in pitch during reaming or implantation that may accompany a femoral split. Up to 50% of femoral fractures go unrecognized at the time of surgery (12). Where there are concerns that fracture may have occurred, the surgeon must extend the approach to inspect the femur directly and/or undertake intraoperative radiographs. If detected intraoperatively, most can be managed with a cable or double wire to close the split (13). It is our practice to back out the prosthesis, place a cable closing the split, and then advance the prosthesis until the split opens prior to final tightening of the cable. If any doubt exists regarding the primary stability of the construct, then an alternative prosthesis should be employed (14,15). The fracture should be bypassed. A reasonable alternative might be a fully coated and distally fixed stem (16).

RECOMMENDED READING

1. Teloken MA, Bissett G, Hozack WJ, et al. Ten to fifteen-year follow-up after total hip arthroplasty with a tapered cobalt-chromium femoral component (tri-lock) inserted without cement. *J Bone Joint Surg Am* 84:2140–2144, 2002.
2. Keisu KS, Orozco F, Sharkey PF, et al. Primary cementless total hip arthroplasty in octogenarians. Two to eleven-year follow-up. *J Bone Joint Surg Am* 83:359–363, 2001.
3. Lehman DE, Capello WN, Feinberg JR. Total hip arthroplasty without cement in obese patients. A minimum two-year clinical and radiographic follow-up study. *J Bone Joint Surg Am* 76:854–862, 1994.
4. Parvizi J, Keisu KS, Hozack WJ, et al. Primary total hip arthroplasty with an uncemented femoral component: a long-term study of the Taperloc stem. *J Arthroplasty* 19:151–156, 2004.
5. Reitman RD, Emerson R, Higgins L, Head W. Thirteen year results of total hip arthroplasty using a tapered titanium femoral component inserted without cement in patients with type C bone. *J Arthroplasty* 18:116–121, 2003.
6. Bourne RB, Rorabeck CH. Porous coated femoral fixation: the long and short of it! *Orthopedics* 26:911–912, 2003.

7. Burkart BC, Bourne RB, Rorabeck CH, Kirk PG. Thigh pain in cementless total hip arthroplasty. A comparison of two systems at 2 years' follow-up. *Orthop Clin North Am* 24:645–653, 1993.

8. Sharkey PF, Albert TJ, Hume EL, Rothman RH. Initial stability of a collarless wedge-shaped prosthesis in the femoral canal. *Semin Arthroplasty* 1:87–90, 1990.

9. Lavernia C, D'Apuzzo M, Hernandez V, Lee D. Thigh pain in primary total hip arthroplasty: the effects of elastic moduli. *J Arthroplasty* 19:10–16, 2004.

10. Vresilovic EJ, Hozack WJ, Rothman RH. Incidence of thigh pain after uncemented total hip arthroplasty as a function of femoral stem size. *J Arthroplasty* 11:304–311, 1996.

11. Schwartz JT Jr, Mayer JG, Engh CA. Femoral fracture during non-cemented total hip arthroplasty. *J Bone Joint Surg Am* 71:1135–1142, 1989.

12. Peak EL, Parvizi J, Ciminiello M, et al. The role of patient restrictions in reducing the prevalence of early dislocation following total hip arthroplasty. A randomized, prospective study. *J Bone Joint Surg Am* 87:247–253, 2005.

13. Fitzgerald RH Jr, Brindley GW, Kavanagh BF. The uncemented total hip arthroplasty. Intraoperative femoral fractures. *Clin Orthop Relat Res* Oct(235):61–66, 1988.

14. Sharkey PF, Hozack WJ, Booth RE Jr, Rothman RH. Intraoperative femoral fractures in cementless total hip arthroplasty. *Orthop Rev* 21:337–342, 1992.

15. Sharkey PF, Wolf LR, Hume EL, Rothman RH. Insertional femoral fracture: a biomechanical study of femoral component stability. *Semin Arthroplasty* 1:91–94, 1990.

16. Parvizi J, Rapuri VR, Purtill JJ, et al. Treatment protocol for proximal femoral periprosthetic fractures. *J Bone Joint Surg Am* 86(Suppl 2):8–16, 2004.

17

The Modular Stem in Developmental Dysplasia of the Hip

David A. Mattingly

INDICATIONS/CONTRAINDICATIONS

Elements of developmental dysplasia of the hip (DDH) occur frequently in primary total hip arthroplasty (THA) (1–6). A review of 75 hips with idiopathic osteoarthritis revealed proximal femoral deformity in 40% of cases and acetabular dysplasia in 39% of hips (4). Variable shape of the femoral canal (canal/flare index) may make it difficult to achieve proximal and distal fit with standard femoral components (7).

While useful in most hips undergoing primary THA, modular femoral stems are especially indicated where proximal femoral deformity is present. Abnormal femoral neck anteversion, previous proximal femoral osteotomy, and small femoral canals are ideal indications for use of a modular femoral stem. Small-diameter stems are frequently required for DDH hips. Press-fit modular stems avoid the problems of thin cement mantels and subsequent cement fracture, while also reducing the probability of cementless stem fracture since the stem itself is not porous coated (8). Torsional stability of modular stems is equivalent to cemented stems, also making it the implant of choice for subtrochanteric osteotomy stabilization for reduction of high-riding DDH (9).

Contraindications to the modular stem are rare but might include extreme femoral canal deformity where cemented or custom stem fixation is more easily achieved.

PREOPERATIVE PLANNING

Detailed history, physical, and radiographic evaluation are required for any patient undergoing primary THA. The history in DDH patients should focus on prior treatments, surgeries, and complications. The patients' disabilities (leg length, fatigue, limp, etc.) and pain patterns should be thoroughly discussed.

Physical examination will often reveal abnormalities in size, range of motion (stiffness or laxity), leg lengths, and prior incisions, which can make surgery more difficult. Surgeries to the contralateral limb (e.g., epiphysiodesis) should be noted. Leg lengths are assessed by tape measure and blocks under the short limb to determine exact discrepancies and what length appears to best balance the pelvis. Thorough preoperative assessment of femoral and sciatic nerve function is essential.

Plain radiographs should include an anteroposterior (AP) projection pelvis and AP and Lauenstein lateral x-rays of the involved hip. Radiographic magnification markers taped to the involved hip allow for an accurate estimate of x-ray magnification, permitting precise femoral canal sizing and templating. Computed tomography (CT) scans are rarely indicated but can provide more accurate assessment of anteversion, femoral canal dimensions, and acetabular bone stock assessment. Scanograms may be useful to more accurately assess limb length inequalities.

SURGERY

The patient is positioned laterally with the affected side up. The underlying leg is placed in flexion to reduce the degree of lumbar lordosis. The trunk and pelvis are appropriately stabilized while the operated leg is prepped and draped free over a radiolucent table to permit possible fluoroscopic evaluation.

Anterolateral, direct lateral, and posterior approaches to the DDH hip can be used. I prefer the posterior approach to avoid scars from prior anterior surgeries (which are common), minimize damage to the abductors, and ease of identifying, protecting, and monitoring the sciatic nerve. The posterior approach can be easily converted to a trochanteric or subtrochanteric osteotomy for stiff or high-riding DDH cases (see Fig. 1).

For thin, flexible hips requiring less than 1 cm limb lengthening, a small incision is made from the midpoint of the vastus tubercle extending proximally and posteriorly for 4 to 6 inches (see Fig. 2). The incision is extended further proximally and distally for larger and stiff patients, especially those requiring trochanteric or subtrochanteric osteotomy or limb lengthening greater than 1 cm. The fascia lata and gluteus maximus are divided in line with the incision. The sciatic nerve is identified by palpation but not dissected. Partial or full release of the gluteus maximus tendon at the linea aspera is performed to prevent tethering of the sciatic nerve during leg manipulations and lengthening. All of the external rotators

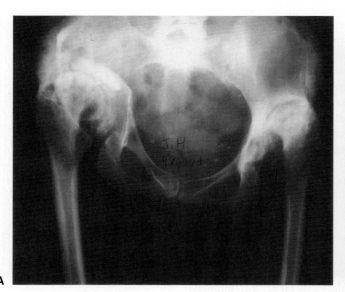
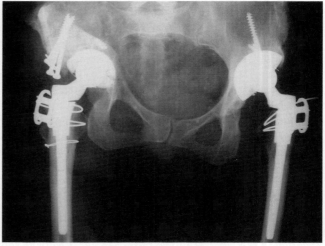

Figure 1. Preoperative **(A)** and postoperative **(B)** AP pelvis x-ray demonstrating transtrochanteric approach required for marked stiffness from prior bilateral iliac osteotomies.

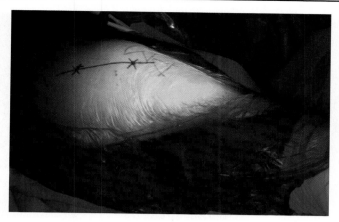

Figure 2. The standard incision is lateral, from the midpoint of the vastus tubercle extending proximally and posteriorly for 4 to 6 inches *(X to X)*. It can be easily extended proximally and distally for more extensile exposure.

are released separately from the posterior capsule and reflected posteriorly to further protect the sciatic nerve, which often lies just lateral to the ischium. While posterior capsulotomy and repair are preferred for Crowe I DDH hips (see Fig. 3), capsulectomy is generally preferred for Crowe II, III, and IV hips, requiring further exposure and limb lengthening. A smooth 7- to 16-inch Steinman pin can be placed in the ischium at the level of the transverse ligament for limb length assessment prior to dislocation.

The hip is dislocated posteriorly if not already severely subluxed or dislocated (Crowe III and IV) (2). The greater and lesser trochanters and femoral head are used as landmarks in conjunction with preoperative templates to determine the level of femoral neck osteotomy (see Fig. 4). When subtrochanteric osteotomy (10) is performed to help reduce the hip (Crowe III and IV), the femoral canal is prepared distally and proximally, and the trial sleeve is positioned in the proximal femur (see Fig. 5). The vastus lateralis is then reflected from the vastus tubercle distally for 6 to 10 cm. The linea aspera is identified, and rotation marks are made on the femur prior to the osteotomy. The iliopsoas tendon is sectioned just proximal to its insertion at the lesser trochanter. A transverse osteotomy is then made distal to the sleeve

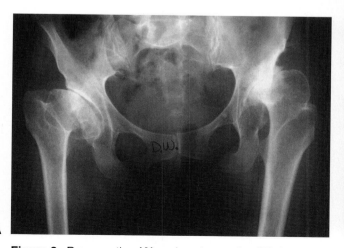
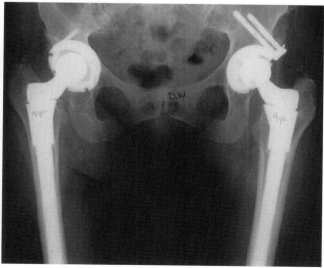

A   B

Figure 3. Preoperative **(A)** and postoperative **(B)** AP pelvis x-ray in patient with Crowe I and Crowe II dysplasia. Acetabular structural autograft is used for the Crowe II hip. Note difference in proximal sleeve placement to accommodate for version differences.

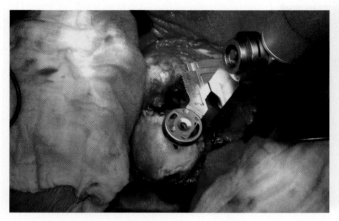

Figure 4. A femoral neck resection template for stem size, neck length, and offset determines the level of initial femoral neck osteotomy.

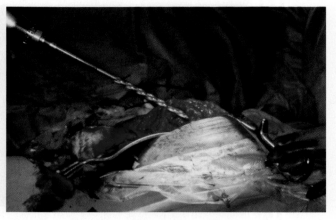

Figure 5. Preparation of the femoral canal is performed prior to subtrochanteric osteotomy.

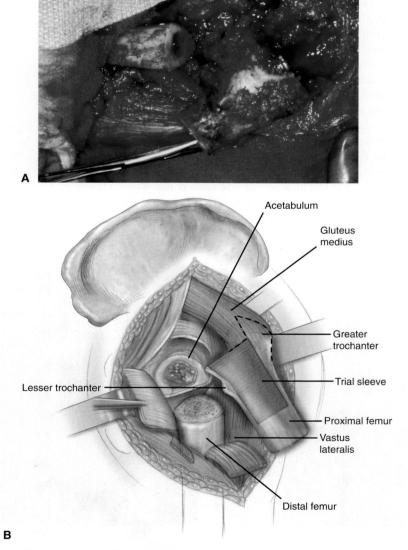

Figure 6. Initial transverse osteotomy distal to the trial sleeve, approximately 3.5 cm distal to the lesser trochanter.

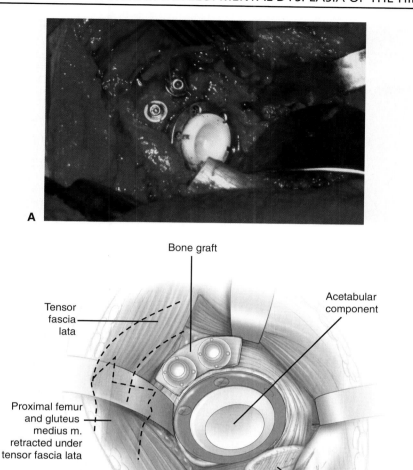

Figure 7. Acetabular exposure is excellent after completion of the osteotomy.

and approximately 3.5 cm distal to the lesser trochanter (see Fig. 6). The acetabulum is then easily exposed by complete capsulectomy and anterior displacement of the proximal femoral fragment and attached abductors (see Fig. 7). If subtrochanteric osteotomy is not performed (Crowe I and II hips), then the capsule is dissected inferiorly until the transverse ligament and true socket are identified. The acetabulum is then prepared and positioned. Acetabular bone deficiencies may require cup placement more medial, higher, or in more abnormal version than desired. The advantage of the modular stem in this setting is that it can easily accommodate to these abnormal socket positions by increasing offset, neck length, or independent version of the stem from the sleeve to maximize myofascial tension, leg length, and stability.

The femoral canal is identified with a box osteotome and canal finder. A three-step milling process then prepares the femoral canal. Step one involves cylindrical diaphyseal reaming until firm endosteal cortical contact is achieved to prepare the distal femur (see Fig. 8). Since DDH femoral canals are often small, begin with the smallest-diameter reamer and increase in 0.5- to 1.0-mm increments. The final reamer should match or be 0.5 mm greater than the minor diameter of the chosen stem. If subtrochanteric osteotomy has been performed, reamers can be placed into the distal bone fragment through the osteotomy site to a depth matching or exceeding the final stem placement after excision of the subtrochanteric fragment.

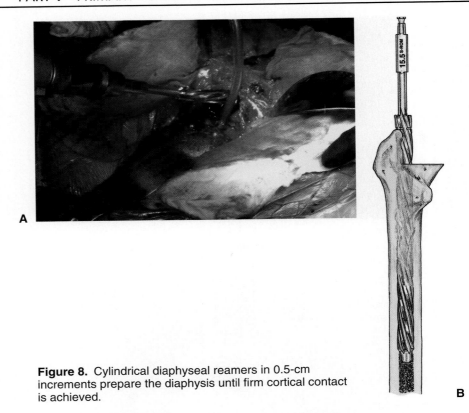

Figure 8. Cylindrical diaphyseal reamers in 0.5-cm increments prepare the diaphysis until firm cortical contact is achieved.

The proximal femur is prepared in two steps. A shaft pilot, matching the minor stem diameter, directs proper placement of the proximal reamers. Conical metaphyseal reamers in 2-mm increments are placed until firm anterior/posterior proximal diaphyseal and metaphyseal contact is obtained without excessive thinning of the proximal endosteal cortex (see Fig. 9). Calcar miller reamers are then used to mill the metaphyseal flare to maximize host bone contact irrespective of sleeve version (see Fig. 10).

Femoral sleeve and stem trials are then placed. There are ten sleeve options for each diameter stem. The trial neck can be rotated in 10-degree increments until desired stem anteversion is achieved (see Fig. 11). Femoral neck and head options are then selected to provide desired leg length and offset.

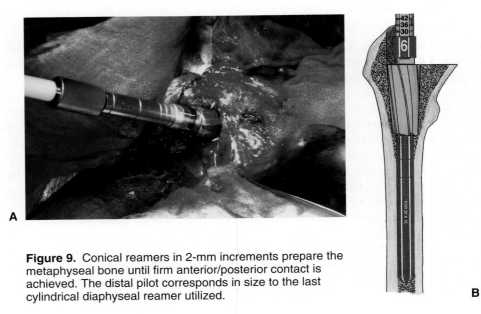

Figure 9. Conical reamers in 2-mm increments prepare the metaphyseal bone until firm anterior/posterior contact is achieved. The distal pilot corresponds in size to the last cylindrical diaphyseal reamer utilized.

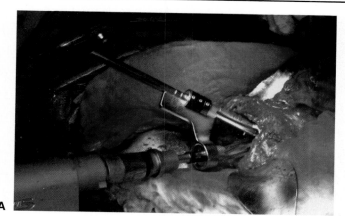

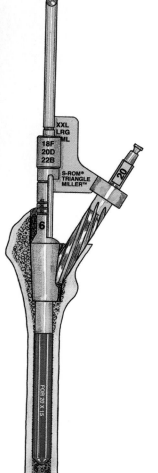

Figure 10. The triangle calcar miller prepares the metaphyseal flare in the version that allows maximum contact with host bone. The distal pilot and proximal cone pilot correspond to the final distal and proximal reamers previously used.

Trial reduction is then performed to assess leg length, stability, combined anteversion, and range of motion. If limb lengthening has been performed, begin the initial reduction with the shortest length and offset trial and slowly increase both as desired. Soft tissue releases of the capsule, gluteus maximus tendon, iliotibial band, tensor

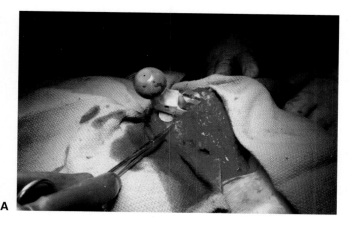

Figure 11. The trial neck assembly can be rotated in 10-degree increments until desired stem anteversion is achieved, independent of sleeve placement.

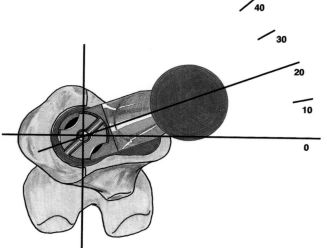

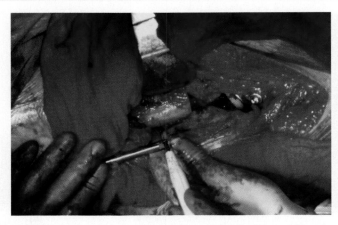

Figure 12. With the trial reduced, distraction of the distal fragment will estimate the amount of distal bone to be resected by measuring overlap between the two fragments.

fascia lata, straight head of the rectus femoris tendon, and iliopsoas tendon are performed until desired tissue tension and leg length are achieved. When subtrochanteric osteotomy has been performed, the trial stem and sleeve are placed into the proximal fragment and reduced into the acetabular component with the leg in full extension. An assistant then distracts the distal fragment, and the amount of overlap between the distal and proximal bone fragments determines the amount of initial subtrochanteric bone to be resected (see Fig. 12). A second transverse osteotomy is then made in the distal fragment. Trial reduction can then be completed, correcting for anteversion abnormalities either through the stem placement or derotation of the osteotomy fragment. A Lohman bone clamp stabilizes the fragments during trial reduction and implant insertion.

Upon trial implant removal, differences in stem and sleeve anteversion are noted. The real sleeve is then inserted into the prepared proximal femur, and the stem is introduced in the proper amount of socket and femoral head of anteversion (see Fig. 13). Final reduction is then performed with a desired combined anteversion of 40 to 45 degrees. If subtrochanteric osteotomy is performed, rotational stability is assessed. Either a unicortical plate or a cortical onlay allograft is applied if the osteotomy is not completely stable rotationally.

POSTOPERATIVE MANAGEMENT

The patient is transferred to a standard orthopaedic bed with a regular pillow between the legs. An AP pelvis and operative hip x-ray are obtained in the recovery room to assess proper implant positioning and to exclude fracture and dislocation. Mobilization begins on the first postoperative day with assisted standing. Drains, if used, are removed on the first postoperative morning. Ambulation with a walker is begun on the first or second postoperative day and progressed to 50% weight bearing with crutches for 4 weeks, followed by weight bearing as tolerated with two crutches for 2 weeks.

REHABILITATION

All patients are re-evaluated at 6 weeks postoperatively. If progress is appropriate, strict hip precautions are eliminated, and progressive range of motion, biking, and strengthening are permitted. I encourage weight bearing as tolerated with a cane for 3 more weeks. All patients are informed that they will make improvements in flexibility, strength, endurance, and gait until 1 to 2 years postoperatively.

Passive resistive exercises are allowed at 3 to 4 months postoperatively, but only light

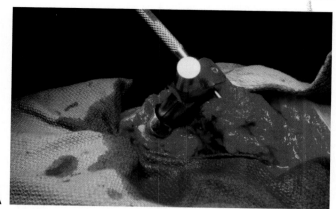

A

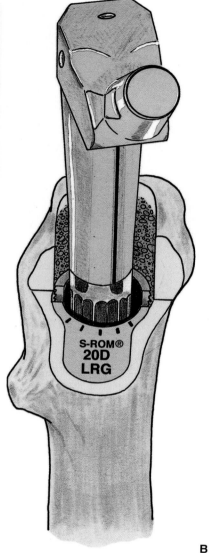

Figure 13. Orientation lines in 20-degree increments on the implanted sleeve are matched to the stem/neck witness mark to assure proper version of the stem/neck during implantation.

B

resistance (10 to 20 lbs) is encouraged. Golf and doubles tennis are allowed at 6 months postoperatively. Low-impact activities are encouraged (walking, elliptical machine, swimming), and running and jumping are discouraged.

For patients undergoing subtrochanteric osteotomy, crutch walking for 10 to 12 weeks is anticipated until the osteotomy is clinically healed. At this point, further rehabilitation as mentioned above is initiated.

COMPLICATIONS

Excessive limb lengthening and nerve palsy are serious potential complications of primary THA in the DDH patient. Accurate preoperative and intraoperative leg length assessment is critical. I prefer to place a leg length pin in the ischium near the desired hip center prior to dislocation. The pin's axial position can be marked on the vastus lateralis with a stitch before dislocation and after reconstruction. Limb lengthening greater than 2.5 cm should be avoided in order to minimize risks of femoral and sciatic nerve palsy. During surgery, limited hip flexion (20 to 30 degrees) and knee flexion (30 to 40 degrees) minimize excess tension on the femoral and sciatic nerves. Femoral and sciatic nerve palsies occur

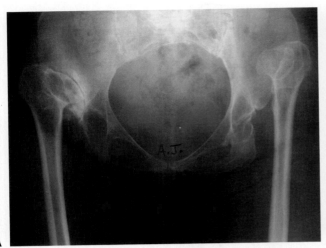 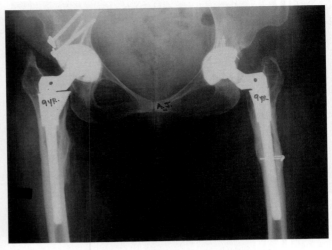

Figure 14. Preoperative **(A)** and 9-year postoperative **(B)** x-rays after bilateral subtrochanteric osteotomies for high-riding DDH.

most frequently in hips with prior surgery, where anterior or posterior scars inhibit nerve excursion during limb lengthening. Careful and gentle retractor placement must be constantly monitored. Finally, for patients undergoing limb lengthening greater than 1.5 cm, an awake test to assess sciatic and femoral nerve function can be performed. Preoperative patient instruction and anesthesia cooperation are required. Sciatic nerve evoked potential monitoring during surgery may also be useful. Other potential complications of DDH surgery include femoral fracture and trochanteric problems. For small femoral canals, power milling is preferred over broaching, and smaller than standard instruments and implants may need to be selected. For short femurs or femurs shortened by subtrochanteric excisional osteotomy, anterior perforation of the femoral bow can be avoided by flexible reaming of the canal or shortening the femoral implant with a metal-cutting device. Trochanteric abutment against the ischium in extension, especially in hips with a high hip center, can be minimized by derotational subtrochanteric osteotomy or trimming of the posterior trochanter and/or lateral ischium. Subtrochanteric osteotomy is preferred over trochanteric advancement with femoral neck shortening in order to avoid problems with trochanteric fixation (nonunion, fibrous union, bursitis).

RESULTS

Since 1992, I have used 120 modular stems for cementless femoral fixation in DDH (Crowe I to IV) hips undergoing primary THA. Complications include three femoral nerve palsies (all resolved), one sciatic nerve palsy (not resolved), two intraoperative fractures treated with cerclage wiring, and one nonrecurrent posterior dislocation. All femoral stems are stable and ingrown. Only one stem has been revised because of periprosthetic fracture at 4 years postoperatively (see Figs. 14 and 15).

Figure 15. Serial x-rays demonstrating versatility of modular stems in femoral deformity and periprosthetic fractures. **A:** Preoperative x-ray demonstrating proximal deformity after femoral osteotomy. **B:** Postoperative x-ray shows proximal sleeve triangle placed laterally to improve host bone contact. A calcar replacement neck was used to accommodate for low neck cut and to equalize leg lengths. **C:** Transverse fracture below stem at 2 years postoperatively after falling from 8 ft staging. **D:** The index stem has been replaced with a longer stem, leaving the original sleeve in place. Flexible reamers can be placed through the sleeve to prepare the distal femur. A cortical onlay graft has been added.

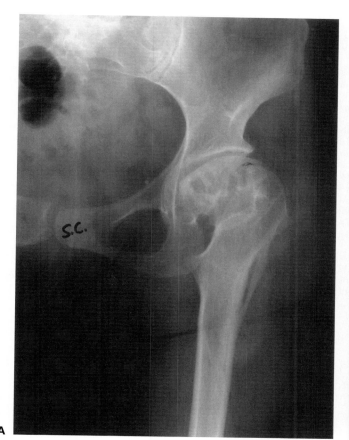

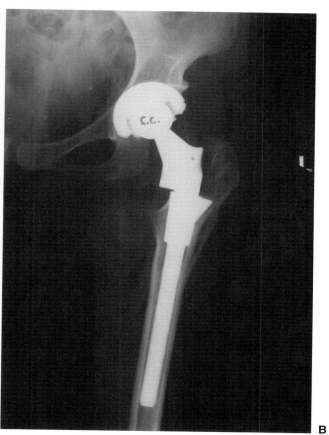

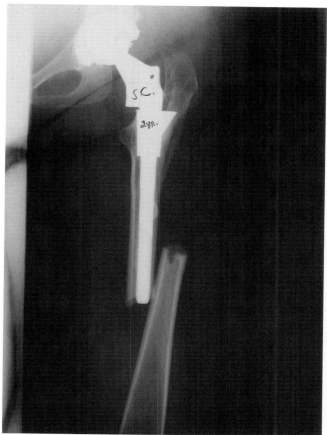

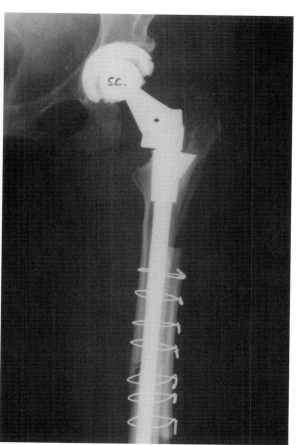

RECOMMENDED READING

1. Anderson MJ, Harris WH. Total hip arthroplasty with insertion of the acetabular component without cement in hips with total congenital dislocation or marked congenital dysplasia. *J Bone Joint Surg Am* 81(3):347–354, 1999.
2. Crowe JF, Mani VJ, Ranawat CS. Total hip replacement in congenital dislocation and dysplasia of the hip. *J Bone Joint Surg Am* 61(1):15–23, 1979.
3. Garvin KL, Bowen MK, Salvati EA, Ranawat CS. Long-term results of total hip arthroplasty in congenital dislocation and dysplasia of the hip. *J Bone Joint Surg Am* 73(9):1348–1354, 1991.
4. Harris WH. Etiology of osteoarthritis of the hip. *Clin Orthop Relat Res* 213:20–33, 1986.
5. MacKenzie JR, Kelley SS, Johnston RC. Total hip replacement for coxarthrosis secondary to congenital dysplasia and dislocation of the hip: long-term results. *J Bone Joint Surg Am* 78(1):55–61, 1996.
6. Sanchez-Sotelo J, Berry DJ, Trousdale RT, et al. Surgical treatment of developmental dysplasia of the hip in adults: arthroplasty options. *J Am Acad Orthop Surg* 10(5):334–344, 2002.
7. Noble PC, Alexander JW, Lindahl LJ, et al. The anatomic basis of femoral component design. *Clin Orthop Relat Res* 235:148–165, 1988.
8. Bobyn JD, Tanzer M, Krygier JJ, et al. Concerns with modularity in total hip arthroplasty. *Clin Orthop Relat Res* 298:27–36, 1994.
9. Ohl MD, Whiteside LA, McCarthy DS, White SE. Torsional fixation of a modular femoral hip component. *Clin Orthop Relat Res* 287:135–141, 1993.
10. Masonis JL, Patel JV, Bourne RB, et al. Subtrochanteric shortening and derotational osteotomy in primary total hip arthroplasty for patients with severe hip dysplasia. *J Arthroplasty* 18(3):68–73, 2003.

18

The Proximal Ingrowth Stem

David W. Manning, Dennis W. Burke,
and Harry E. Rubash

INDICATIONS/CONTRAINDICATIONS

Proximally porous coated femoral implants were introduced as an alternative to cemented and fully porous coated uncemented implants over 15 years ago. Many different stems with porous ingrowth/ongrowth surfaces (fiber metal, sintered beads, grit blasting, or hydroxyapatite) limited to the proximal one third or less of the implant have achieved excellent results with regard to loosening and survivorship at midterm follow-up (see Table 1) (1–11). Stable bony ingrowth/ongrowth of these proximally porous coated stems is dependent upon pore size (50 to 250 μm), initial fixation (micromotion <50 μm), and intimate contact with host bone (prosthesis/bone gap <50 μm) (12,13).

In theory, bony ingrowth/ongrowth of proximally porous coated femoral implants provides a lasting dynamic fixation and an attractive option for young patients. At midterm follow-up, many proximally porous coated femoral implants have results comparable to cemented implants (Table 1) (1–11,14,15). Transfer of weight-bearing force to metaphyseal bone in a well-fixed proximally porous coated implant may minimize the proximal femoral stress shielding seen with fully porous coated implants. Proximally porous coated implants are ideally indicated for young patients and active older patients with adequate bone stock (Dorr type A or B) undergoing total hip arthroplasty (see Fig. 1). Better alternative procedures and implant choices exist for patients with sepsis, metabolic bone disease, a history of radiation to the hip, severe deformity, and Dorr type C bone.

For the purposes of classification, proximally porous coated stem designs are considered as *tapered stems* when the cross-sectional anatomy of the stem is a two- or three-dimensional taper over its entire length or as *cylindrical stems* when the cross section changes from a two- or three-dimensional taper proximally to a cylinder in the diaphyseal portion of the stem (see Fig. 2). Cylindrical stems with a proximal three-dimensional taper may be considered *anatomic cylinders* or *nonanatomic cylinders,* depending on whether or not the prosthetic neck has a built-in version requiring left- or right-sided application. This classification groups stems on the basis of implant geometry, the mode of initial fixation, and the technique of implantation regardless of differences in metallurgy, type of porous surface, or presence of a collar. Simply stated, tapered stems achieve stable fixation solely in the metaphy-

Table 1. *Results with Various Proximally Porous-coated Femoral Components*[a]

Study[b]	Stem	Design Parameters	Follow-up	Stable Ingrown	Thigh Pain	Survivorship
Romagnoli (10)	CLS	Ti, collarless, 100% grit blast, 3D taper	>10 y (10 to 16)	97%	NC	90% at 14 y
Kawamura (6)	PCA	CoCr, collarless, sintered beads, anatomic	12 y (10 to 14)	88%	36%	94.9% at 14 y
McLaughlin (8)	Taperloc	Ti, collarless, plasma spray, taper	10 y (8 to 12.5)	96%	6%	95% at 10 y
Hellman (4)	Omnifit	CoCr, collarless, sintered beads, 2D taper	119 mo (61 to 150)	97.4%	3.9%	96.1% at 10 y
Archibeck (1)	Anatomic hip	Ti, collarless, fiber metal, anatomic	10 y (8 to 11)	100%	9%	100% at 10 y
Sinha (11)	Multilock	Ti, collar, fiber metal, distal flutes nonanatomic	78 mo (60 to 117)	96%	8%	97% at 10 y
Laupacis (7)	Mallory head	Ti, collar, plasma spray, 3D taper	6.3 y (5 to 8.6)	100%	NC	99% at 6 y
Smith (17)[b]	Many stems	Second-generation cement	18.2 y (17 to 20)	NA	NC	81% at 20 y

[a]CLS, cementless locking stem; 2D, two-dimensional; 3D, three-dimensional; Ti, titanium; NC, not considered; PCA, porous coated anatomic; CoCr, cobalt chrome; NA, not applicable.
[b]Patients all ≤50 years old.

seal region of the femur, while cylindrical stems have added rotational stability provided via interference fit in the diaphysis. This chapter deals predominantly with cylindrical-type proximally porous coated implants.

PREOPERATIVE PLANNING

Radiographs of the pelvis and hip should be carefully evaluated with regard to type and severity of disease (e.g., osteoarthritis, rheumatoid arthritis, avascular necrosis, Paget disease). Preoperative templating of radiographs provides an assessment of implant size, type, neck length, and offset; the location of the femoral neck cut; and need for restoration of limb length as discussed in Chapter 14. Specifically, in choosing to use a proximally porous coated cylindrical stem, radiographs are reviewed with emphasis on bone stock (Dorr type A or B) and location and severity of the femoral bow.

SURGERY

The patient is positioned in the lateral decubitus position with the operative side up after the administration of anesthesia. It is critical that all pressure points and traction sites be well padded and protected to prevent neurologic injury at such sites as the axilla and the fibular head. The operative extremity is prepped and draped, leaving the iliac crest to the midthigh visible. Note that flexion of the down hip aids in stabilizing the patient in the lateral position but is associated with flattening of the lumbar spine and flexion of the pelvis. These positional alterations must be accounted for during final component positioning, assessment of range of motion, and stability testing.

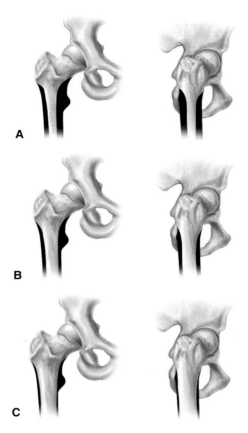

Figure 1. Sketch of Dorr A-, B-, and C-type femurs. Note the thick cortices and fluted shape of the metaphyseal region in Dorr type A femur. Dorr type C femur has thin cortices with an expansive proximal diaphysis and loss of flute shape. Dorr type B has preservation of cortices but some loss of fluted shape. (After LaPorte DM, Mont MA, Hungerford DS. Proximally porous-coated ingrowth prostheses: limits of use. *Orthopedics* 22(12):1157, 1999.)

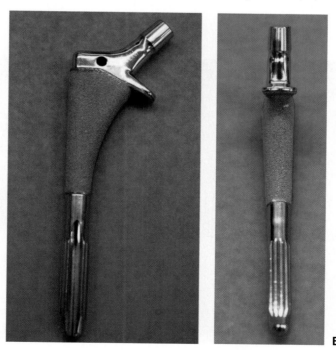

Figure 2. Anterior-posterior and lateral projections of a three-dimensional nonanatomic cylindrical proximally porous coated stem. The proximal portion is a three-dimensional taper while the distal portion is fluted. Note the stem has neutral version and can be used for either a left or right hip.

We routinely and successfully use proximally porous coated implants through a variety of surgical approaches to the hip. For convention, the discussion and images in this chapter are referable to the posterior-lateral approach. The incision is centered over the greater trochanter, extending 3 to 6 cm both proximally and distally. The proximal arm of the incision parallels the posterior boarder of the gluteus medius muscle while the distal arm is centered over the lateral aspect of the femur. The fascia lata is divided sharply in line with the incision, and the gluteus maximus muscle belly is split in line with its fibers. With progressive internal rotation of the hip, the external rotator musculature is put on stretch and dissected from the intertrochanteric line. The external rotators and capsule are reflected in separate layers and tagged for later repair.

Recessing the posterior 5% to 10% of the gluteus medius off the posterior greater trochanter allows visualization of the piriformis tendon all the way to its insertion at the piriformis fossa. This maneuver permits maximal tendon length for later reattachment. The tendon is freed from the underlying capsule and taken sharply from bone. Likewise, the capsule is reflected off the base of the femoral neck with attention to preservation of length (see Fig. 3). Repair of shortened external rotators and/or capsule may cause a postoperative external rotation contracture of the hip.

Femoral neck osteotomy is performed at the preoperatively determined length. Femoral reconstruction follows acetabular reconstruction by first clearing any residual soft tissue from the piriformis fossa and successively opening the femoral canal with a box osteotome and Charnley awl. The piriformis fossa is the superficial landmark most directly in line with the femoral canal and marks the appropriate site for opening the proximal femoral canal.

Retraction of the recessed posterior 5% of the abductor mechanism permits placing the box osteotome in a posterior and lateral position so that it removes the bony insertion site of the piriformis tendon (see Fig. 4). The preoperative anteroposterior (AP) hip radiograph shows the degree to which the trochanter overhangs the femoral canal and indicates the amount of trochanteric bone that must be removed to ensure adequate lateralization of the opening to the femoral canal (see Fig. 5).

Failure to achieve the desired lateral opening to the canal commonly results in varus positioning and undersized femoral stems. Intraoperatively, varus positioning of an

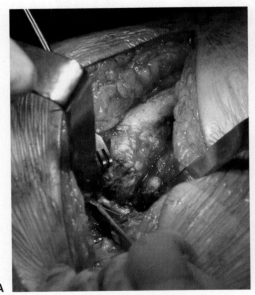
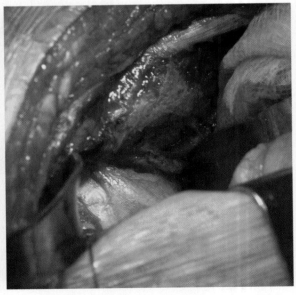

A   B

Figure 3. A: The recessed posterior 5% of the gluteus medius insertion to the greater trochanter and the underlying intact piriformis tendon. **B:** The posterior hip capsule after the piriformis and other external rotators have been dissected from the intertrochanteric line. *(continues)*

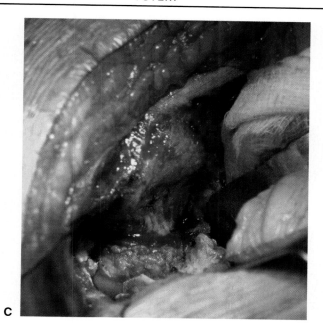

C

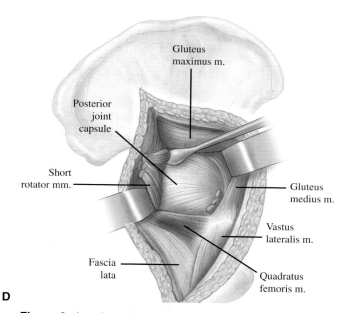

Gluteus
maximus m.

Posterior
joint
capsule

Short
rotator mm.

Gluteus
medius m.

Vastus
lateralis m.

Fascia
lata

Quadratus
femoris m.

D

Figure 3. *(continued)* **C:** The exposed hip once the capsule has also been dissected from the intertrochanteric line. Note no soft tissue remains on the posterior femur as all length was preserved for later repair. **D:** Schematic diagram of the posterior anatomy of the hip. (**D** after Hoppenfeld S. *Surgical Exposures in Orthopaedics: The Anatomic Approach.* 2nd ed. Philadelphia: JB Lippincott Co; 1994: 380.)

undersized femoral component should be suspected when the final implant choice is more than one size smaller than predicted during preoperative templating. Confirmation of adequate lateralization may be obtained by palpating the femoral endosteal transition from diaphyseal to metaphyseal bone. The transition should be smooth. Persistence of a metaphyseal ridge indicates inadequate lateralization.

The femur is prepared by a combination of broaching the metaphysis and reaming the proximal diaphysis. The two processes are performed independently but ultimately prepare the femur to accept a single-size implant. Hence, reaming and broaching are done successively for each increasing size in order to prevent mismatching the metaphysis and

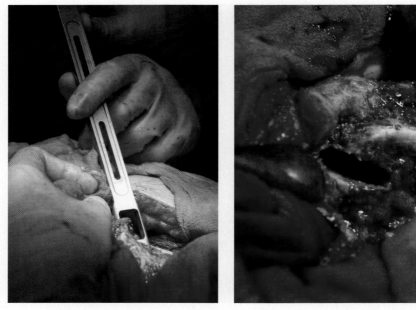

A   B

Figure 4. Opening of the proximal femoral canal with box osteotome. Note the lateral nature of the opening necessary to gain direct in-line access to the canal.

diaphysis. It is extremely important to fully understand the sizing options of the chosen implant, as several manufacturers offer implants with multiple different combinations of metaphyseal and diaphyseal sizing.

The goal of reaming is to machine the endosteal walls of the proximal diaphysis to create a cortical cylinder that can be engaged by the slightly oversized splines/flutes of the final implant and ultimately provide rotational stability. During the reaming process, minimal endosteal cortical bone is removed with straight, sharp reamers. The anterior lateral bow of the femur is encountered during reaming with straight reamers and is best navigated by

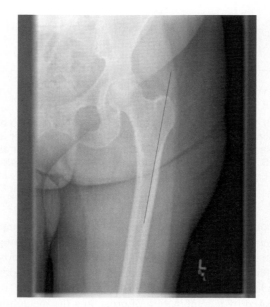

Figure 5. Anterior-posterior radiograph of the hip depicting the magnitude of trochanteric overhang. Trochanteric bone medial to the superimposed line must be removed in order to gain straight access to the canal. Failure to remove this bone may result in varus malpositioning and undersizing of the prosthesis.

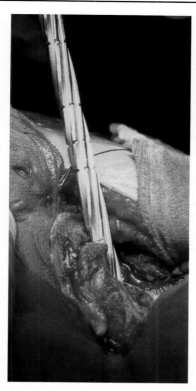

Figure 6. Reaming of the femoral canal with straight reamers. Posterior and lateral pressure aids in negotiating the femoral bow. Note the lateral nature of the reamer and the removal of trochanteric bone.

applying steady posterior and lateral pressure. The final size is signaled by an increased pitch of the power reamer and an increased tactile "chatter" (see Fig. 6). Reaming is usually performed in a line-to-line fashion up to the anticipated final implant diameter. *Familiarity with specific manufacturer recommendations is necessary, as some implants vary with respect to reaming guidelines.*

The goal of broaching is to machine the femoral metaphysis to receive the largest-bodied implant in 15 to 20 degrees of anteversion. In arthritis associated with developmental dysplasia or slipped capital femoral epiphysis, the patient's native femoral neck anteversion may be distorted. Referencing the ipsilateral tibia best assesses appropriate implant version. Each successive broach should be implanted flush with the osteotomized surface of the femoral neck in the desired amount of anteversion. Changing version during the broaching process creates a bony envelope with suboptimal dimensions and suboptimal prosthesis/bone contact. The final size is determined when a properly lateralized broach makes contact with cortical bone in the calcar region. Cortical contact is usually first observed in the anterior medial portion of the neck (see Fig. 7). Manually rotating the final broach should *not* result in visible motion at the bone-prosthesis interface.

Anatomic and nonanatomic cylindrical proximally porous coated designs differ in geometry in the metaphyseal region of the stem, and the broaches for each system reflect these differences. Anatomic stems are designed for right and left use, have larger metaphyseal flares, and have built-in versions that must be accounted for. Nonanatomic stems are straight two- or three-dimensional tapers proximally with neutral version and are intended for use in either left or right hips. As a result, the bodies of anatomic stems may more frequently match the native femoral version and more completely fill the metaphysis. We routinely use nonanatomic, three-dimensional, cylindrical, proximally porous coated stems for the benefit of decreased implant and equipment inventory.

Trial reduction and stability testing are performed prior to implanting the final prosthesis. Forcible reduction maneuvers should be avoided as they can lead to fracture.

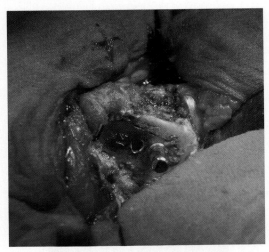

Figure 7. Final broach placement. Note the lateral nature of the broach's shoulder and the anterior medial cortical contact. This broach is appropriately sized, fully seated, and without micromotion during manual rotation.

We define minimal acceptable stability as full flexion without dislocation, a minimum of 45 degrees of internal rotation at 90 degrees of flexion without dislocation, and a minimum of 30 degrees external rotation at 20 degrees hyperextension without dislocation. Dislocation prior to minimal acceptable stability necessitates component repositioning.

The final implant is first seated by hand in the predetermined amount of anteversion and fully lateralized. The distal flutes or splines engage the endosteum once the implant is two thirds of the way down, leaving the implant only 3 to 4 cm proud (see Fig. 8). Changing the implant version at this point should be very difficult. Thus, that the appropriate version is in use must be ensured before further imposition of the implant. The remainder of the implant is impacted by a series of moderate mallet blows. A change in pitch or a visible halt to progress indicates that the implant is completely seated (see Fig. 9).

An implant is likely to be undersized in its cylindrical portion if it is easily implanted by hand so that less than 3 to 4 cm are proud. A larger trial implant should be inserted to assess the distal sizing. The cylindrical portion of the implant is likely larger than the prepared

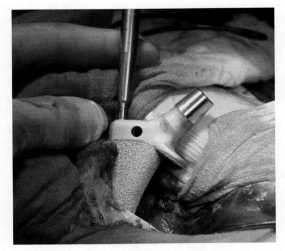

Figure 8. The prosthesis has been manually inserted 3 to 4 cm proud. The distal flutes have engaged the endosteal surface of the proximal diaphysis and provide resistance to further seating. The remainder of the prosthesis must be inserted with mallet blows. Note the lateral positioning of the prosthesis into trochanteric bone.

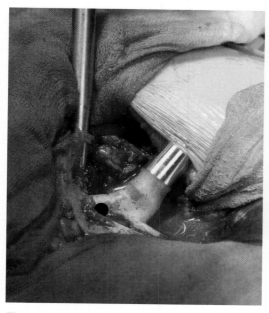
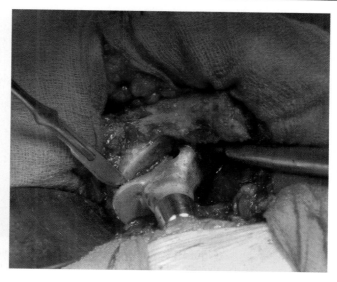

A   **B**

Figure 9. The prosthesis is fully seated and stable to rotational testing. The prosthesis is appropriately lateralized, is canal filling, and has complete collar-calcar contact as indicated by the inability to pass a blade between bone and prosthesis.

canal if the implant cannot be manually implanted to this depth. If this is the case, then it may be necessary to repeat the reaming process to upsize the distal endosteal cylinder. When malleting the final implant into position, femoral fracture should be suspected when slow progress is followed by rapid advance.

Prosthetic collar contact with the bony calcar should not be misinterpreted as evidence of appropriate final seating of a well-sized prosthesis. Undersized components achieve prosthetic collar contact with calcar bone but may remain rotationally unstable. Micromotion with rotational stress indicates instability.

Before wound closure, the posterior capsule is sutured through drill holes to the intertrochanteric line, and the piriformis tendon is sutured to the reflected posterior portion of the gluteus medius (see Fig. 10). The capsule and piriformis should be repaired with the hip in 15 degrees of internal rotation to avoid producing an external rotation contracture.

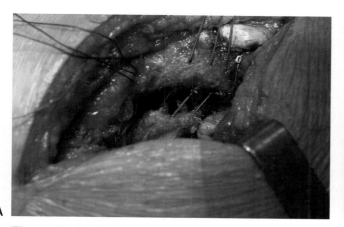
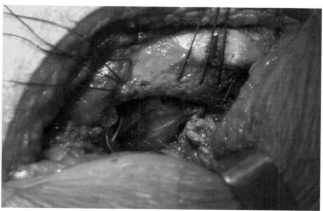

A   **B**

Figure 10. A: The posterior capsule is sutured through drill holes in the posterior intertrochanteric line. **B:** The suture is pulled taut and tied with the hip in 15 degrees of internal rotation. The piriformis is repaired to the reflected 5% of the posterior gluteus medius insertion.

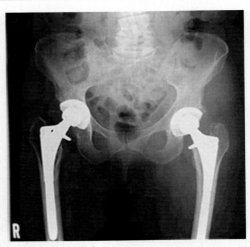

Figure 11. Immediate postoperative radiograph of left hip replacement with nonanatomic cylindrical stem. The right hip was replaced 3 years earlier and shows some calcar rounding, streaming trabeculae, greater trochanteric osteopenia, and slight nondivergent lines at the noningrowth surface. These findings are all consistent with a stable, ingrown stem at 3 years.

POSTOPERATIVE MANAGEMENT

The patient is transferred to a standard orthopaedic unit and routinely monitored for 3 to 4 days. Mobilization begins on the first postoperative day under the supervision of a certified physical therapist and includes partial weight bearing with an assistive device. Posterior hip precautions are observed, but adequate posterior capsule and piriformis repairs obviate the need for abduction braces in our practice. Drains, if used, are discontinued at 24 to 48 hours. Intravenous antibiotics are used for 24 hours to protect against potential gram-positive skin pathogens. Pharmacological and mechanical prophylaxis is used to prevent venous thrombosis.

Partial weight bearing with an assistive device is continued for 6 weeks. At 6 weeks, assistive devices are weaned under the supervision of outpatient physical therapists, and full weight bearing is permitted. Pharmacological prophylaxis for venous thrombosis is continued for 3 weeks postoperatively. Posterior hip precautions are observed for 3 months.

Routine follow-up visits are scheduled for 6 weeks, 3 months, 6 months, and annually postoperatively. Routine radiographs are obtained at each visit. Specific radiographic changes continue to appear for several years in association with bony ingrown, proximally porous coated, cylindrical stems. The anticipated changes include calcar rounding, greater trochanteric osteopenia, trabeculae streaming toward ingrowth surfaces, nondivergent radiolucencies about noningrowth surfaces, and proximal diaphyseal cortical hypertrophy (see Fig. 11) (1,4,6,11,14).

COMPLICATIONS

Complications germane to hip surgery in general also apply to total hip arthroplasty performed using cylindrical proximally porous coated implants. These complications include venous thrombosis, pulmonary embolism, bleeding, infection, dislocation, limb length discrepancy, and limp. Complications specifically related to proximally porous coated implants include the following.

Fracture

Fracture may occur at the greater trochanter, the calcar, or the diaphysis of the femur during implantation. Fracture of the greater trochanter may be related to overaggressive lateralization or to broach impingement during removal. Nondisplaced fractures with an intact tissue sleeve may be treated with non–weight bearing for 6 weeks and an abduction orthosis. Displaced fractures require fixation with wires and/or a plate as well as non–weight bearing. Calcar splits can be related to oversizing, inadequate broaching for the chosen implant size, or failure to match the implant's version to the prepared version. Calcar splits may be treated simply with a cerclage wire and protected weight bearing provided that adequate rotational stability is achieved in the diaphyseal portion of the construct. Shaft fractures require fixation with a combination of wires and plates and prolonged non–weight bearing until adequate healing is radiographically observed.

Malposition

Malposition may be with regard to version or varus/valgus. Improper version usually results in instability and is detected during stability testing. Increasing the anteversion leads to increased posterior stability, and decreasing the anteversion leads to increased anterior stability. If changes in implant version result in micromotion with torsion, then alternate reconstruction options like cemented femoral arthroplasty may be necessary. Implant valgus malposition is unlikely, but varus malposition is common. Varus positioning is due to inadequate lateralization of the femoral component and may result in undersized implants and instability.

Thigh Pain

Thigh pain, more commonly associated with fully porous coated devices, may occur in proximally porous coated devices. Treatment is difficult for painful ingrown prosthesis and is centered on activity modification. Loose prostheses should be revised (1–10,16).

Failure of Bony Ingrowth/Ongrowth

Failure of bony ingrowth/ongrowth may be a combination of mechanical (poor initial stability) and biologic factors (history of radiation or metabolic bone disease). The source of failure should be addressed at the time of revision (12,13).

Lysis

Osteolysis is a well-described process of particle-induced, cell-mediated bone loss. Bone loss should be limited to the "effective joint space" or wherever lysis-inducing particles may gain access to bone. Prostheses with a complete biologic purse string of osseous integration with the prosthetic ingrowth/ongrowth surface should prevent particle access to the femoral endosteum and limit distal osteolysis (1–11).

RECOMMENDED READING

1. Archibeck MJ, Berger RA, Jacobs JJ, et al. Second-generation cementless total hip arthroplasty: eight to eleven year results. *J Bone Joint Surg Am* 83(11):1666–1673, 2001.
2. Bourne RB, Rorabeck CH, Patterson JJ, et al. Tapered titanium cementless total hip replacements: a 10 to 13-year followup study. *Clin Orthop Relat Res* 393:112–120, 2001.
3. Cimbrello EG, Pardos AC, Madero R, et al. Total hip arthroplasty with use of the cementless Zweymuller alloclassic system: a 10 to 13 year follow-up study. *J Bone Joint Surg Am* 85(2):296–303, 2003.
4. Hellman EJ, Capello WN, Feinberg JR. Omnifit cementless total hip arthroplasty: a 10-year average followup. *Clin Orthop Relat Res* 364:164–174, 1999.
5. Hofmann AA, Feign ME, Klauser W, et al. Cementless primary total hip arthroplasty with a tapered, proximally porous-coated titanium prosthesis: a 4 to 8 year retrospective review. *J Arthroplasty* 15(7):833–839, 2000.
6. Kawamura H, Dunbar MJ, Murray P, et al. The porous coated anatomic total hip replacement: a 10 to 14 year follow-up study of a cementless total hip arthroplasty. *J Bone Joint Surg Am* 83(9):1333–1338, 2001.

7. Laupacis A, Bourne R, Rorabeck C, et al. Comparison of total hip arthroplasty performed with and without cement: a randomized trial. *J Bone Joint Surg Am* 84(10):1823–1828, 2002.

8. McLaughlin JR, Lee KR. Total hip arthroplasty with an uncemented femoral component: excellent results at ten-year follow-up. *J Bone Joint Surg Br* 79(6):900–907, 1997.

9. Purtill JJ, Rothman RH, Hozack WJ, et al. Total hip arthroplasty using two different cementless tapered stems. *Clin Orthop Relat Res* 393:121–127, 2001.

10. Romagnoli S. Press-fit hip arthroplasty: a European alternative. *J Arthroplasty* 17(4 suppl 1):108–112, 2002.

11. Sinha RK, Danton DS, Yeon HB. Primary total hip arthroplasty with a proximally porous-coated femoral stem. *J Bone Joint Surg Am* 86(6):1254–1261, 2004.

12. Burke DW, O'Connor DO, Zalenski EB, et al. Micromotion of cemented and uncemented femoral components. *J Bone Joint Surg Br* 73(1):33–37, 1991.

13. Pillar RM, Lee JM, Maniatopoulos C. Observations on the effect of movement on bone ingrowth into porous-surfaced implants. *Clin Orthop Relat Res* 208:108–113, 1986.

14. Martell JM, Pierson RH, Jacobs JJ, et al. Primary total hip reconstruction with a titanium fiber-coated prosthesis inserted without cement. *J Bone Joint Surg Am* 75(4):554–571, 1993.

15. Mulroy WF, Estok DM, Harris WH. Total hip arthroplasty with use of so-called second-generation cementing techniques. *J Bone Joint Surg Am* 77(12):1845–1852, 1995.

16. Engh CA Jr, Culpepper II WJ, Engh CA. Long term results of use of the anatomic medullary locking prosthesis in total hip arthroplasty. *J Bone Joint Surg Am* 79:177–184, 1997.

17. Smith SW, Estok DM II, Harris WH. Total hip arthroplasty with use of second-generation cementing techniques. An eighteen-year-average follow-up study. *J Bone Joint Surg Am* 80(11):1632–1640, 1998.

19

The Cemented Acetabulum

Amar S. Ranawat and Chitranjan S. Ranawat

INDICATIONS/CONTRAINDICATIONS

Cemented acetabular fixation has fallen out of favor in the U.S. marketplace over the last decade as there has been a marked shift to cementless fixation. The reasons for this are multifactorial but include both unacceptably high rates of loosening associated with cemented metal-backed sockets (see Fig. 1) and the relative ease of insertion of press-fit components. As a result, an entire generation of orthopaedic surgeons in this country has not been exposed to the technique of cemented fixation of an all-polyethylene cup. Nonetheless, it remains the overwhelming mode of acetabular fixation worldwide. The reasons for this are simple: Cemented all-poly sockets are inexpensive, they are approximately one third the cost of their noncemented counterparts and, using proper technique and appropriate indications, they are durable (see Fig. 2).

At the Ranawat Orthopaedic Center in New York, the indications for cemented total hip arthroplasty with an all-polyethylene acetabular socket include all patients greater than 60 years of age with osteoarthritis of the hip. We reserve the use of press-fit components for patients with excessive acetabular bleeding after reaming, extensive cyst formation, and/or weak cancellous bone such as in inflammatory arthropathies, dysplasia, or protrusio deformities. The use of cement is also generally contraindicated in patients with significant cardiopulmonary disease to minimize embolization secondary to cement pressurization. Using these criteria, 20-year survivorship of cemented all-poly sockets is 98%.

PREOPERATIVE PLANNING

Evaluate all patients with history and physical examination and proceed to radiographic analysis. At our center, all hip patients are evaluated with a hip series that consists of an anteroposterior (AP) pelvis including the proximal one-third femora, a

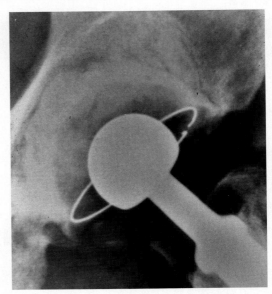

Figure 1. Evidence of radiographic loosening of an all-poly cup with early demarcation in all three zones.

standard AP view of the affected hip, a false profile view of the affected hip, and AP and lateral views of the lumbar spine.

Once indicated for total hip arthroplasty, counsel all patients with regard to fixation techniques and alternative bearing surfaces in addition to the risks of potential perioperative complications.

As the final step prior to surgery, it is imperative to template the hip. Draw a line connecting the bottom of the teardrops on the AP pelvis. Mark a point 1 cm lateral to the most inferior point of the teardrop. Draw a 45-degree line from this point toward the outer edge of the acetabulum. Determine where this line crosses the lateral margin of the acetabulum (i.e., inside the bone/outside the bone/flush with the bone). Take into account any osteophytes or cysts. Use manufactured templates to estimate socket size in both AP and false profile views to preserve bone where possible and avoid overmedialization. Determine the center of rotation (COR) of the femoral head. Measure the distance from the superior aspect of the lesser trochanter to the COR, also known as the LTC distance. Next, identify the center of the femoral canal. Determine leg length discrepancies, offset, canal diameter, and neck osteotomy site using manufactured templates. Record the measurements for intraoperative comparison.

SURGERY

The surgical technique as described by the senior author has been well documented. As mentioned previously, hypotensive, epidural anesthesia (defined as mean arterial blood pressure ≤50 mmHg) is mandatory to achieve a dry cancellous bed to allow for cement intrusion during pressurization.

Current design parameters allow for a high-walled, highly cross-linked polyethylene component with a 28-mm inner diameter to mate with a chromium-cobalt femoral head (see Fig. 3).

Exposure is accomplished through the posterior approach to facilitate acetabular visualization, which is further enhanced by release of the insertion of the gluteus maximus tendon, release of the reflected head of the rectus femoris, and excision of the labrum (see Figs. 4 and 5). After trapezoidal capsulotomy, an Aufranc retractor is placed just inferior to the transverse ligament at the level of the obturator foramen. Attention is given to the identification and preservation of the transverse ligament, which aides in containment and

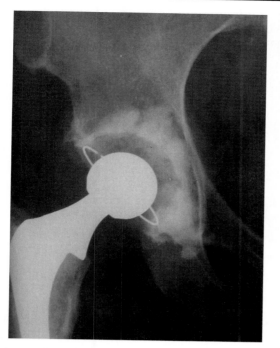

A

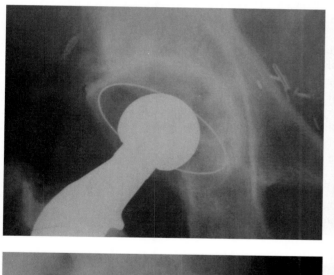

B

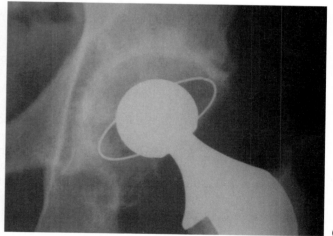

C

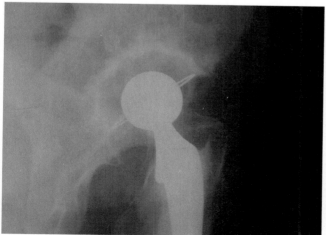

D

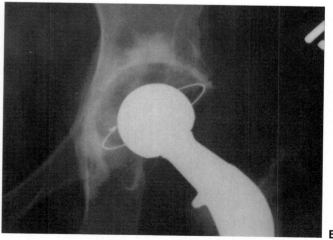

E

Figure 2. Five examples of excellent cement interdigitation in all three zones.

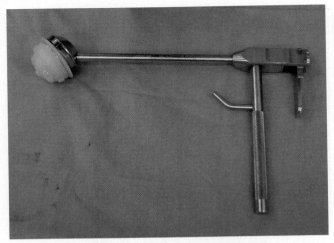

Figure 3. Highly cross-linked polyethylene and cup holder.

pressurization of cement. A curved C-retractor is placed anteriorly, bringing the femur forward and out of the field of view. A Steinman pin is placed superiorly to retract the gluteus medius muscle. The exposure is completed with a narrow, 90-degree bent Hohmann retractor placed in the ischium in the interval between the capsule and labral remnant (see Fig. 6).

Circumferential reaming commences in a stepwise fashion until the blush of cancellous bleeding bone is noted in both anterior and posterior columns where the pubis and ischial tuberosity meet the pelvis. Medialization to the inner mantle is avoided in order to preserve medial cancellous bone. Trial fitting using a hemispherical device allows for optimization of orientation (40-degree lateral opening and 15-degree anteversion) and assessment of cement mantle (trial should spin easily between two fingers to accommodate for adequate thickness of cement mantle) (see Fig. 7).

Multiple fixation holes are burred into the superior dome in the area of the cancellous bone of the posterior column, and two larger cavities are created in the pubis and ischium to facilitate macrointerlock (see Fig. 8). Pulsatile lavage is used to remove blood and fat debris, and the bed is dried with sponges and pressure (see Fig. 9). Heated cement is allowed to cure to a doughy consistency during the setting phase (see Fig. 10). Cement is then introduced

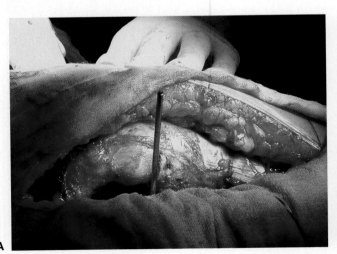

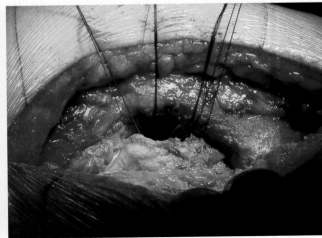

A   B

Figure 4. Posterior exposure.

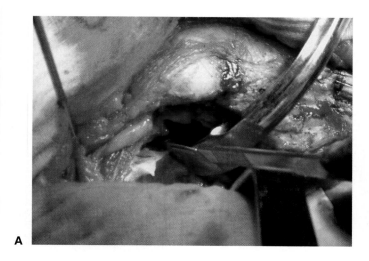

A

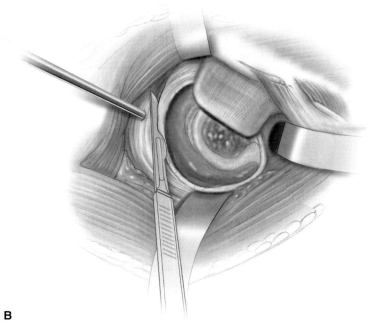

B

Figure 5. Release of reflected head of rectus femoris.

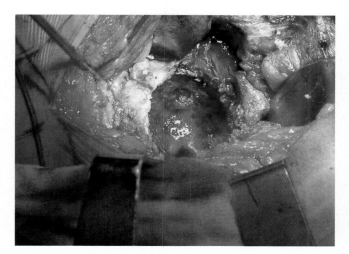

Figure 6. Acetabular exposure with retractors.

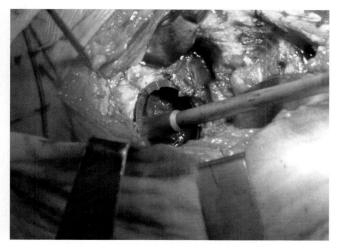

Figure 7. Acetabular trial (should spin easily).

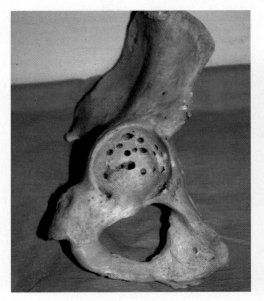

Figure 8. Multiple fixation holes.

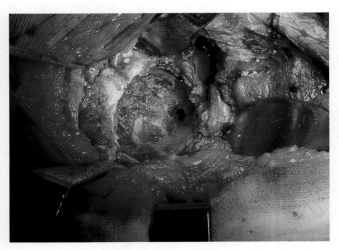

Figure 9. Dry cancellous bed.

into the bony cancellous bed and pressurized using a special bulb syringe device to enhance microinterlock via cement intrusion (see Figs. 11 and 12). Care is taken to remove excess cement from the inferior teardrop area prior to insertion of the all-poly cup (see Fig. 13). The cup is inserted with a cup holder, engaging inferiorly first and then in a medial-superior direction (see Fig. 14). Cement is reinforced over the superior edge with the finger, and final positioning is achieved with the cup holder. Removal of the cup holder allows for circumferential inspection, final adjustments of orientation, and removal of excess cement. The cup is held in place with medial pressure, and the cement is allowed to polymerize (see Fig. 15).

Attention can now be turned to the femur for preparation of femoral component cementation as described elsewhere.

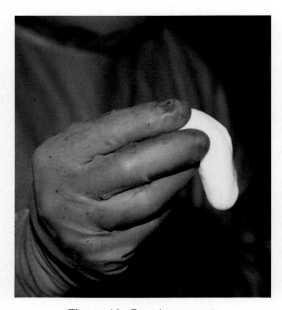

Figure 10. Doughy cement.

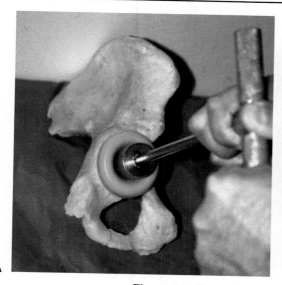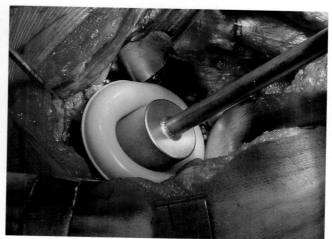

A   B

Figure 11. Pressurization with bulb syringe.

POSTOPERATIVE MANAGEMENT

The postoperative total hip protocol at our institution uses a multimodal pain management program combined with immediate weight bearing as tolerated. Deep venous thrombosis prophylaxis relies on operative time less than 1 hour, early ambulation, mechanical compression, and warfarin sodium (Coumadin). All patients receive Doppler ultrasound on postoperative day 3. Patients with negative tests are placed on aspirin; otherwise they are treated appropriately. Average hospital length of stay is less than 4 days. With this protocol, the majority of patients are walking unassisted and without limp by 6 weeks.

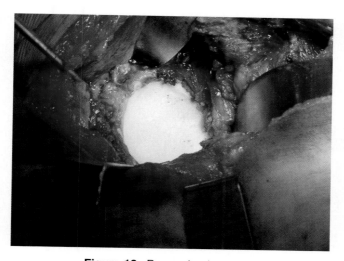

Figure 12. Pressurized cement.

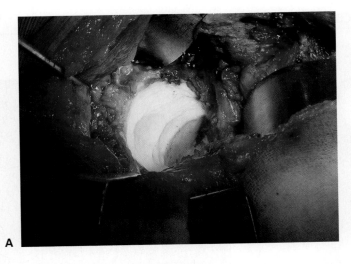

A

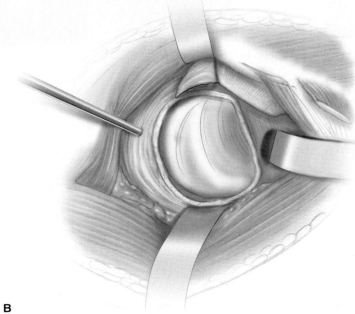

B

Figure 13. Elevation of cement out of teardrop.

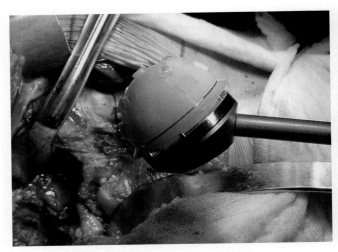

Figure 14. Insertion of cup with holder.

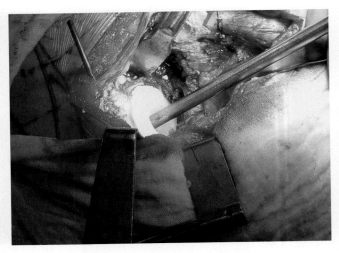

Figure 15. Awaiting polymerization.

Table 1. *Failure Rate—Cemented Cups*

Author, Date	Prosthesis	Hips	Follow-up Minimum	Revision Rate (%)
Stauffer, 1982	Charnley	231	10	3
Ranawat, 1988	Mixed (old)	50	10	2
Ranawat, 1988	Mixed (new)	50	5	0
Ranawat, 1995	Mixed	236	5	0.8
Severt, 1991	Mixed	75	4	5.3
Ritter, 1992	Charnley	238	10	4.6
Wroblewski, 1993	Charnley	193	18	3
Mulroy, 1995	CAD, HD-2	105	10	5
Delee, 1976	Charnley	141	Mean 10	NR (9)
Cornell, 1986	Mixed	101	4	2
Older, 1986	Charnley	153	Mean 11	2
Poss, 1988	Mixed	267	11.9	3.1
Fowler, 1988	Exeter	426	11	3.9
McCoy, 1988	Charnley	32	14.4	3
Kavanagh, 1989	Charnley	333	15	NR (14)
Hozack, 1990	Charnley	590	Mean 6.8	0.6

RESULTS

The long-term results of cemented all-poly sockets are excellent, especially within a defined indication. Revision rates at 10 to 20 years vary between 2% and 14% for osteoarthritis (see Table 1). Similarly, radiographic loosening over the same time period ranges from 6% to 23%. Nonetheless, confusion has arisen regarding their durability since many studies focusing on the long-term survivorship of cemented cups were often confounded with differing designs, diagnoses, and definitions of failure. Using the historical literature, if one were to eliminate 32-mm heads, metal-backed sockets, rheumatoid arthritis, developmental dysplasia of the hip, and revisions from consideration, the long-term results of cemented all-poly cups are impressive. In fact, our published data support an 88% survivorship of 236 hips with cemented all-poly cups at 15 years for all comers, which increases to 98% survivorship of 160 hips at 20 years for osteoarthritis alone (see Figs. 16 and 17).

Using direct compression molded polyethylene, wear rates have been documented as low as 0.075 mm/year. As a result, 10-year follow-up data in 235 consecutive hips have yielded no clinical failures (see Fig. 18).

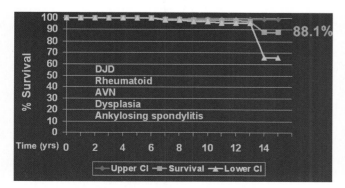

Figure 16. Fifteen-year cemented cup survivorship, all sockets (*N* = 236).

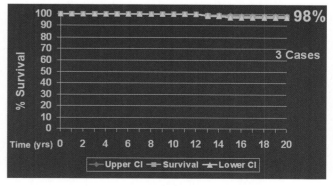

Figure 17. Twenty-year cemented cup survivorship, only degenerative joint disease (*N* = 160).

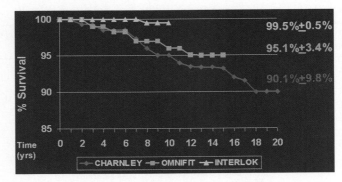

Figure 18. Ten-year cemented cup survivorship, direct compression molded.

RECOMMENDED READING

1. Creighton MG, Callaghan JJ, Olejniczak JP, et al. Total hip arthroplasty with cement in patients who have rheumatoid arthritis. A minimum ten-year follow-up study. *J Bone Joint Surg Am* 80:1439–1446, 1998.
2. Herberts P, Malchau H. How outcome studies have changed total hip arthroplasty practices in Sweden. *Clin Orthop Relat Res* 344:44–60, 1997.
3. Jasty M, Goetz DD, Bragdon CR, et al. Wear of polyethylene acetabular components in total hip arthroplasty. An analysis of one hundred and twenty-eight components retrieved at autopsy or revision operations. *J Bone Joint Surg Am* 79:349–358, 1997.
4. Malchau H, Herberts P, Ahnfelt L. Prognosis of total hip replacement in Sweden. Follow-up of 92,675 operations performed 1978–1990. *Acta Orthop Scand* 64(5):497–506, 1993.
5. Ortiguera CJ, Pulliam IT, Cabanela ME. Total hip arthroplasty for osteonecrosis: matched-pair analysis of 188 hips with long-term follow-up. *J Arthroplasty* 14(1):21–28, 1999.
6. Ranawat CS, Beaver WB, Sharrock NE, et al. Effect of hypotensive epidural anaesthesia on acetabular cement-bone fixation in total hip arthroplasty. *J Bone Joint Surg Br* 73:779–782, 1991.
7. Ranawat CS, Deshmukh RG, Peters LE, Umlas ME. Prediction of the long-term durability of all-polyethylene cemented sockets. *Clin Orthop Relat Res* 317:89–105, 1995.
8. Ranawat CS, Peters LE, Umlas ME. Fixation of the acetabular component. The case for cement. *Clin Orthop Relat Res* 344:207–215, 1997.
9. Ranawat CS, Rothman RH. All change is not progress. *J Arthroplasty* 13:121–122, 1998.
10. Schmalzried TP, Kwong LM, Jasty M, et al. The mechanism of loosening of cemented acetabular components in total hip arthroplasty. Analysis of specimens retrieved at autopsy. *Clin Orthop Relat Res* 274:60–78, 1992.
11. Sochart DH, Porter ML. The long-term results of Charnley low-friction arthroplasty in young patients who have congenital dislocation, degenerative osteoarthrosis or rheumatoid arthritis. *J Bone Joint Surg Am* 79:1599–1617, 1997.

20

The Press-fit (Ingrowth) Socket

Douglas E. Padgett and Alejandro González Della Valle

Acetabular component fixation is crucial to the long-term success of any total hip arthroplasty. Successful acetabular fixation with acrylic cement requires exacting techniques of bone preparation and anatomic placement (1). While initial fixation is excellent, longer-term loosening has been noted by many. Loosening of a cemented socket appears to be a biologic occurrence with macrophage- and cytokine-induced osteolysis. While clearly polyethylene plays a role, particulate polymethylmethacrylate has been implicated as well. Cementless acetabular fixation has become attractive because of its ease of use as well as its clinical track record of success (2,3). Socket placement can be adjusted to available host bone location, and cranial placement (the so-called high hip center) does not appear to adversely effect results. In addition to socket location, intraoperative flexibility such as the ability to change orientation after initial insertion, the use of modular liners for stability, and the use of adjuvant screw fixation for supplement lend support for uncemented socket fixation.

INDICATIONS/CONTRAINDICATIONS

Predictable biologic fixation involves two aspects: the implant and host biologic response. The implant requisites include a biologically friendly surface, intimate host bone–implant apposition, and rigid implant stability. The host requirement for press-fit (ingrowth) fixation involves a process of biologic incorporation akin to that of fracture healing. The initial phases include the formation of hematoma adjacent to the porous substrate, which then undergoes a transformation from fibrous tissue to woven bone and ultimately to mature lamellar bone (see Fig. 1). Therefore, there is a need for healthy bone tissue; patients with adequate pelvic support and healthy bone are candidates for press-fit fixation on the socket side. In our hands, this represents the overwhelming majority of patients.

Conversely, any condition that would alter the process of biologic fixation would raise doubts over the predictability of press-fit fixation. These conditions include severe metabolic bone disease (i.e., osteomalacia), irradiated bone (i.e., post pelvic irradiation), metastatic disease, and perhaps the setting of pelvic Paget disease.

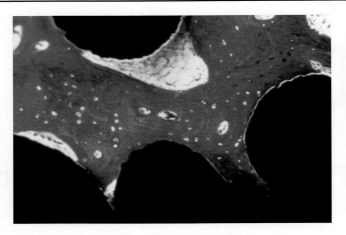

Figure 1. Histology of an ingrown uncemented prosthesis after 6 months demonstrates pore filling with mature lamellar bone in intimate contact with the metallic implant.

PREOPERATIVE PLANNING

The specifics of the evaluation and indications for surgery have been presented earlier. It is anticipated that the history of the patient's symptoms, appropriate findings on physical examination, and confirmatory radiographic findings support the performance of total hip arthroplasty. Laboratory analysis paying particular attention to hematocrit, coagulation status, and chemistry profile can never be emphasized enough. We have on several occasions identified patients with myeloma, coagulopathies, and other significant medical morbidities simply on the basis of these exams.

Preoperative radiographic evaluation includes an anteroposterior (AP) radiograph centered on the pubis and true AP and lateral of the affected hip. Socket-specific parameters include the determination of acetabular location, the presence of socket dysplasia, acetabular osteophytes, segmental bone loss, and the presence and location of subarticular cysts. Templating begins with drawing the interteardrop line. The teardrops are the most consistent radiographic feature least sensitive to pelvic rotation. From the base of the teardrop, a 40-degree line is drawn to the superolateral margin of the acetabulum. This represents desired acetabular component insertion. At this point, acetabular overlays are placed: Templates should be placed with the inferior border of the cup approximating the base of the teardrop and angulated on the 40-degree inclination line. The size of the template should reach the subchondral bone of the acetabulum, but the medial extent of the template should not violate Kohler's line (ilioischial line). We prefer to draw the outline of the anticipated cup directly on the radiograph (see Fig. 2) (6).

A recording of the size of anticipated socket, the new center of rotation, and the relative amount of uncovering (if any) of the implant is important. In cases of dysplasia, it is not uncommon to have 20% of the socket covered. An appropriate template for the femoral component is now performed (6).

SURGERY

General Principles

While "minimally invasive surgery" or less invasive procedures are becoming the trend, the long-term success of total joint arthroplasty is contingent upon the precision and accuracy with which we place our components. In general terms, as wide exposure as necessary to allow accurate socket preparation and insertion is encouraged. We tend to favor the posterolateral approach because of its more anatomic dissection and the general

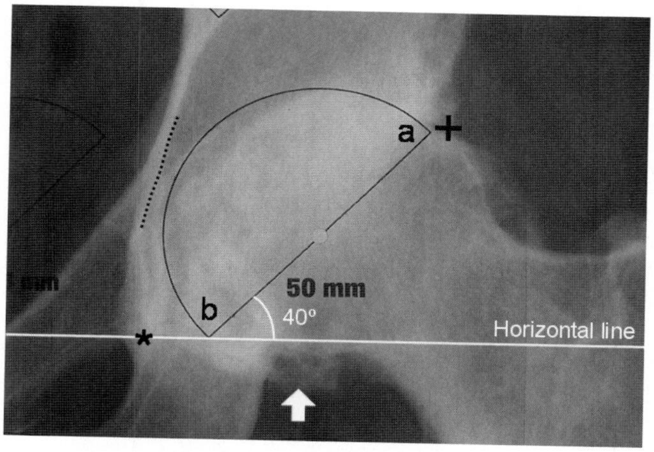

Figure 2. After drawing a horizontal line (*white line*) through the base of the teardrops, the cup should be sized so that when the template is placed with cup opening at 40 degrees of inclination, the inferior border of the cup is level with the reference line and the medial border approximates the ilioischial line (*dotted line*), providing adequate lateral coverage with minimum removal of the supportive subchondral bone. The acetabular silhouette should be drawn on the radiograph with a soft pencil. The relationship between the superolateral margin of the bony acetabulum (*plus*) and the superolateral border of the shell (*a*) should be reproduced during cup insertion. Reproducing the relationship between the inferomedial border of the shell (*b*) and the base of the teardrop (*asterisk*) is helpful in optimizing cup positioning as well and avoids accidental vertical placement of the shell. Osteophytes to be removed after cup insertion should be recorded (*white arrow*).

ability to make it more extensile as needed. While the specifics of the posterolateral approach were discussed in Section II, the key in our minds is the ability to translate the femur anteriorly. Inability to get the femur forward will limit exposure and may impede the use of reamers and socket implantation.

There are two maneuvers that greatly facilitate anterior translation when encountering difficulty. The first is to perform a partial release of the femoral insertion of the gluteus maximus tendon. The second is to release the reflected head of the rectus tendon off the superior acetabulum. These two gestures will get the femur forward.

Primary Osteoarthritis

We try to identify all osteophytes suspected from radiographic analysis. The labrum must be completely resected at this time. Infolded labral tissue will prevent both reamers and the socket component from fully seating. At times, the outer surface of the labrum is calcified and cannot be excised until after initial reaming. This is verified at the check prior to component insertion. Prior to reaming, remove the pulvinar to identify the medial aspect of the acetabulum (see Figs. 3–5). Often, a medial acetabular osteophyte is present, and reaming through this osteophyte should proceed until the true medial wall is encountered. We also will identify the entrance into the obturator foramen. This area is the region of the radiographic teardrop. Socket placement will be judged relative to this point. It is not uncommon for there to be bleeding from this point. This is the ascending branch of the obturator artery, and it should be cauterized. At this time, reaming to the outer table of the medial wall is performed. When doing this via the posterolateral approach in a patient lying in the lateral decubitus position, the reamer will be perpendicular to the floor. Once the medial wall is reached, the reamer angle is changed to proceed in 40 degrees of abduction and 20 to 25 degrees of anteversion. Medial reaming should proceed with caution. Sharp reamers and soft bone are a recipe for disaster. Acetabular preparation is based upon the patient remaining in the lateral decubitus position. Verify this: Pelvic shifting is quite common, and adjustments need to be made accordingly.

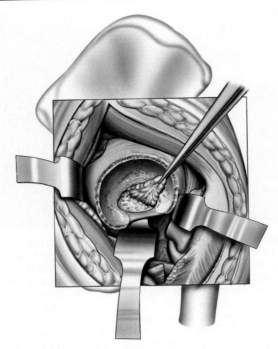

Figure 3. Prior to reaming, remove the pulvinar to identify the medial aspect of the acetabulum.

Concentrically larger hemispherical reaming then proceeds with the reamers oriented to the desired component position. Reaming to size occurs when subchondral bone is exposed, and healthy bleeding host bone is visualized. At this point, the acetabular bed should be inspected for subchondral cysts, which are curetted and packed with graft, and any soft tissue such as retained labrum, which might interfere with socket seating. The ultimate size implant to insert is based upon surgeon preference. Underreaming by 1 to 2 mm has been promoted as a way of enhancing initial component stability. In general, we favor this technique. We currently use a porous shell with limited screw holes (a "cluster hole" shell) (3). This socket allows visual inspection to confirm that the cup is completely

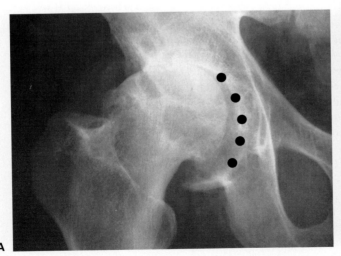
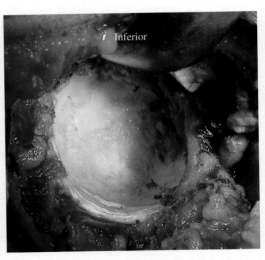

Figure 4. When a medial osteophyte is present (*dotted line*), the teardrop is covered. Reaming through the medial osteophyte to expose the teardrop is mandatory to restore the anatomic center of rotation.

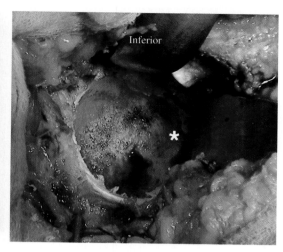

Figure 5. The medial osteophyte has been removed, and the base of the teardrop is clearly visualized (*asterisk*). An Aufranc retractor has been placed distal to it.

seated medially. In addition, if socket stability is questionable, adjuvant screw insertion in the "safe zones" can be performed (4).

If the acetabular component is being held up because of dense sclerotic acetabular rim bone, ream the rim of the socket with the reamer matching the component size. This peripheral ream will enable the socket to be seated. If the socket seems "less stable" than desired, the use of an adjuvant screw is warranted.

Once the real component is inserted, verification of position using a commercial socket holder is useful. We have found that on average, these devices give useful information regarding abduction angles, assuming that the patient has not rotated during the procedure. Identify and remove all peripheral osteophytes. Verify socket position relative to the "teardrop" (the entryway into the obturator foramen) (Fig. 5). Cephalad placement of the cup is common, and this may lead to overall shortening. Significant cephalad placement may need to be adjusted on the femoral side. The provisional liner or the final liner (polyethylene, metal, or ceramic) is inserted at this time, and femoral preparation is begun.

Developmental Dysplasia

Ingrowth socket use has made the performance of total hip arthroplasty in the patient with dysplasia much easier to perform. Historically, cemented socket fixation required superolateral bone graft insertion and cementation of an all-polyethylene cup (1). With cementless fixation, two options for socket reconstruction are available: traditional anatomic placement at the level of the teardrop with bulk autogenous/allograft bone graft placed superiorly or the use of a porous implant at a higher hip center.

In situations of significant dysplasia (Crowe III or IV), the degree of bone loss is estimated from the preoperative radiograph and verified intraoperatively. The defect is almost always anterosuperior, and the supporting lateral lip of the acetabulum is deficient (see Fig. 6). The amount of coverage needed can be estimated by initially using a hemispherical reamer *at the level of the teardrop* (see Figs. 7–9). We will prepare the bed at this level and note the amount of uncovering of the reamer shell. At this time, grafting is performed. Host femoral head is an excellent source of graft for this area. The femoral head is denuded of any remaining articular cartilage with the use of a high-speed burr. A matching surface is sculpted on the pelvic side using either a burr or a small acetabular reamer. The femoral head is then initially fixed with larger-diameter K-wires or Steinmann pins. Do not place

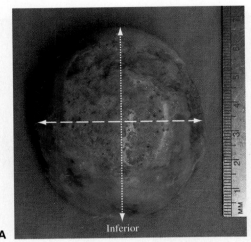
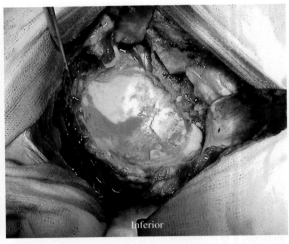

A   B

Figure 6. In the dysplastic femoral head the anteroposterior diameter *(dashed line)* is smaller that the cephalocaudal diameter *(dotted line)*. Ideally, a small-diameter cup (slightly larger than the anteroposterior diameter) should be templated and implanted in a near-anatomic position.

any screws at this time, as the site of fixation often needs to be changed because of reaming of graft. Once the graft is in place, we use a high-speed burr to contour the general shape of the graft and then insert the reamers. If graft position and reamer position appear anatomic, fix the graft with at least two cancellous screws with washers (see Fig. 10). The actual cementless shell can be inserted at this time. We favor the use of at least one adjuvant screw for support. Because of the nature of this reconstruction, delayed weight bearing until 2 months is recommended.

The alternative method of reconstruction is the "high hip center." In this type of reconstruction, a smaller-diameter shell is placed directly upon host bone, resulting in often

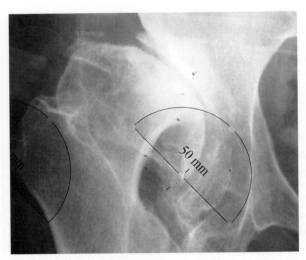

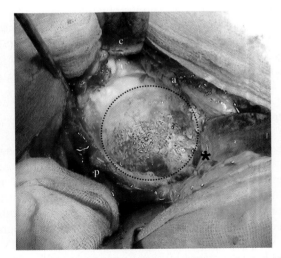

Figure 7. Small-diameter cup templated in a near-anatomic position. Though the lateral cup seems excessively uncovered, the well-developed posterior wall in the dysplastic acetabulum will generally allow for adequate coverage in the posterolateral aspect of the acetabulum. Depending on the coverage achieved, cup fixation can be supplemented with screws, coverage can be optimized with a bulk autograft of the patient's femoral head, or the cup can be positioned slightly proximally (the so-called "high-hip-center technique").

Figure 8. After clearly identifying the teardrop *(asterisk)* and placing a retractor distally, reaming should be done in the anatomic or near-anatomic position *(dotted line)*. In the dysplastic acetabulum, the anterior wall *(a)* is usually deficient, and the C-retractor *(c)* should be placed in a more cephalic position. The well-developed posterior wall *(p)* generally allows for adequate coverage of a small cup.

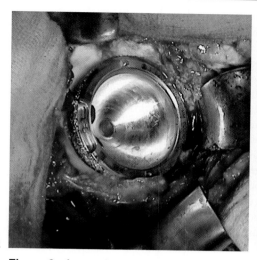
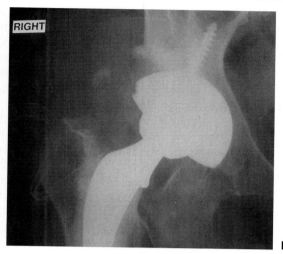

Figure 9. A cup placed in a near-anatomic position. When less than 30% of the cup is uncovered, the fixation can be supplemented with screws. (Courtesy of Dr. Eduardo A. Salvati.)

complete host bone coverage. However, since the defect of bone is superior, the socket is reamed into the remaining host bone at a more cephalad level. This greatly impacts leg lengths, and appropriate intervention on the femoral side needs to be made. The keys to success of the high hip center are as follows:

1. Recognition of the need to place the implant higher, but size is usually small because of the narrowing dimensions of the pelvis as one proceeds upward.
2. Care in placing the component high but not lateral. Lateralization of the socket in a high hip center can compromise abductor function of the hip and has been associated with lateral breakout due to insufficient support (1).

Protrusio Acetabulum

Acetabular protrusio presents several challenges to the reconstructive surgeon. This condition is often seen in inflammatory arthritis (i.e., psoriatic arthritis), and bone strength

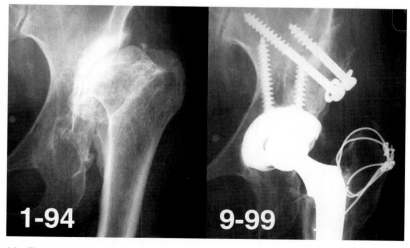

Figure 10. Total hip arthroplasty in a severely dysplastic hip performed with the use of a bulk autograft, which shows radiographic incorporation 5 years after surgery. (Courtesy of Dr. Eduardo A. Salvati.)

may be compromised. Protrusio can be detected radiographically by the observation of the femoral head lying medial to Kohler's line. There are two practical considerations in dealing with protrusio: difficulty in dislocation and volumetric loss of bone medially. Depending upon the degree of protrusio, exposure may be difficult. In cases of protrusio, we do not hesitate to perform an in situ neck osteotomy for exposure. The osteotomy should be subcapital: Once the femur is dislocated, the neck resection level can be adjusted. At this point, the femoral head can be removed with a periosteal elevator or a skid.

Acetabular preparation in protrusio is unique in that "medialization" is not required. Use the small-diameter reamer to simply remove any remaining articular cartilage and soft tissue. Focus acetabular reamer size on obtaining peripheral rim fit! Ignore the fact that the reamer is not in contact medially. Ensure that there is superior dome contact. The femoral head is denuded of bone, morcelized in a bone mill, and the bone chips introduced into the medial defect. Compaction of the bone and contour with the reamer on reverse should fill the void. The appropriate-sized socket component is then inserted. Adjuvant screw fixation is recommended (see Fig. 11). Despite the use of bone graft, we permit early weight bearing as tolerated when performing this technique in protrusio. We believe that compression on the graft will lead to better graft consolidation.

Posttraumatic Degenerative Joint Disease

The major obstacles encountered during acetabular reconstruction following trauma are difficulty of exposure, the presence of hardware, and pelvic deformity or bone loss. Exposure is often complicated because of prior incisions that may or may not be extensile coupled with scarring and ectopic bone formation. Surgical exposure must be carefully planned so as to be able to gain access to all aspects of the acetabulum, including the possibility of having to remove previously placed pelvic plates or screws. We prefer to leave hardware in place unless it compromises socket preparation or is encountered during the reaming process (see Fig. 12). Extensive dissection during periacetabular fixation can lead to vascular compromise of the bone. Take notice of bone viability evidenced by bone bleeding. Sclerotic nonbleeding bone may necessitate the use of a cemented socket.

While volumetric loss of bone is rare following trauma, fracture and subsequent fixation may affect host socket orientation. Preoperative assessment of the amount and orientation

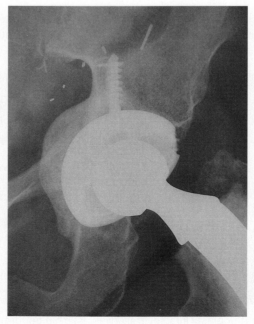

Figure 11. Acetabular reconstruction in protrusio, utilizing medial morcellized autograft and an uncemented cup with peripheral press fit and supplemented with a screw.

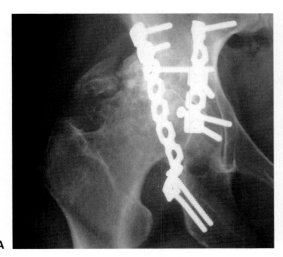
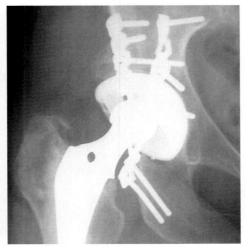

A   B

Figure 12. Total hip arthroplasty after acetabular fracture. The hardware that will not contact or jeopardize the positioning and fixation of the acetabular cup should be left in place. (Courtesy of Dr. Eduardo A. Salvati.)

of pelvic bone stock can be determined by the use of computerized tomography. However, intraoperative landmarks may be obscured, and therefore placement of reamers and the component may be confusing. If the exact orientation of the socket is unclear, preparation of the femur first may give guidance. We will insert the femoral trial and use this to help guide the direction of acetabular preparation.

Postarthrodesis

Total hip arthroplasty following arthrodesis may present one of the greatest challenges to the adult reconstructive surgeon (see Fig. 13). Prior incisions, the presence of hardware,

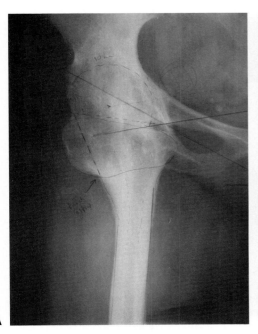
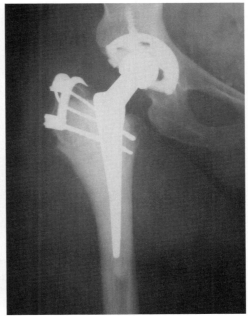

A   B

Figure 13. Ankylosis of the hip. The joint space disappeared, and there are trabeculae crossing from the femur to the iliac bone. There is severe osteopenia in the femoral head, iliac bone, and greater trochanter. The teardrop image is present.

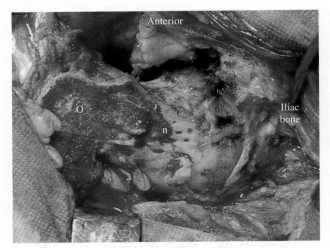

Figure 14. A trochanteric osteotomy *(O)* in a fused hip secondary to ankylosing spondylitis allows exposure of the anterior, superior, and posterior neck *(n)*, required to perform a neck osteotomy in situ.

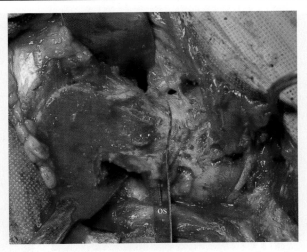

Figure 15. An oscillating saw *(OS)* is used to perform the osteotomy in situ.

bone loss, deformity of bone, and soft tissue contractures all contribute to the complexity of this case. The specifics of acetabular preparation include exposure, determination of femoral neck osteotomy, and locating and preparing the host acetabular bed. The exposure for a takedown may necessitate a trochanteric osteotomy or slide simply for exposure purposes (see Figs. 13 and 14). The type and location of the osteotomy should be planned preoperatively on the basis of some identifiable landmark (the vastus ridge is often used). Following exposure, the neck osteotomy is performed (see Figs. 13 and 15). As in doing any in situ neck, it is better to err on the high side. At this point, the femur is translated away from the acetabulum, and following the placement of acetabular retractors, socket preparation begins (see Fig. 16). The key to acetabular preparation is the identification of the medial wall (see Fig. 17). In many instances, the fibrofatty pulvinar remains intact and is used as a guide. Ream

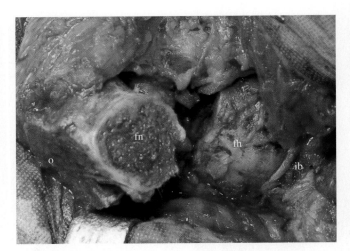

Figure 16. After performing the in situ osteotomy of the femoral neck *(fn)*, the femur can be mobilized, and the acetabular area can be exposed in the standard fashion. Here, o, trochanteric osteotomy; fh, fused femoral head; ib, iliac bone.

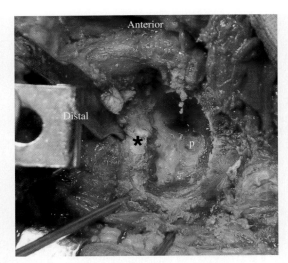

Figure 17. The fused head has been reamed. It is now possible to identify the base of the teardrop *(asterisk)* and the soft tissue attachments in the pulvinar *(p)*, thus judging the depth of reaming. Because of the osteopenia in the acetabulum and lack of supportive subchondral bone, reaming should be done with extreme caution, intraoperative radiographs may be obtained, and ancillary screw fixation is often required.

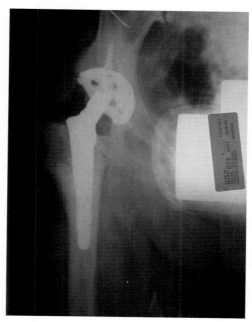

Figure 18. Intraoperative radiograph during conversion of an ankylosed hip demonstrates the position of the cup and stem.

medially until the pulvinar is encountered. At this point, concentrically larger reamers are used until adequate coverage and position are obtained. Obtain an intraoperative radiograph at this point (see Fig. 18). Exact location within the pelvis is often confusing, and the radiograph ensures proper position. Implantation proceeds using guides as previously described. Often, the bone quality is less than robust, and the use of adjuvant screws is common.

POSTOPERATIVE MANAGEMENT/REHABILITATION

In general, postoperative management is going to be dictated more by type of femoral reconstruction rather than acetabular reconstruction. Weight-bearing status may be influenced by stability of the construct, the use of supportive bone graft, and whether an osteotomy was performed. For the vast majority of cases, immediate weight bearing is recommended usually with the first 24 hours following surgery. Assistive devices are utilized as required, with our own bias being toward transition to cane or forearm crutches as rapidly as possible. Range of motion exercise will be influenced by surgical approach with avoidance of flexion greater than 90 degrees and no internal rotation for the initial 8 weeks following surgery.

Unique postoperative considerations pertaining to complex acetabular reconstruction include the possibility of heterotopic ossification and soft tissue contractures, particularly in the posttraumatic and postarthrodesis patient. Patients felt to be at high risk for heterotopic bone are clearly in the posttraumatic group, especially if there is preexisting heterotopic bone. Excision of the heterotopic ossification at the time of reconstruction and prophylaxis is recommended. We prefer single-dose radiation with Cerrobend (lead shield) blocking over any porous surface and any osteotomy site. This regimen has been shown to be effective.

Soft tissue contractures are best addressed early by specifically tailoring a physical therapy program. Most problematic are flexion contractures and limited rotation. Having the patient work on prone extension exercises as well as encouraging early hip flexion coupled with external rotation (so-called "figure four position") is both safe and highly effective. Emphasize the need to perform these activities at home several times a day and not just when at therapy.

RESULTS

Cementless hemispherical acetabular components have been utilized for almost 20 years. The original technique of insertion utilized line-to-line reaming and supplemental use of screws or spikes. Martell et al. reported on the results of this first-generation technique and found loosening rates of 2% at a mean of 7 years. Clearly, fixation appeared to be reliable. With time, the technique of preparation and insertion evolved to employing the underreaming technique and avoidance of supplemental screws. We demonstrated that at 5-year follow-up there is secure, predictable fixation in cups inserted without holes, relying on press fit for initial stability (3). As we now accumulate data with greater than 10- to 15-year follow-up, fixation remains predictable. However, as we continue to follow these groups, particle-induced osteolysis appears to be the prime source of concern. The trend for increasing rates of osteolysis in a time-dependent fashion points out the continued need for reevaluating alternative bearing surfaces and improvements in the articulation.

COMPLICATIONS

Complications related to press-fit socket use are extremely rare. The major risks are related to technical errors during preparation and insertion. Sharkey et al. have reported acetabular fracture during cementless socket insertion in a multicenter study (5). These fractures can be the result of undersized reaming, and particularly in osteopenic bone component impaction, care should be taken to avoid overzealous cup impaction in soft bone. In these situations, line-to-line reaming and adjuvant screw insertion are recommended.

Instability after total hip arthroplasty can often be the result of component malposition. Acetabular positioning is influenced by several factors including pelvic bone loss, osteophytes, and sclerotic bone, as well as patient positioning on the operating table. The key to avoidance of malposition is to identify acetabular landmarks such as the teardrop or superior dome and use these to help guide component abduction angle. Version angles can be aided with the use of commercial guides applied to the cup during insertion. However, absolute reliance on the use of external guides is not recommended, and intraoperative trial reduction to assess alignment is key.

While the routine use of supplemental screws for fixation in primary total hip arthroplasty is becoming less common, complications related to screw placement are best managed by avoidance of the danger zones as described by Wasielewski et al. (4). Familiarity with the safe quadrants for screw placement is mandatory for all surgeons performing uncemented acetabular surgery and will certainly reduce the risk of neurovascular injury.

RECOMMENDED READING

1. Johnston RC, Brand RA, Crowninshield RD. Reconstruction of the hip. *J Bone Joint Surg Am* 61:639–652, 1979.
2. Clohisy JC, Harris WH. The Harris-Galante porous-coated acetabular component with screw fixation. An average ten year follow-up study. *J Bone Joint Surg Am* 81:66–73, 1999.
3. Gonzalez Della Valle A, Zoppi A, Peterson M, Salvati E. Clinical and radiographic results associated with a modern, cementless modular cup design in total hip arthroplasty. *J Bone Joint Surg* 86(9):1908–2063, 2004.
4. Wasielewski RC, Cooperstein LA, Kruger MP, Rubash HE. Acetabular anatomy and the transacetabular fixation of screws in total hip arthroplasty. *J Bone Joint Surg Am* 72:501–508, 1990.
5. Sharkey PF, Hozack WJ, Callaghan JJ, et al. Acetabular fracture associated with cementless acetabular component insertion: a report of 13 cases. *J Arthroplasty* 14(4):426–431, 1999.
6. Gonzalez Della Valle A, Slullitel G, Piccaluga F, Salvati E. The precision and usefulness of preoperative planning for cemented and hybrid total hip arthroplasty. *J Arthroplasty* 20(1):51–58, 2005.

PART VI

Revision Total Hip Arthroplasty

21

Principles, Planning, and Decision Making

R. Stephen J. Burnett, Aaron G. Rosenberg,
and Robert L. Barrack

INDICATIONS AND CONTRAINDICATIONS

The concept of "surgical indication" can be defined as the situation where a patient will benefit from a specific surgical intervention in such a way, and with sufficient likelihood, that warrants the specific risks involved in the intervention. Contraindications would connote the opposite: the risks involved and/or the likelihood of the intervention's failure to achieve the desired results outweigh the expected benefit of the intervention. Particularly in revision surgery, the term "indications" actually represents the end point of a complex decision-making process that must be carried out by the medical practitioner in conjunction with the patient. The primary requirement for the clinician must be the ability to carefully evaluate the patient's complaints and clinical condition and to arrive at a diagnosis. Knowledge of the treatment options available allows the surgeon to consider the overall utility of these choices and to help educate the patient, and it allows the surgeon and patient to choose an appropriate treatment. This may require the full range of the surgeon's analytical and communication skills.

The term "indications" carries a sense of certainty that may not be present in many surgical settings. Wide variations in the regional performance of multiple routine surgical techniques demonstrate that specific applications of many interventions are not universally agreed upon. Thus, while carrying the ring of specificity, the term "indications" is rarely as straightforward as the term is generally understood and frequently used. In reality, the term often means simply that the surgeon's thinking process has led to the conviction that the patient will be better off with surgery.

While in general the generic thought processes required for making a decision as to the indications for any type of surgical procedure are essentially identical, there are differences in the primary and revision settings that may lead to an alteration in the thinking process that leads the clinician to decide that surgical intervention is warranted. One of the main differences is the fact that in contemplating revision surgery, a bridge has already been crossed; the surgeon is no longer dealing with a "virgin" hip, and the gravity of the decision of crossing the bridge from nonreplacement options to elimination of the native head and neck has been recognized. This, in some respects, makes the decision to surgically intervene somewhat more palatable to the patient who has, in most cases, new or continued complaints relative to the arthroplasty. On the other hand, revision surgery is often performed with less confidence in the underlying diagnosis, is less predictable, and has a higher complication rate than primary surgical interventions, and these factors may make the decision to intervene more difficult. Ultimately, these contradictory features may balance out, and so an even "trade-off" occurs. This concept of "trade-off" is an important one used in many models of decision making and can be a useful technique for the surgeon and patient to consider when making difficult choices.

A simple example of one of the many "trade-offs" the surgeon must consider prior to recommending the performance of any elective surgical procedure is the relative risk of perioperative events, which carry with them significant morbidity or mortality. The surgeon contemplating any elective surgical intervention must essentially compare the potential long-term benefits of symptom reduction and/or improved function versus the short-term risks of death and other complications that may potentially occur following surgery. This is no less true for revision than for primary hip arthroplasty, and evaluation of the "trade-offs" involved in any decision can be simple or complex.

A simple example of the type of trade-offs that may require consideration is the use of intervention for deep venous thrombosis (DVT) prophylaxis, where the benefits of thrombosis and embolism reduction may be accompanied by an increased risk of bleeding complications. As more data accumulate on the risks and benefits of various forms of prophylaxis, the surgeon is able to make more rational and better decisions about the "indications" for specific methods of prophylaxis.

Decision Making

Surgical decision making represents a fascinating and complex subset of the processes commonly undertaken to determine whether or not active intervention—and more specifically, what type of intervention—is in the best interests of the patient. Of course, this needs to be evaluated and compared with the option of *not intervening*, which requires an understanding of the natural history of the disease process involved and its implication for future health and the need for potential future medical or surgical interventions. Unfortunately, many of the factors related to quality of life, as well as the specific outcomes related to a given intervention and their likelihood of occurring following the chosen intervention, are based on scanty data.

Although there is a burgeoning literature devoted to the thought processes involved in medical decision making, there is no consensus on the specific methods that are most appropriately used to determine when a specific intervention is indicated. The medical decision-making process is far from uniform and, in different settings, requires different analytical skills. Diagnostic decision making differs in many respects from therapeutic decisions, and decisions of "consequence" (where potential risks and complications are high and outcomes are not reliable) can stress even the most experienced decision maker.

At the least, medical decision making requires consideration of the potential risks and benefits of a particular intervention as applied to a specific patient and subsequent comparison with other potential courses of action. A simple risk to benefit ratio can be considered by remembering that the risks are a sum—the sum of all of the potential medical and surgical risks faced by the patient. The medical risks may be best determined by an internist familiar with the physiologic burden imposed on the patient with revision surgery. In some cases, it is important for the surgeon to accurately describe these burdens for the internist to accurately assess the medical risks involved. To these risks must be added the general and specific risks of the surgical exercise, accounting for the specific features of the patient's pathology, the technical feasibility and the complexity of the reconstruction, and the skills of the surgical team.

Conversely, the benefit is not a sum but a difference: the difference between the potential outcome that may be achieved by the revision and the current state of the patient due to their pain and/or functional disability. The better the current status of the patient, the less likely that the improvement from surgical intervention will yield a high figure in the "benefits" column. Thus, the more compromised the patient's prerevision condition, the more likely that a large benefit would result from a successful intervention. Determining the likely clinical consequence of successful reconstruction provides the end point from which the preoperative disability must be subtracted to arrive at the relative benefit of the procedure.

More complex decision making involves situations where the trade-offs are more numerous and the data are less clear. Consider a case pertinent to revision surgery. A patient with a clearly loose acetabular component is being revised for persistent, severe, and incapacitating groin pain. The femoral component is well fixed radiographically and clinically at the time of surgery. It is in an acceptable, but not ideal, position in terms of overall hip stability following revision of the acetabular component. There is a fixed femoral head, and while stability is good, it is not perfect, and had the patient required femoral component revision, increasing leg length, improving anteversion, and increasing head size would be available options. However, removal of the well-fixed femoral component will take additional time and may result in bone loss or femoral shaft fracture, and the revision may not achieve adequate fixation. In addition, removing the current component may increase blood loss, and the incidence of postoperative infection.

The potential complexity of the revision scenario can be better understood by envisioning alteration of the variables, by altering the degree of hip stability noted after revision of the acetabulum with the old femur by some amount, or by imagining the new femoral component as providing only a 50% increase in hip stability and a 20% chance of failure to get adequate femoral fixation if revision is chosen as an appropriate option.

This particular decision involves only one factor in the revision process, which may include dozens of other considerations—some of which may be addressed preoperatively and some which may only arise intraoperatively. As opposed to primary hip arthroplasty, the potential number of factors to be considered in this type of decision can be significantly larger. This increases the relative complexity of the surgical decision-making process in revision hip arthroplasty. The type of "apples and oranges" comparison of both short- and long-term risks and potential complications with the expected short- and long-term benefits of a specific intervention is common in reconstructive surgical practice and keeps much of actual surgical decision making in the realm of heuristic rather than algorithmic problem-solving.

Evaluating the Factors

The indications for revision surgery are related to pain or functional disability caused by diagnoses that may be corrected by revision surgery. That is, the symptoms must be directly caused by an identified problem that is likely to be corrected by the revision procedure. Exploratory surgery for symptoms that are not well identified as having specific component-related causes is not likely to improve the patient's symptoms. Specific diagnoses that may indicate revision include: mechanically loose components, recurrent dislocation, biomechanical abnormalities of the reconstruction, sepsis and periprosthetic fracture, and/or advanced wear and its sequelae. All of these conditions represent good reasons to revise a hip arthroplasty. In isolation, however, the mere presence of symptoms and clearly identified associated pathology do not allow the use of the term "indicated." That is a more complex decision-making process, which must take into account a thorough review of the patient in their entirety.

An underlying assumption in most surgical decision making—and one predicated on the relative unpredictability of surgical outcomes, particularly in the elective setting—is that nonsurgical treatment should be attempted prior to proceeding with surgery. This may include the use of assistive devices for ambulation, weight loss, systemic or local medications, and physiotherapy and activity modification to make symptoms more tolerable for the patient. However, in some settings, the symptoms, physical findings, and x-ray changes are severe enough to warrant consideration of revision even if the patient has had no prior conservative treatment.

While making a diagnosis is an essential part of evaluating the patient's need for surgical intervention, it is not the diagnosis per se that indicates the need for or advisability of revision surgery. Loose components may cause little in the way of symptoms. Revision for loosening may well be indicated in the symptomatic patient but may not be in the asymptomatic patient. However, despite the paucity of symptoms, an additional indication for revision surgery must include the scenario where failure to revise may lead to a more complex surgical revision or compromise of the revision procedure if the surgery is delayed until symptoms force the surgeons or the patient to consider surgical intervention. This scenario is usually predicated on the prediction of tissue loss. In particular, progressive loss of bone is an important part of the natural history in many cases and must be factored into any decision-making process where the surgeon counsels or agrees with delaying intervention. Factors such as the presence of known wear generators, the speed of lesion progression, and its size and anatomic importance may all influence the surgical decision.

In many cases, determining whether or not revision surgery is indicated or contraindicated involves several interrelated steps involving the consideration of multiple factors. The first step is to make a diagnosis. While some patterns of failure are typical and relatively easy to diagnose, others are more subtle, and the surgeon who treats these problems should have access to a specific protocol that will allow appropriate testing to assist in the making of an accurate diagnosis.

The diagnosis itself carries with it several essential elements that contribute to the decision-making process. First is the natural history implied by the diagnosis. It is only by understanding the likely consequences of leaving the patient untreated that a reasonable comparison can be made with various treatment options. If leaving the patient with their symptoms is not likely to lead to the development of additional symptoms (nor is it likely to make any future intervention, if needed, more difficult), then it is relatively safe to choose a conservative course. Specifically, cases where the patient's medical conditions place them at substantial risk, where the psychological factors or patient expectations are unrealistic, or where there has been adequate accommodation and adaptation of the patient to their symptoms without putting future options in jeopardy may warrant a conservative course. In patients requiring revision for problems that are not currently causing symptoms (progressive osteolysis or accelerated polyethylene wear), it may be necessary to demonstrate to the patient that surgical treatment is needed, though it will not result in the relief of symptoms or improve function and indeed may carry substantial potential risks and potential complications. In this setting, the surgeon must clearly explain to the patient the natural history of the anticipated failure mode and the likelihood of symptoms developing in the future.

A second factor of note is the degree of disability, as well as the level of activity and associated symptom severity caused by the pathology. This will vary by patient and by diagnosis but gives essential information regarding the potential utility gained by elimination or minimization of the symptoms produced by revision. While pain and functional disability are the most significant complaints prior to revision, in most cases, symptoms are activity related. When symptoms are clearly amenable to activity modification and where revision is not ideal because of age, comorbidities, or other specific anatomic factors, the surgeon should opt for conservative treatment. An obvious and clear-cut example would be a younger individual who has what appears by all diagnostic measures to be a well-fixed and functioning arthroplasty who has athletic activity–limiting symptoms only with very vigorous athletic endeavors. If the individual has little or no symptoms with activity modification, then activity limitation would be a more reasonable course than proceeding with revision because of the potential difficulty involved in revising components that are already well fixed and the relatively small benefit that will be obtained.

Another confounding factor may center on specific anatomic abnormalities of soft tissue or bone that would place the patient at substantial increased risk from the surgical procedure itself and the technical feasibility of performing an adequate surgical reconstruction. For example, revision in the face of severe bone loss, the need to remove massive amounts of well-fixed intrapelvic cement, or the presence of severe soft tissue deficits may alter the equation. Again, the risks of surgery must be balanced with the patient's symptoms and the likelihood that symptoms will be ameliorated by the revision.

Of course, all interventions must be evaluated against the background of the patient's general health and personal expectations. Thus, the first major step, in addition to establishing a diagnosis, is to simultaneously establish the overall health status of the patient. The presence of substantial comorbidities may preclude the use of surgical intervention in all but the most incapacitated of patients. Certainly, the risks of perioperative mortality following surgical intervention must be carefully weighed against the expected functional improvement and pain relief that can be expected with any type of surgical intervention.

As an example, consider first a relatively young, otherwise healthy individual with a known radiographically and clinically loose cemented total hip arthroplasty (THA). Living with the disability of the failed implant because of social obligations, the patient must be carefully followed for the development of bone loss regardless of symptoms. However, let us now imagine that the implant becomes infected after extraction of an abscessed tooth. The patient is now septic with fever, has an elevated white blood cell count, and has shaking chills with hypotension. There is little room for questioning the indications for emergency revision of the hip (either in one or two stages) in this scenario.

On the other hand, consider an asymptomatic 56-year-old patient who, at a 9-year routine follow-up visit, demonstrates linear acetabular wear and mild trochanteric osteolysis with an otherwise well-fixed and well-functioning hybrid total hip replacement. Surgical intervention may well be indicated here. Now consider the same patient with severe cardiomyopathy with the need for continuous oxygen and a cardiac ejection fraction of 21%. Here the situation is dramatically different.

The severity of the symptoms and the amount of pain and/or functional disability must be carefully evaluated in order to decide on the advisability of revision. Pain is usually easily quantitated but should be accompanied by a sense of frequency and the degree of disability it produces in addition to a thorough understanding of the activities that cause and relieve the pain. Functional disability is more complex and less often associated with specific reliable revision indications. These problems may range from stiffness to recurrent dislocation, from leg length discrepancy to persistent limp due to failure to reestablish appropriate mechanics. Here again, the decision-making process will be improved by determining the specific type of functional handicap experienced by the patient, as well as the frequency and severity of symptoms.

The decision to proceed with revision hip arthroplasty may be relatively simple or extremely complex. In either case, in order to make such decisions, the surgeon must not only accurately assess the multiple patient-related factors as noted above but also adequately judge his own skills, experience, and resources with regard to any particular procedure. While hard data may not be available, an approximation of outcomes and risks will prove quite useful. Even on an informal basis, this type of thinking can assist the surgeon in looking at all of the factors in a complex decision-making scenario and may also aid in communicating with the patient all of the potential risks and benefits involved in complex clinical settings with regard to specific interventions.

PREOPERATIVE PLANNING

Although THA is successful operation in over 90% of patients, revision surgery is becoming increasingly more common due to the increased number of joint replacements performed with broader indications. Establishing an accurate diagnosis is the first step in successful planning for revision total hip arthroplasty (RTHA). Details of the patient's history, review of symptoms, and physical examination help ensure that an accurate diagnosis is formulated. A detailed history of the patient's prior surgeries and perioperative treatments should be obtained. A history of prior hip surgery (trauma, internal fixation, or infection) should alert the surgeon to consider the case as a revision, often requiring further information for planning. Hospital records from previous operations may provide clues to a patient's diagnosis. Records that list implanted components can be especially helpful. The patient should be questioned for "red flags" in the history, including persistent postoperative drainage, multiple surgical procedures, or evacuation of a hematoma.

Specific data obtained from the history and physical examination, however, are crucial in the preoperative planning process. The review of systems particularly is important. Patients having RTHA frequently are elderly and have associated medical comorbidities that require evaluation and occasionally treatment and medical optimization before any surgery is performed. Any potential source of future or concurrent infection must be identified during the review of systems so that this may be addressed appropriately in advance. Urological disorders are frequently encountered in this population. Men with prostate disease or women with recurrent urinary tract infections or incontinence should be evaluated by a urologist preoperatively. Patients should have dental examinations in advance of surgery, so that any potential or ongoing dental infections can be treated prophylactically. This is not only a potential source of infection but also a potential perioperative complication of fractured teeth and aspiration during intubation in patients in whom general anesthesia is considered. Patients with chronic venous stasis ulcers, absent pulses, or prior lower extremity vascular bypass surgery should be evaluated by a vascular surgeon. A history of cardiac bypass surgery, angioplasty, or stenting often requires a preoperative stress test or preoperative cardiac catheterization. When advanced cardiovascular or respiratory monitoring is indicated, coordination with an anesthesiologist (and the intensive care unit) is necessary pre- and postoperatively to ensure that the appropriate monitoring equipment and personnel are available to manage such patients.

Obtaining an accurate history particularly is important in the preoperative planning process. The preoperative ambulatory status is important to determine. Patients who have been immobilized because of chronic or recurrent dislocations, periprosthetic fractures, explantation of an infected THA, severe pain, or chronic disability may be immobile for a period and are particularly prone to thromboembolic events (pulmonary embolism, DVT). In such patients, it may be prudent to obtain preoperative screening for DVT. If a DVT is present, preoperative treatment may be advisable before an elective revision procedure. If a semiurgent procedure is necessary, such as in the case of a periprosthetic fracture or chronic dislocation, it may be advisable to insert an inferior vena cava filter, proceed with the surgery, and defer anticoagulation to the postoperative period. Failure to detect a proximal DVT in the setting of major hip revision surgery may place a patient at risk for catastrophic intra- or postoperative thromboembolism.

Preoperatively, ruling out infection is an important step in planning for every patient having revision surgery. Most episodes of deep sepsis associated with a THA may be diagnosed from careful history and physical examination alone. Certain historic factors suggest infection, including a history of a previous delayed wound healing, persistent drainage, a prolonged course of postoperative antibiotics, or a history of night pain—particularly if it is relieved by antibiotics. Patients should be questioned specifically as to whether they have been or are currently taking antibiotics. Prior to performing a hip aspiration, antibiotics should be discontinued for at least 4 weeks to improve the sensitivity of this test. Hip aspiration generally is used selectively rather than on a routine basis. Despite preoperative aspiration and laboratory testing, the diagnosis of infection may not be ruled out completely until the time of surgery. In such cases, intraoperative tissue sampling may be necessary to gather additional information to determine the likelihood that infection is present. It is prudent to plan for intraoperative frozen sections by alerting the pathology department in advance and ensuring that they are familiar with the specific requirements for frozen analysis for a total joint infection.

Historic factors can influence the decision on implant selection. Patients who have had previous high-dose pelvic irradiation likely are not good candidates for porous-coated implants. Cemented all-polyethylene acetabular components with or without a protrusio ring probably are a better choice in this scenario. This is more commonly seen in primary THA, but it also is seen occasionally in RTHA.

Patients with a history suggestive of subluxation or dislocation require special preparation and preoperative planning. Patients who have a history of popping, clicking, or a sensation of the hip coming in and out of the joint may be having subluxation. If there is a questionable history of subluxation and dislocation, it is advisable to plan for a preoperative fluoroscopic evaluation before proceeding with a revision procedure. In patients who have documented dislocations, and where the components seem well positioned, a fluoroscopic evaluation also is valuable. In planning for revision in this setting, it is advisable to have special implants available, such as large heads, constrained liners, and bipolar components (see Fig. 1).

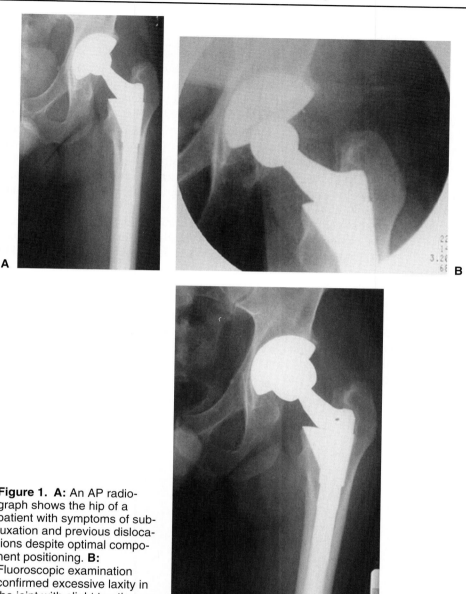

Figure 1. A: An AP radiograph shows the hip of a patient with symptoms of subluxation and previous dislocations despite optimal component positioning. **B:** Fluoroscopic examination confirmed excessive laxity in the joint with slight traction on the extremity. **C:** Revision to a larger, longer head completely resolved the symptoms of instability.

Patients should be questioned about the location and nature of the pain that they are experiencing because it may influence the preoperative plan. Groin pain is more typical of an acetabular side problem—such as polyethylene wear debris synovitis or acetabular component loosening—and if this is present, particular attention should be given to exposing the entire rim of the acetabulum to detect micromotion at the interface between the component and host bone. Similarly, pain that is well localized to the thigh and that is worse with startup (getting out of a chair) or going up and down stairs is more typical of femoral component failure and loosening. Methods of detecting occult loosening on the femoral side that have been suggested include the use of dynamic computed tomography (CT) scanning with the hip in internal and external rotation or the intraoperative use of a torque wrench.

Physical Examination

The first useful step in the physical examination is to observe the patient's gait. A marked Trendelenburg gait indicates that the abductor musculature is nonfunctional due to paralysis or loss of continuity. If the trochanter seems intact radiographically, a preoperative electromyogram may be advisable to determine whether denervation of the abductor musculature has occurred. If revision is being considered for instability and the patient has absent or nonfunctional abductors, he or she particularly is prone to recurrent dislocations, and special components such as a constrained liner or large head should be considered (see Fig. 2). It is useful to have the patient lie on the unaffected side and test the ability to effectively abduct against gravity and against resistance to further objectively assess abductor function. If the trochanter is detached or migrated, instruments and implants to reattach the trochanter should be available for surgery (see Fig. 3).

After observation of gait, inspection of the wound is important. Planning of the operative incision relative to previous incisions is an important consideration. Wound necrosis is less common in the hip than in the knee, but it does occasionally occur. Generally, it is not advisable to make a second parallel incision, particularly one that is parallel to a previously posteriorly placed incision.

The next item of the physical examination is to test the patient's range of motion actively and passively. Patients who have a partially or completely ankylosed hip or patients with medial migration or protrusio may require a more extensile exposure. If a trochanteric osteotomy or a trochanteric slide is planned, trochanteric reattachment equipment and implants must be available. Extremes of passive motion should be avoided in order not to precipitate an iatrogenic dislocation. Occasionally, with an intrapelvic dislocation or intrapelvic migration

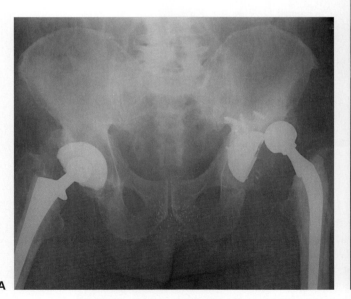

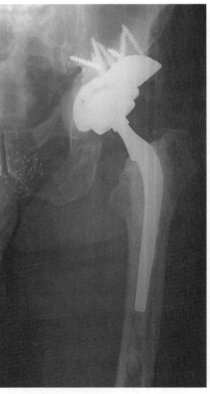

A   **B**

Figure 2. A: AP radiograph of a left THA with chronic instability and prior acetabular bulk structural allograft. The cup placement is vertical with limited anteversion. **B:** Postoperative AP radiograph following revision. A trabecular metal structural augment was utilized in order to allow placement of the revision cementless cup in a more horizontal position. A modular exchange to a larger head diameter was also performed to improve stability.

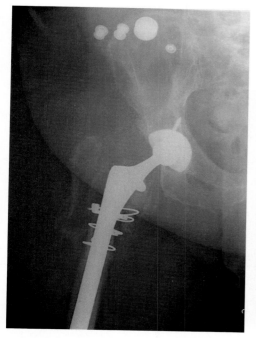
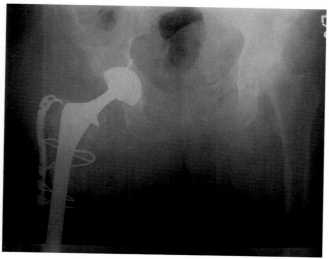

A

B

Figure 3. A: AP radiograph of a THA with an escape of a prior extended trochanteric osteotomy. Specialized trochanteric cable plates with cable fixation and the option to retension cables during application has provided a useful adjuvant to complex trochanteric problems. **B:** Postoperative radiograph with fixation of the osteotomy.

of a loose component, an alternative surgical approach such as the ilioinguinal approach must be considered and planned for at the time of revision surgery (see Fig. 4).

Measurement of limb length should be a standard part of the physical examination, and this also is relevant to preoperative planning. Limb lengthening frequently occurs during a revision procedure. In cases where lengthening of several centimeters is anticipated, it particularly is important to evaluate the neurovascular status of the limb, preoperatively. Partial sciatic palsy is the most common nerve injury occurring in THA. At least partial recovery can be expected in 70% to 80% of cases, with the remainder frequently displaying dissatisfaction with their surgery. Somatosensory evoked potentials (SSEPs) may be considered intraoperatively. In these cases, a preoperative SSEP usually is obtained as a baseline for intraoperative changes that may occur. It also is important to focus preoperatively on the examination of the lumbar spine. Patients with lumbar radiculopathy or spinal stenosis probably are at higher risk for nerve palsy (double-crush phenomenon), particularly if lengthening or traction on the nerve is anticipated. In patients with absent pulses or previous vascular bypass surgery, the operative approach may be modified to minimize kinking of the femoral vessels or grafts. Intraoperative heparin therapy and vascular assessment prior to and immediately after surgery also may be advisable in these patients. Vascular injury is most frequently associated with the use of screws for fixation of structural grafts, acetabular components, and protrusio rings or cages. An understanding of the acetabular quadrant system is crucial in minimizing these potentially catastrophic complications.

Radiographic Examination

A review of an adequate set of radiographs is an important step in planning for revision THA. A low anteroposterior (AP) radiograph of the pelvis is useful in determining relative length by comparing the interischial line with a fixed point on the lesser trochanter. Radiographic measurements should be correlated with findings on physical examination.

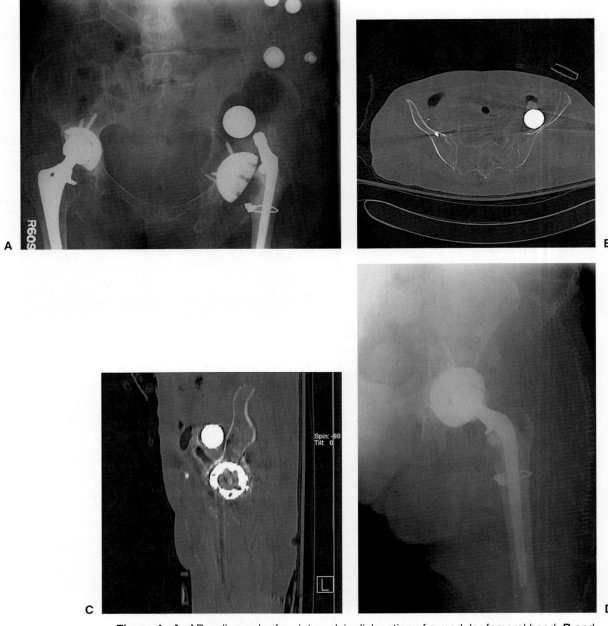

Figure 4. A: AP radiograph of an intrapelvic dislocation of a modular femoral head. **B** and **C:** Axial and sagittal CT scans confirm intrapelvic location of the modular head. **D:** Post-operative radiograph following revision surgery that required both an ilioinguinal surgical approach to remove the head and a standard posterolateral approach to revise the modular polyethylene component.

Judet views are useful for assessing acetabular bone stock and the interface between implant and bone. Lucent lines and osteolytic lesions frequently are more apparent on a Judet view than on an AP radiograph (see Fig. 5). A cross-table lateral radiograph of the acetabulum is useful for assessing the acetabular version, which particularly is important for suspected instability. The shoot-through lateral radiograph also is useful for templating the acetabulum to ensure that the shell diameter estimated on the AP view will fit without reaming away the anterior and posterior walls and for assessing for retroacetabular osteolysis involving the posterior column.

Anteroposterior and lateral radiographs of the femur are necessary to assess the femoral component and any cement that is present. The radiograph must extend beyond the tip of

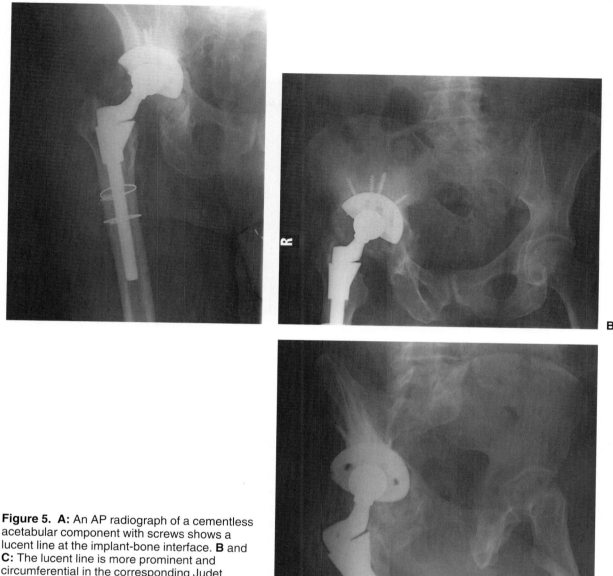

Figure 5. A: An AP radiograph of a cementless acetabular component with screws shows a lucent line at the implant-bone interface. **B** and **C:** The lucent line is more prominent and circumferential in the corresponding Judet views.

the component and any cement that is present (see Fig. 6). When there has been a previous fracture or osteotomy or other surgical procedure on the femur, it is advisable to obtain AP and lateral radiographs of the entire femur. Radiographs of the femur should be scrutinized to assess for areas of perforation, thinning, or osteolysis. Areas of extreme thinning or bone loss also may require strut allograft bone for support. It also is important to assess the bow of the femur on the lateral view particularly if a stem greater than 6 to 7 inches of length may be used or in shorter patients where the bow of the femur may be encountered even with primary cementless femoral component stem lengths. To assess the bow of the femur, a table-down or Lowenstein lateral radiograph is more accurate than the traditional frog leg lateral radiograph.

On the acetabular side, it is important to evaluate the intrapelvic cement or components. Components that are medial to Köhler's ilioischial line may require additional evaluation. A CT scan can define the proximity of major vascular structures to host bone, cement, screws, or acetabular components and may be helpful; however, metal-backed components may cause distortion of the imaging, and angiography occasionally may be necessary to evaluate vascular structures (see Fig. 7).

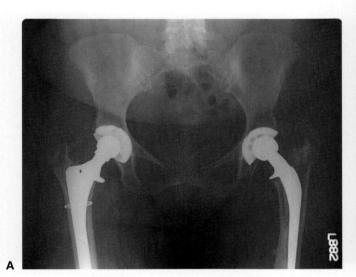
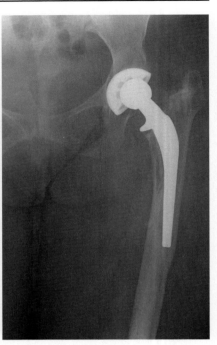

Figure 6. A: AP pelvis radiographs show a symptomatic subsided and loose cemented stem. **B:** The extent of the cement column and femoral remodeling is visualized on a longer AP view of the femur.

Heterotopic ossification (HO) should be graded on plain radiographs. The presence of Grade 3 or Grade 4 HO should alert the surgeon to the possible need for prophylactic radiation or medication. This may be encountered in the setting of prior trauma (acetabular fracture with internal fixation) or surgery to the hip (see Fig. 8). To prevent recurrent HO, radiation must be administered either preoperatively or within 48 hours postoperatively to be most effective, and this must be planned and coordinated with the radiation oncology department. Cementless components and trochanteric osteotomies should be shielded to minimize the risk of nonunion or failure of ingrowth. It is helpful to provide the radiation therapist with diagrams or references regarding shielding of components because some may not be familiar with this method.

Identification of the components that are in place is an important part of the preoperative planning process. This particularly is true if one or more components may be left in place. It is crucial that the characteristics and design of a retained component are well known so that the component is compatible with the component with which it is mated. A review of a large series of revisions revealed that at least one component is retained at least half the time, making this an important consideration in revision planning. The most accurate information is the company implant record in the patient's medical record. It is common to place copies of the stickers from the actual components that were implanted into the patient's medical record, so that detailed information including the sizes, manufacturer, and lot numbers are obtainable. On the acetabular side, for example, if the components are well fixed and aligned, it may be appropriate to perform a liner exchange procedure for polyethylene wear and osteolysis. The appropriate modular liner should be available. This may require special tools to remove and reinsert a second liner and/or a new locking mechanism (see Fig. 9). The locking mechanism may be damaged, and it may not be advisable to reinsert a second liner. In such a case, an all-polyethylene liner should be available, which can be cemented into the well-fixed acetabular implant. Seating the liner, avoiding rim elevation, and scoring the back of the liner with a high-speed burr may improve cement interdigitation and fixation.

On the femoral side, it is important to know whether the stem is a fixed head (monoblock) or modular design. If the stem is monoblock, it is important to know the

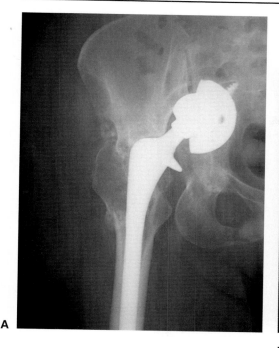

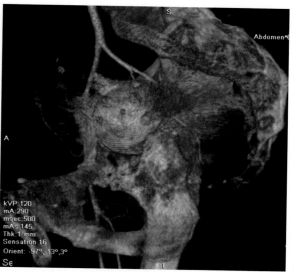

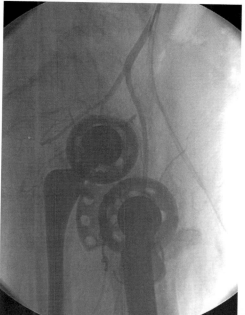

Figure 7. A: AP radiograph of a loose acetabular component with intrapelvic migration. **(B)** A preoperative three-dimensional CT scan with reconstruction and **(C)** an angiogram of the internal iliac artery were obtained, which showed the close proximity of the acetabular screws and implant to the vascular structures.

diameter of the head in the event that it may be retained so that the appropriate acetabular component liners may be available (see Fig. 10). If the stem is modular, the appropriate modular heads and trials should be available in case the head is damaged, which frequently is the case. In addition, longer head lengths (or offset liner options) frequently are necessary to restore tissue tension and stability after acetabular revision. Many implant manufacturers have more than one modular head taper available, so it is important to know which components are in place.

Acetabular components of specific design and manufacturers may have screws that require special screwdrivers for removal. If a cementless shell is well fixed and must be removed because of malposition or infection, special osteotomes are available that can remove porous-coated ingrown components with minimal bone damage. More commonly,

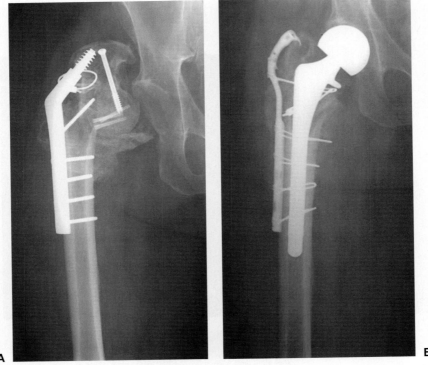

Figure 8. A: Preoperative AP hip radiograph showing prior trauma and failed internal fixation of a femoral head and reverse oblique intertrochanteric fracture, with persistent dislocation. There is heterotopic bone bridging the inferior acetabulum to the femur. **B:** Six months' postoperative revision to a right hip hemiarthroplasty, trochanteric osteotomy, and internal fixation. Postoperative radiotherapy with shielding of the femoral component and osteotomy was performed to minimize the risk of recurrence of the heterotopic ossification.

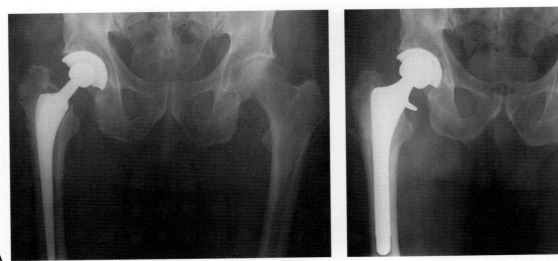

Figure 9. A: Preoperative AP radiograph of a right THA with aseptic loosening of the femoral component and a well-fixed cementless acetabular implant. **B:** AP radiograph at 6 months following revision of the femoral component to a fully porous coated stem and modular liner exchange. A new locking mechanism was inserted at the time of modular revision of the polyethylene liner.

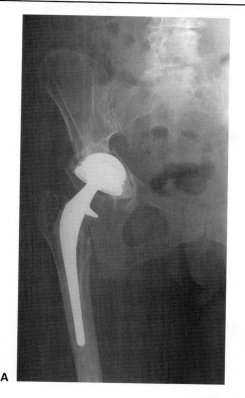

A

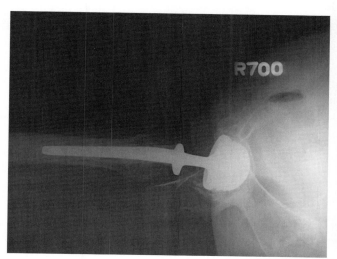

B

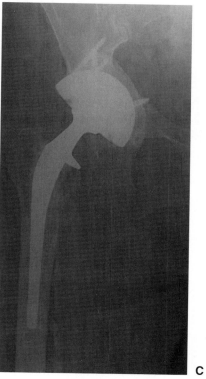

C

Figure 10. A: Preoperative AP hip radiograph shows the right hip with a loose acetabular component with an associated protrusio defect. The femoral component is a well-fixed monoblock Harris design 2 stem (HD-2, Howmedica, NJ) with a 26-mm head. **B:** Cross-table lateral radiograph showing a narrow anterior column and contained acetabular defect. **C:** Postoperative radiograph following acetabular revision to a large cementless cup with screw fixation and allograft cancellous graft impacted medially. A 26-mm modular polyethylene liner for this shell was used, and the monoblock stem was retained.

in a well-fixed cementless acetabular implant with a proven track record and appropriate orientation/version, a modular liner exchange or cementing in a new liner may be performed. On the femoral side, well-fixed cementless components may require special equipment for removal such as high-speed burrs or trephines. A well-fixed, cementless, fully porous coated stem may require sectioning of the stem and trephining, which requires numerous high-speed carbide cutting tools and trephines. Similarly, cementless acetabular component removal may be facilitated with sharp curved osteotomes that match the diameter of the implant (see Fig. 11). If a modular component is present, special tools may be necessary to disassemble or retrieve modular portions of the component (see Fig. 12). Removing well-fixed cemented stems may be facilitated by special equipment such as ultrasonic tools that require advance planning because most hospitals do not own such special equipment.

Radiographs should be reviewed not only to identify the components but also to determine the adequacy of the component positioning and fixation status. This should then be correlated with the findings at the time of surgery. A review of sequential plain radiographs is the most accurate means of estimating the fixation status. Radiographs also should be reviewed for the location and extent of osteolytic lesions. The treatment of osteolysis is dealt with elsewhere, but for planning purposes, it should be noted that large amounts of

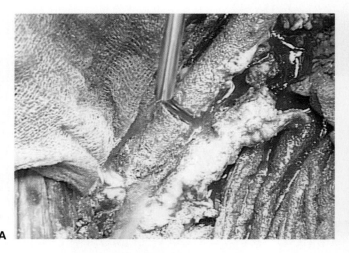

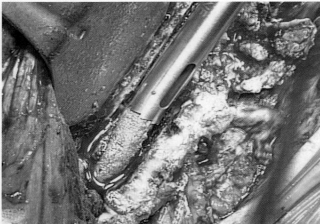

A   B

C

Figure 11. A: Intraoperative photograph using a high-speed carbide disc-cutting wheel to cut across a well-fixed cobalt chrome femoral stem. **B:** Trephining over the distal portion of a transected fully porous coated stem to remove the stem. **C:** Explant Acetabular Cup Removal System (Zimmer, Warsaw, IN) removal instrumentation for removing a well-fixed cementless acetabular implant.

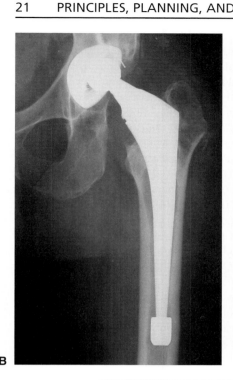
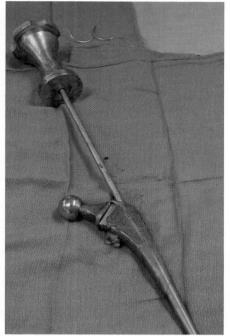
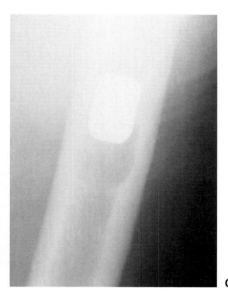

A, B   C

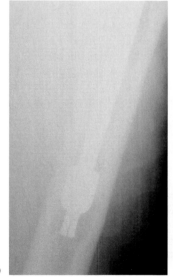
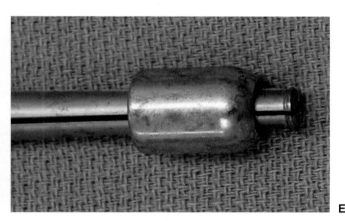

D   E

Figure 12. A: A preoperative radiograph of a cementless stem with a modular distal bullet tip that requires specific removal instruments to facilitate extraction. **B:** Stem extraction leaves the distal bullet remaining within the canal. **C:** Radiograph of distal bullet tip once stem has been removed. **D** and **E:** Extraction of the bullet with the appropriate three-prong device, which expands once the instrument is screwed into the bullet, allowing safe removal.

bone graft or bone graft substitutes or both frequently are necessary to treat lytic lesions at the time of RTHA. After general review of the radiographs, planning for the actual implantation of components occurs during the process of templating.

Laboratory Tests

Once the surgeon has performed an initial history, physical examination, and radiographs, often adjunctive testing may be required in order to establish or confirm a definitive diagnosis. Blood testing is frequently performed preoperatively, most commonly to assess for possible infection related to the THA. The hemoglobin/hematocrit and mean cell volume can uncover anemia and direct preoperative treatment or further investigations. Malnutrition is a risk factor for infection and should be corrected preoperatively if possible, before elective surgery. Preoperative nutritional status may be evaluated using serum protein levels and total lymphocyte count. Serum total protein, albumin and prealbumin, and transferrin are useful preoperative markers of nutritional status in patients undergoing total joint arthroplasty. The white blood cell count (WBC), while routinely performed in the complete blood count, is rarely elevated even in the presence of obvious infection in THA and is unreliable to assess for infection in THA. The erythrocyte sedimentation rate (ESR) is a nonspecific inflammatory marker that normalizes between 6 and 12 months after THA surgery. Several studies have reported that using a cutoff of an ESR >30 mm/hour provides increased sensitivity and specificity in the diagnosis of infection in THA. The C-reactive protein (CRP) is an acute phase reactant that increases normally within hours of surgery and returns to normal within 3 months following THA. The sensitivity/specificity of this measurement when a CRP of >10 mg/dL is chosen has been studied in infected revision THA. Most useful is the combination of these two measurements of a CRP >10 and an ESR >30; values that are below these or in the normal range are most useful in excluding infection in THA, while elevation of both increases the probability of sepsis.

Hip aspiration improves the accuracy in diagnosing infection when the ESR and CRP are elevated. While a sensitivity of 67% to 92% and specificity of 94% to 97% are reported, the usefulness of this test is primarily in combination with history, exam, and ESR and CRP measurements. Aspiration and arthrography may be useful to define pseudocapsule, joint space extension, and sinus tracts in the setting of infection.

The use of nuclear medicine imaging may occasionally be useful in evaluating the painful THA preoperatively. To differentiate infection from loosening more accurately, 111In leukocyte scans have been combined with complementary 99Tc sulfur colloid imaging. The 99Tc sulfur colloid has similar uptake to 111In-labeled WBC in normal bone; however, its uptake is inhibited by infection. This complementary scan improves the sensitivity and specificity in diagnosing infection from aseptic loosening of implants in THA.

Templating

Careful preoperative templating of an adequate set of radiographs is a crucial portion of preoperative planning for revision THA. The sequence of steps is analogous to primary THA and begins on the acetabular side. A porous-coated hemispheric component is used most commonly. The first step is to place an acetabular template against host bone to maximize coverage and attempt to place the inferomedial edge adjacent to the teardrop. Some degree of proximal migration frequently occurs because of bone loss. Fortunately, this frequently is offset because a larger component is used, which in many cases brings the center of rotation back close to normal. It is helpful to place the same size template that is planned on the AP view on a shoot-through lateral to ensure that the size selected will fit on both views. Overreaming can remove most or all of the bone of the anterior and posterior rim, making it difficult to obtain a press-fit. When the component has been placed in the desired position, the degree of uncoverage laterally should be determined. Minor degrees of as much as 20% generally can be ignored. When 20% to 40% of uncoverage is present, structural graft occasionally may be used, and distal femoral allograft generally is preferred. When contact of the porous-coated component with less than 50% to 60% host bone is anticipated, an antiprotrusio cage and structural bone graft should be available. If pelvic discontinuity is suspected, a CT scan may be helpful. Radiographic signs of pelvic discontinuity include a visible fracture line through the anterior and posterior columns, medial translation of the inferior aspect of the hemipelvis relative to the superior aspect (seen as a break in the Köhler line), and rotation of the inferior aspect of the hemipelvis relative to the superior aspect (seen as asymmetry of the obturator rings) on a true AP radiograph. A protrusio cage can be used in this scenario; however, alternatives such as posterior column plates also should be available.

After the acetabular side has been templated, the center of rotation is marked, and the femoral templating is planned around this center of rotation. As in the primary situation, restoring hip biomechanics is the ultimate goal, which is achieved by restoring leg length, offset, and center of rotation. The center of rotation is the most difficult to replicate because it is dependent on placement of the acetabular component, which often is nonanatomic because of bone loss. Specifically, with larger revision cup diameters, the center of rotation moves proximally. Eccentric, oblique, anteverted, or other special liner options may be useful, especially in the case of a jumbo acetabular component, in order to restore the center of rotation to a more anatomic level. Special femoral components must also be available to restore length and offset when there is a nonanatomic center of rotation. This frequently requires calcar replacements and stems with increased offset. It is important to have appropriate radiographs to determine offset. Typically, the hip should be internally rotated 15 degrees to compensate for the typical amount of femoral anteversion and to accurately reflect the offset of the femur. This brings the femoral neck to a plane 90 degrees to the radiograph and more accurately depicts the femoral offset and the area of the intertrochanteric region, which allows for more accurate femoral templating. If the affected hip cannot be rotated internally by this amount, it may be useful to template off the nonaffected side. The center of rotation is raised vertically by the amount of lengthening that is planned. Generally, only approximately two thirds of shortening is corrected at the time of surgery to avoid excessive tissue tension. When there is significant distortion in offset or length, or both, it also may be advisable to template off the nonoperative side. In such a case, the center of rotation should be transposed from the operative side to the nonoperative side, and the femoral side templating can proceed around that point, more normally reproducing length and offset.

The femoral template is then placed over the center of rotation of the acetabular component at the level of the plus zero head to allow for sizing above or below this point. Generally, a stem length is chosen that will bypass any femoral defects by two to three canal diameters. For extensively coated stems, an area of direct cortical contact with porous coating over approximately 6 cm is desirable. The stem diameter that most effectively achieves this is selected. Attention then is directed to the proximal fill and the point of contact with the collar relative to the available calcar bone. Invariably, there is some degree of bone loss in the area of the lesser trochanter, and frequently it is necessary to place a component on the lesser trochanter. As a general rule, this requires a 15-mm adjustment in vertical height. Most systems have calcar replacements that allow for replacement of 15- to 30-mm length. Bone loss to the top of the lesser trochanter generally requires a 15-mm calcar replacement (see Fig. 13). If more than 30- or 40-mm length must be restored, other options include proximal femoral replacement or an allograft prosthetic composite. If there is a cortical shell of bone for several centimeters proximally, followed by a short or narrow isthmus beyond this point, the situation is not ideal for cemented or cementless conventional stems. In this setting, impaction grafting may be considered. This requires an array of bone-grafting instruments and implants that requires additional planning, including surgeon education.

It is important to template the radiographs on a lateral view. Stem lengths greater than 175 mm frequently impinge on the anterior cortex distally. Longer stems frequently require a bow to avoid eccentric reaming or perforation (see Fig. 14). The AP radiograph also must be reviewed for varus remodeling of the proximal femur. This frequently necessitates an extended osteotomy to safely insert a long, cementless stem and occasionally may require a transfemoral osteotomy (Fig. 14). Templating of a cemented stem requires provision for room for a cement mantle that should be approximately 2 mm circumferentially. In addition, it generally is desirable to have contact between the cement mantle and relatively healthy bone for several centimeters. It is difficult to introduce a cemented stem longer than 160 to 180 mm without eccentric cement mantles and abutment of the cement tip on the femoral cortex. It generally is desirable to avoid

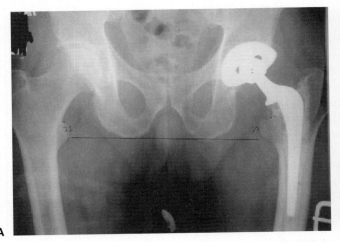

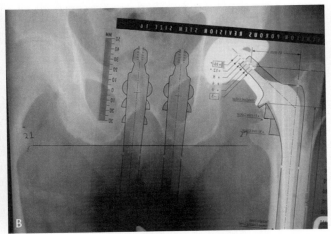

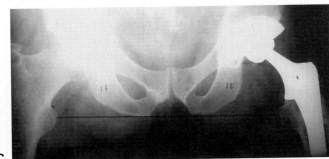

Figure 13. A: An AP radiograph shows a loose cemented stem with the operative side measuring 6 mm short radiographically. **B:** The template indicates that a 15-mm calcar replacement set on the lesser trochanter will restore limb length. **C:** A postoperative radiograph shows restoration of leg length with a 15-mm calcar replacement.

cementing stems beyond the isthmus because of the difficulty with cement pressurization and with subsequent revision of such stems.

Discussion

Adequate preoperative planning is the first and most important step in the successful completion of RTHA. The many challenges facing the surgeon usually exceed those of primary THA. A complex primary THA may require a similar preoperative planning process. Although the surgery may be complex in RTHA, the planning process should be organized and consistent. This should consist of a history and review of systems to ensure an accurate diagnosis and physical examination to take into account the unique findings of each patient. Careful review of a complete series of radiographs, implant records, and adjunctive laboratory testing or imaging follows the clinical encounter. Ruling out infection should be a part of every RTHA preoperative plan. Templating a clear plan for selection of implants, instruments, and other equipment and bone graft is essential to a successful outcome. Removal of well-fixed implants often requires specialized instruments that may not be immediately available. A backup plan or second line of reconstructive options should always be considered and in place prior to surgery. Communication with the operating room team in advance of surgery will help facilitate an efficient surgery. Using such an organized approach helps provide for more specific informed consent to the patient and family and prepares the surgeon and the operative team for the surgery. This helps reduce the operative time, minimize the risk of complications, and improve the chances of success for an RTHA procedure.

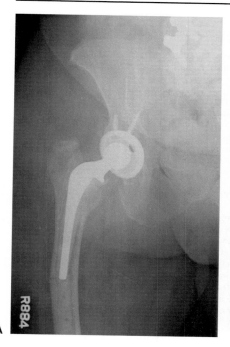

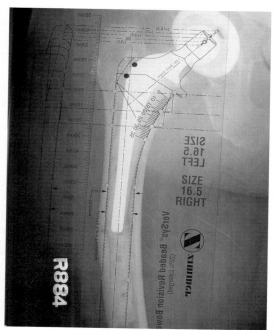

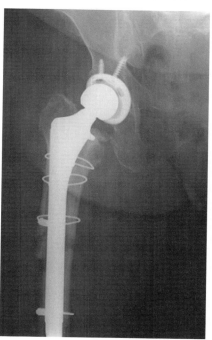

Figure 14. A: Preoperative radiograph showing a right THA with aseptic loosening of a cemented stem. There is varus remodeling of the femur, with an associated fracture, and templating **(B)** shows that a long cementless stem inserted without an osteotomy will result in perforation. **C:** Postoperative radiograph: a revision of the femoral component requiring an extended trochanteric osteotomy. The varus remodeling necessitated completion of a transfemoral osteotomy to allow the bowed stem to pass into the distal canal. There is strut allograft reinforcement of the osteotomy sites.

RECOMMENDED READING

1. Abernathy CM, Hamm RM. *Surgical Intuition: What It Is and How To Get It.* Philadelphia: Hanley & Belfus; 1995.
2. Baron J. *Thinking and Deciding.* Cambridge: Cambridge University Press; 2000.
3. Barrack RL. Preoperative planning for revision total hip arthroplasty. In: Steinberg ME, Garino JP, eds. *Revision Total Hip Arthroplasty.* Philadelphia: Lippincott Williams & Wilkins; 1998: 151–165.
4. Barrack RL, Harris WH. The value of aspiration of the hip joint before revision total hip arthroplasty. *J Bone Joint Surg Am* 75(1):66–76, 1993.
5. Berry DJ, Lewallen DG, Hanssen AD, et al. Pelvic discontinuity in revision total hip arthroplasty. *J Bone Joint Surg Am* 81(12):1692–1702, 1999.
6. Brown TE, Larson B, Shen F, Moskal JT. Thigh pain after cementless total hip arthroplasty: evaluation and management. *J Am Acad Orthop Surg* 10(6):385–392, 2002.

7. Della Valle CJ, Bogner E, Desai P, et al. Analysis of frozen sections of intraoperative specimens obtained at the time of reoperation after hip or knee resection arthroplasty for the treatment of infection. *J Bone Joint Surg Am* 81(5):684–689, 1999.

8. Fehring TK, Rosenberg AG. Primary total hip arthroplasty: indications and contraindications. In: Callahan JC, Rosenberg AG, Rubash HE, eds. *The Adult Hip.* Philadelphia: Lippincott–Raven Publishers; 1997: 893–898.

9. Jacobs JJ, Kull LR, Frey GA, et al. Early failure of acetabular components inserted without cement after previous pelvic irradiation. *J Bone Joint Surg Am* 77(12):1829–1835, 1995.

10. Kronick JL, Sekundiak T, Paprosky WG. Proximal femoral deformity secondary to loosening and osteolysis: the effect on reimplantation. *J Arthroplasty* 12(2):226–227, 1997.

11. Levitsky KA, Hozack WJ, Balderston RA, et al. Evaluation of the painful prosthetic joint: relative value of bone scan, sedimentation rate, and joint aspiration. *J Arthroplasty* 6(3):237–244, 1991.

12. Maloney WJ, Herzwurm P, Paprosky W, et al. Treatment of pelvic osteolysis associated with a stable acetabular component inserted without cement as part of a total hip replacement. *J Bone Joint Surg Am* 79(11):1628–1634, 1997.

13. Mancuso CA, Salvati EA, Johanson NA, et al. Patients' expectations and satisfaction with total hip arthroplasty. *J Arthroplasty* 12(4):387–396, 1997.

14. Pellegrini VD Jr, Gregoritch SJ. Preoperative irradiation for prevention of heterotopic ossification following total hip arthroplasty. *J Bone Joint Surg Am* 78(6):870–881, 1996.

15. Rothman RH, Hozack WJ. Early complications. In: Rothman RH, Hozack WJ, eds. *Complications of Total Hip Arthroplasty.* Philadelphia: WB Saunders; 1988: 14–30.

16. Spangehl MJ, Masri BA, O'Connell JX, et al. Prospective analysis of preoperative and intraoperative investigations for the diagnosis of infection at the sites of two hundred and two revision total hip arthroplasties. *J Bone Joint Surg Am* 81(5):672–683, 1999.

17. White RE. Evaluation of the painful total hip arthroplasty. In: Callahan JC, Rosenberg AG, Rubash HE, eds. *The Adult Hip.* Philadelphia: Lippincott–Raven Publishers; 1997:1377–1386.

22

Component Removal

Craig J. Della Valle

INDICATIONS/CONTRAINDICATIONS

The decision to remove loose components is often the primary indication for revision total hip arthroplasty (THA). However, when one of the components is well fixed, the decision-making process becomes more complex. While several reports have suggested that the repeat revision rate for well-fixed cementless and cemented femoral and acetabular components retained at the time of a revision procedure is acceptable, several factors must be considered when determining whether or not well-fixed components should be revised. First and foremost, the surgeon must decide preoperatively and intraoperatively how the retention of a well-fixed component will affect the overall stability of the revision construct. With instability rates of up to 20% reported after isolated component revision, even in experienced hands, preventing instability has become a critical goal for the revision hip surgeon.

Well-fixed Femoral Components

When addressing the femoral side, the surgeon first must determine intraoperatively if the anteversion of the component is appropriate to provide acceptable stability; retroverted components almost always require revision. The second important issue relates primarily to well-fixed femoral components with nonmodular heads. Nonmodular femoral heads limit the ability to create the offset and length that may be needed for a stable reconstruction. Although various liner options are available for most modern acetabular shells (including offset, eccentric, oblique, and elevated rim) if adequate stability cannot be obtained, the femoral component may need to be removed. An additional option is the use of a constrained liner; these devices, however, are associated with increased stress at the interface between the revision acetabular shell and host bone and can fail catastrophically (see Fig. 1). Gross damage to a nonmodular femoral head is another indication for the removal of a well-fixed femoral component, as wear of the bearing surface would be

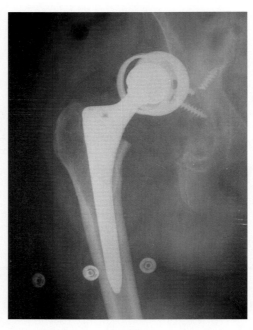

Figure 1. Catastrophic failure of acetabular component with a constrained liner.

adversely affected. Similarly, consideration should also be given to removing well-fixed stems with gross damage or severe corrosion of the Morse taper.

An additional consideration is whether or not a larger-diameter femoral head (greater than 36 mm) can be mated to the Morse taper that is in place. Larger-diameter femoral heads are associated with more favorable head-neck ratios and a substantial increase in the range of motion that decreases the possibility of impingement and appear to have dramatically decreased the rate of instability following revision THA. One of the potential options when a nonmodular 28-mm femoral head is in place or when larger-diameter femoral heads are not compatible with the Morse taper that is in place is the use of a tripolar construct. This technique mates a 40-mm outer diameter, 28-mm inner diameter bipolar head with a standard 28-mm head and effectively creates a large-diameter articulation when one is not commercially available (see Fig. 2). Final indications for the removal of a well-fixed cementless femoral implant include distal osteolysis in a first-generation cementless design with noncircumferential porous coating.

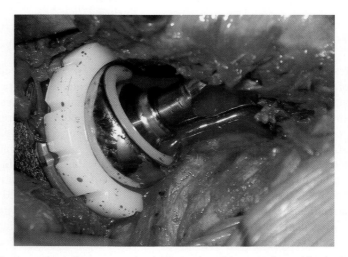

Figure 2. Tripolar articulation; a standard 28-mm head is mated to a bipolar head with a 40-mm outer diameter, a 28-mm inner diameter, and a 40-mm liner.

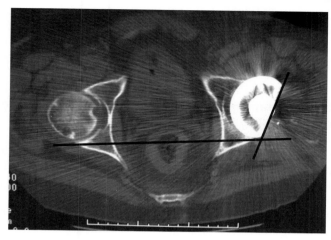

Figure 3. CT scan of the pelvis showing retroversion of the acetabular component.

Well-fixed Acetabular Components

Although well-fixed cemented all-polyethylene acetabular components have been associated with an acceptable rate of repeat revision if retained, as previously discussed, femoral head options are typically limited in these situations, and these components are generally removed so that larger-diameter femoral heads can be utilized. Removal of such components is typically straightforward, as is the subsequent reconstruction.

When considering the retention of a well-fixed cementless acetabular component, the first consideration is component position. Components that are inadequately anteverted or outside the acceptable range of inclination (between 35 and 55 degrees of cup abduction) should be removed. As the intraoperative judgment of acetabular anteversion can be problematic, a preoperative computed tomography (CT) scan can be useful in this regard (see Fig. 3). The next consideration is that of the types of replacement liners available. Although a new liner can oftentimes be cemented into a well-fixed shell, smaller-diameter components, shells that are shallow, or shells that have a thick wall may not be amenable to this technique. In addition, when confronted with components that have known problems with a poor polyethylene liner locking mechanism, strong consideration should be given to cementing a replacement liner into the shell. If significant osteolysis is present, the decision to retain or remove the shell can be complex as well. In general, it is my preference to retain well-fixed components even if significant osteolysis is present since removal in these situations can lead to large defects that can be difficult to reconstruct. A final consideration is the removal of well-fixed cementless acetabular components with poor intermediate to long-term survival rates (such as first-generation hydroxyapatite-coated cups).

PREOPERATIVE PLANNING

Adequate preoperative planning is critical to a successful outcome in revision THA. The most important portion of this evaluation includes definitive identification of the components that are in place. Specific extraction devices are oftentimes available and critical to the safe extraction of well-fixed components. Similarly, preoperative identification of the surface finish of well-fixed cemented femoral components can be critical as certain components (such as those with polymethylmethacrylate precoating) may frequently require the use of an extended trochanteric osteotomy to remove safely. If components are to be retained, both trial and replacement femoral heads and liners should be available. Furthermore, the identification of in situ components allows for appropriate decision making in regard to the removal of components with known problems. If the removal of a well-fixed, extensively coated femoral component is a possibility, specialized instruments will be required as described in the following sections.

SURGERY

Patient Positioning, Draping, Surgical Approach, and Organization of the Operating Room

Position the patient in the lateral decubitus position, taking care to rigidly secure the pelvis to the operating room table, perpendicular to the floor. Great care is taken to pad the down chest and the underside of the down leg, which is typically placed in a slightly flexed position. The lower extremity is prepped from the iliac crest proximally to just above the knee distally and draped free to ensure that a full range of motion can be obtained to adequately test stability (see Fig. 4). Prior skin incisions are typically used to avoid wound-healing problems. My preference is to use a posterior approach to the hip as it is extensile both proximally and distally, allows for access to the posterior column of the pelvis if needed, and is compatible with an extended trochanteric osteotomy if required. Adequate exposure is necessary, and the femur must be sufficiently mobilized to allow for circumferential acetabular exposure. A large operating room is generally used with adequate space for multiple tables given the large number of instruments and trials often required.

Removal of Modular Femoral Heads

After the hip has been exposed, dislocate the femoral head from the acetabulum. Modular femoral heads should be removed to assist with exposure and to allow for their exchange. Remove the femoral head with care so as not to damage the Morse taper, particularly if the femoral component is to be retained. This is most easily accomplished by placing a specially designed wedge beneath the modular junction and impacting the wedge in place, which will disengage the Morse taper (see Fig. 5). A footed impactor can also be utilized; however, this may damage the Morse taper. If the femoral head is nonmodular and the femur is to be retained, perform an anterior capsulectomy to retract the femoral head anterior to the acetabulum in a soft tissue pocket.

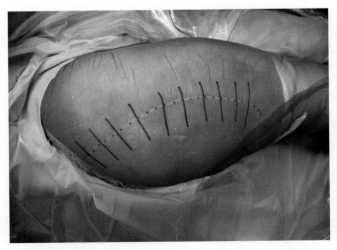

Figure 4. The extremity has been prepped and draped with the entire extremity free to allow for stability testing. The prior skin incision has been clearly marked and will be utilized for the approach.

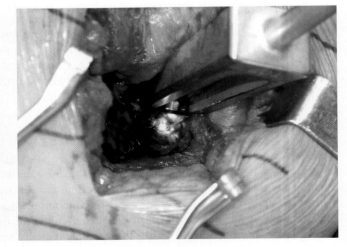

Figure 5. Place a wedge-shaped tuning fork between the modular femoral head and the stem to remove it without damaging the Morse taper.

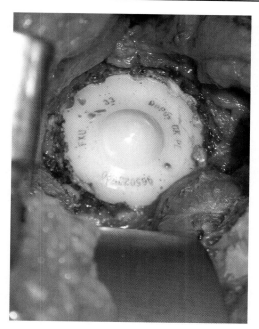

Figure 6. Exposure of acetabular component.

Removal of Cemented Acetabular Components

The extraction of a well-fixed, cemented all-polyethylene acetabular component is typically straightforward. After adequate retraction of the femur anteriorly (see Fig. 6), an osteotome, saw, or high-speed burr can be used to cut the component into quarters (see Fig. 7). Conventional curved acetabular osteotomes are then used to break up the cup, which is

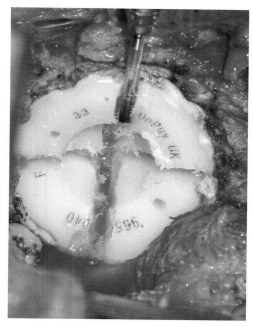

Figure 7. The cemented polyethylene cup is quartered with a pencil-tipped, high-speed burr.

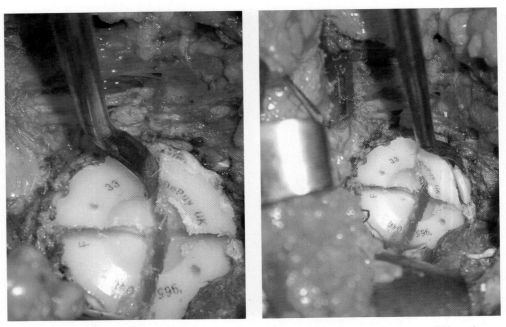

Figure 8. Place a curved acetabular osteotome into the cuts made in the cup **(A)** and behind the cup itself **(B)** to remove the component.

easily removed in pieces (see Fig. 8). Retained cement is removed either with hand osteotomes, curved cement removal instruments, or a high-speed burr (see Fig. 9). Large pockets of cement are most easily removed by cutting them into smaller pieces with a high-speed burr. Retained cement lug holes, which are often made in the ischium, pubis, and ilium, can be extracted by placing a small threaded Steinmann pin into the center of the lug, bending the exposed tip of the pin and using it as a handle to extract the retained cement. It is not necessary (and, in fact, it may be dangerous) to remove large pieces of cement that are beyond the medial wall of the acetabulum, as these may be adherent to intrapelvic vascular structures. Removal of these cement masses must be done with great caution and may require separate intrapelvic exposure as described in Chapter 5 on intrapelvic exposures.

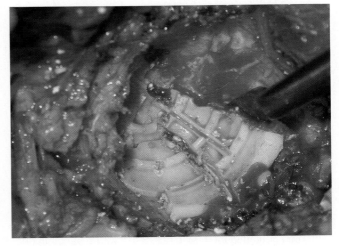

Figure 9. Removal of cement using a curved acetabular osteotome.

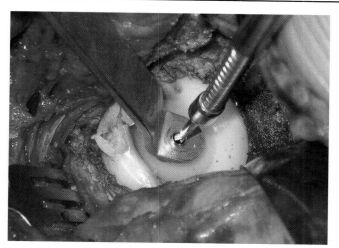

Figure 10. Drill a hole in the center of the polyethylene liner.

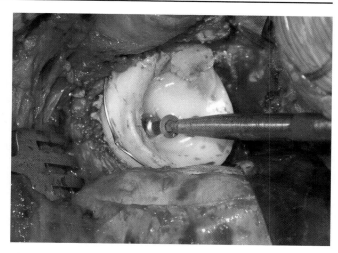

Figure 11. Place a screw into the hole to disengage the polyethylene liner.

Removal of Cementless Acetabular Components

Removing a well-fixed cementless acetabular component begins with removing the polyethylene liner. If the locking mechanism cannot be easily defeated, the majority of liners can be removed by drilling a hole in the center (see Fig. 10) and then inserting a tap or 6.5-mm screw into the hole, thereby levering out the polyethylene liner (see Fig. 11). Any screws that are present are then removed. If the screws are stripped, the head is burred off within the shell with a metal-cutting burr so that osteotomes can be placed around it and the screw shaft can be removed with a broken screw removal trephine or with pliers after the shell has been extracted.

Traditional techniques for removal of the cup itself usually involve the use of curved osteotomes placed around the cup. Although commonly used, this technique has been associated with significant bone loss, particularly if the removed component is in close proximity to the teardrop, and thus many surgeons prefer the Explant system cup remover (Zimmer, Warsaw, IN). This system uses a femoral head substitute as a fulcrum attached to sized, curved blades that match the curvature of the component. This combination fixes the motion of the blade to precisely disrupt the interface between the component and the surrounding host bone. A "short" blade is used first, followed by a longer blade to completely disrupt the interface (see Figs. 12 and 13).

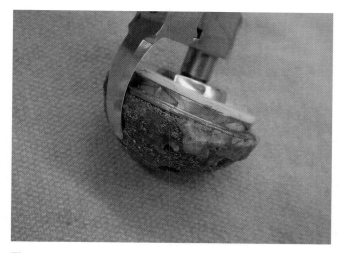

Figure 12. Precisely sized blade to disrupt the interface between the ingrowth surface and the component.

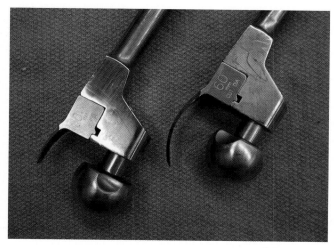

Figure 13. "Short" and "long" blades of the Implex cup remover.

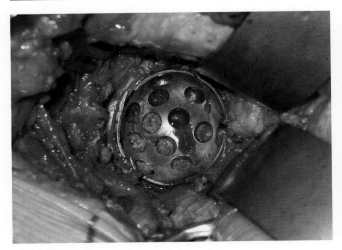

Figure 14. Obtain wide exposure of the component to enable access circumferentially.

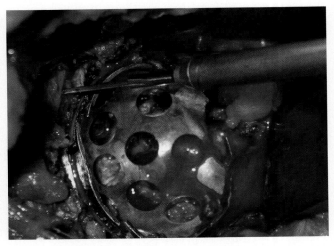

Figure 15. Use a pencil-tipped, high-speed burr to make a trough around the component.

Use is facilitated by carefully exposing the periphery of the cup in its entirety with a pencil-tipped burr to create a trough around the component (see Figs. 14 and 15). The extracted liner (or an appropriately sized trial) is placed back into the component, and an appropriately sized blade is selected on the basis of the outer diameter of the component. It is imperative to know the precise outer diameter of the cup that is being removed (either from a review of prior operative notes or by reading the size off of the inner surface of the cup that is being removed) if this technique is utilized. The short blade is first used around the entire periphery of the component by firmly rotating it around the cup. This is followed by the longer blade, which is passed in the same motion (see Fig. 16). The component typically then easily rotates out with minimal loss of host bone (see Fig. 17).

Removal of Cemented Femoral Components

The first step in removing any well-fixed femoral component is complete clearance of overhanging soft tissue, bone, and cement (if present) from the lateral shoulder of the femoral component to allow for extraction and to prevent fracture of the greater trochanter; a high-speed burr is often helpful in this regard (see Figs. 18 and 19). My preference for removing

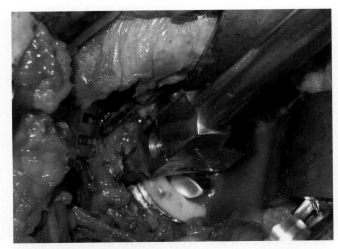

Figure 16. The blade of the cup remover is placed into the trough created with the burr and passed around the component in a firm, circular motion.

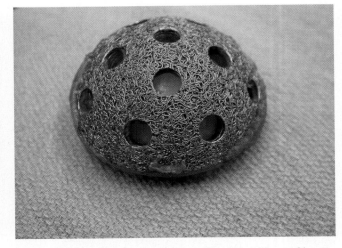

Figure 17. Removed component with minimal loss of host bone stock.

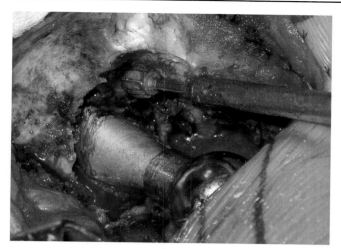

Figure 18. A high-speed burr is used to debride overhanging bone, cement, and soft tissue from the lateral shoulder of the prosthesis to aid with extraction.

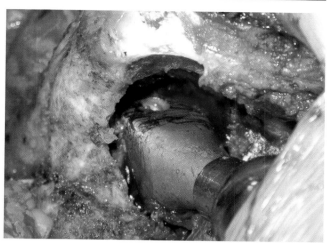

Figure 19. Following thorough debridement at the base of the greater trochanter, the entire lateral shoulder of the prosthesis is visible.

well-fixed cemented femoral components includes the use of an extended trochanteric osteotomy. Although covered elsewhere in depth, certain points are worthy of mention. The osteotomy is most easily accomplished after the component has been removed; if the component has a polished surface, the component is easily tapped out of the cement mantle by placing a footed impactor at the base of the component after all of the surrounding soft tissue and any overhanging bone and cement have been cleared (see Fig. 20). However, roughened or precoated components may require the use of this osteotomy to remove these components, which are tightly bonded to the cement mantle. The distal extent of the osteotomy is carefully templated preoperatively to ensure adequate length. The length of the osteotomy is based on the length of the revision femoral component used for the subsequent reconstruction. The osteotomy is made of adequate length to allow for 5 to 6 cm of press fit of an extensively coated stem distal to the osteotomy (see Fig. 21).

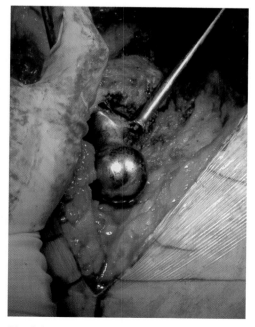

Figure 20. A footed impactor is used to tap the component out of the cement mantle after all soft tissue has been cleared from around the stem.

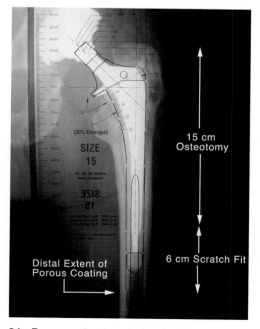

Figure 21. Preoperative templating for the use of an extended trochanteric osteotomy for removing a cemented femoral component.

After the osteotomy is opened, remove the femoral component by disrupting the interface between the femoral component and the cement mantle with a high-speed pencil-tipped burr. Well-fixed cement is most easily removed by dividing it into smaller pieces with a high-speed burr and then extracting the pieces with hand instruments.

Removal of distal cement can be approached with a "drill and tap" technique or with the use of ultrasonic tools. To use the drill and tap technique, drill a hole in the center of the cement mantle (to a depth of approximately 1 cm) using a cement drill; it is critical to be centered, and a canal light can be introduced to ensure appropriate placement of the hole. These drills come in various diameters. Follow this by inserting a tap into the cement mantle. Once the tap is anchored firmly, it is reverse malleted out, extracting a cylinder of cement (see Fig. 22). This procedure is repeated until the final plug is removed.

Ultrasonic tools (commonly known as Orthosonics System for Cemented Arthroplasty Revision [OSCAR]) work by melting the cement mantle and then extracting it in small segments. Cortical bone responds differently to these ultrasonic tools, and thus audible and tactile feedback allows the surgeon to differentiate the two, thereby decreasing the risk of femoral canal perforation. Endoscopic cameras have been added to some of these systems to allow for direct visualization down the femoral canal. This technique is most useful, in my experience, when combined with an extended trochanteric osteotomy to remove long cement mantles (see Fig. 23). Various tips are available, including tips to penetrate or "pierce" the cement mantle and tips to scrape cement off of the sides of the femoral canal (see Fig. 24). The tip of the instrument should not be allowed to contact any metallic surfaces, as this will damage the handset. Once the desired tip has been selected, place gentle pressure on the handset until the tip has advanced approximately 5 mm, release the power, and then withdraw the handset 1 or 2 seconds later once the melted cement has solidified so that it can be removed (see Fig. 25).

Removal of Proximally Coated, Cementless Femoral Components

The removal of a well-fixed, proximally coated femoral component can be performed with or without trochanteric osteotomy. Prior to removing a proximally coated stem, it is

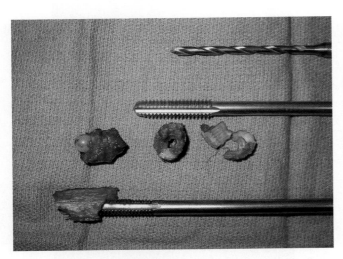

Figure 22. A cement drill (top) is first used to make a pilot hole in the cement mantle. Next, a tap is inserted (middle), and then once firmly anchored, the tap is reverse malleted out to withdraw the retained cement (bottom).

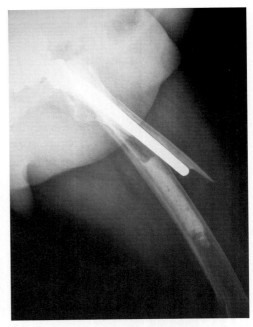

Figure 23. Ultrasonic cement removal devices are most useful in cases where a long cement mantle is present distally.

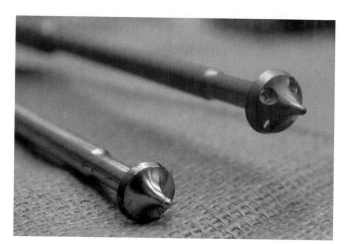

Figure 24. "Scraper" *(left)* and "Piercer" *(right)* tips for the OSCAR.

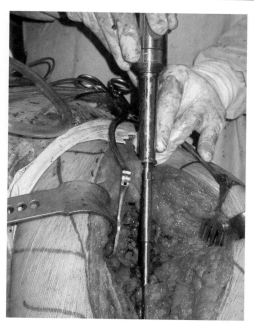

Figure 25. The handset of the OSCAR is advanced into the cement mantle to remove the distal cement plug or scraped along the sides of the femoral canal to remove retained cement.

important to identify the exact make and model of femoral component to be removed. While these devices primarily depend on an in- or ongrowth surface present on the proximal portion of the stem to obtain long-term fixation, many have a bioreactive surface (such as corundumized surface blasting) on the more distal portions of the stem that becomes well bonded to the host bone and, if present, the use of an extended trochanteric osteotomy may be needed for safe removal. Furthermore, components made from titanium, even if devoid of a bioreactive surface more distally can become strongly bonded to the surrounding host bone, making extraction equally challenging.

Removal without an Extended Trochanteric Osteotomy. Completely clear any existing soft tissue and bone from the lateral shoulder of the femoral component; this is critical for extraction without damaging the greater trochanter (Figs. 18 and 19). Next, disrupt the interface between the femoral component and the host bone anteriorly, posteriorly, and laterally with the use of a small, high-speed pencil-tipped burr. If a collar is present medially, it can be cut off with a high-speed metal-cutting burr to allow access to the interface between the prosthesis and host bone medially. Thin osteotomes are then passed in this same interval until the interface between the ingrowth surface and the host bone has been disrupted circumferentially (see Fig. 26). The stem is then removed with a large slap hammer attached to a universal removal device or by using the extraction hole, which is commonly present proximally.

Removal with an Extended Trochanteric Osteotomy. Completely clear out all soft tissue and bone overhanging the lateral shoulder of the prosthesis. The length of the osteotomy to be used is determined preoperatively by templating as previously described; typically, the osteotomy is 12 cm in length (as measured from the tip of the greater trochanter) if a 6-inch revision femoral component is to be used and 16 cm in length if the desired length of the revision femoral component is 8 inches in length. These lengths allow for 4 to 6 cm of press fit distal to the osteotomy if a fully porous coated or tapered, distally fitting device is used.

Measure out the length of the osteotomy and perform the initial cut from the base of the greater trochanter distally with a saw or pencil-tipped burr. The lateral fragment should

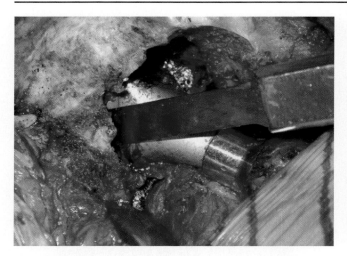

Figure 26. Disrupt the interface between the ingrowth surface and the host bone with a thin osteotome.

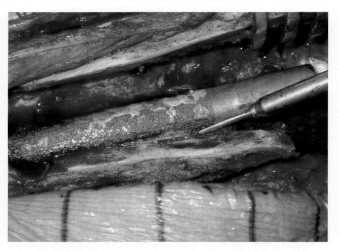

Figure 27. Disrupt the interface between the stem and the host bone with a high-speed burr once the extended trochanteric osteotomy has been performed.

encompass approximately one third of the diameter of the proximal femoral shaft. More details on performance of this technique can be found in Chapter 4. Once the osteotomy is opened, the lateral border of the prosthesis is clearly visible (see Fig. 27). Use a high-speed, pencil-tipped burr to disrupt the interface between the femoral component and the host bone both anteriorly and posteriorly (Fig. 27). Next, place a Gigli saw around the medial portion of the stem to disrupt the medial interface (see Fig. 28); this process can take some time and often requires multiple Gigli saws, as they break easily. Once the entire interface is disrupted medially, the component is easily removed by hand.

Removal of Extensively Coated, Cementless Femoral Components

The removal of an osseointegrated extensively coated femoral stem requires time and patience to avoid severe damage to the surrounding bone stock. An extended trochanteric osteotomy is mandatory for safe removal, and the length of the osteotomy performed is templated preoperatively as previously discussed; in general, longer osteotomies are needed when removing this type of implant (as opposed to a proximally coated or cemented implant) given the difficult nature of their removal.

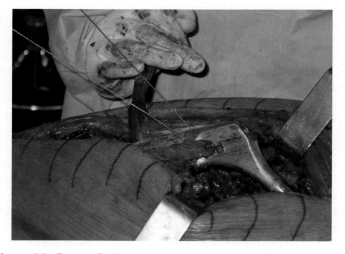

Figure 28. Pass a Gigli saw around the medial border of the stem.

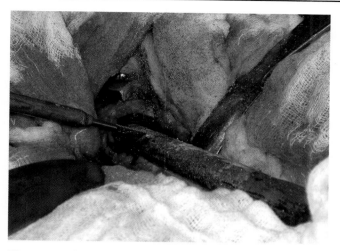

Figure 29. Cut the stem just proximal to the distal extent of the extended trochanteric osteotomy site with a metal-cutting burr; note the liberal use of laps to protect the soft tissues and to facilitate removal of metallic debris.

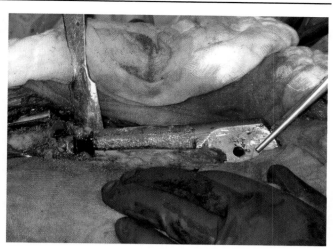

Figure 30. The stem has been cut, and the proximal portion is removed.

After the osteotomy is completed, disrupt the interface between the femoral component and the surrounding host bone anteriorly and posteriorly using a high-speed, pencil-tipped burr (Fig. 27). Pass a Gigli saw around the medial border of the stem to disrupt this interface (Fig. 28); as previously noted, multiple Gigli saws are often required, as they break easily. Cut the femoral component just proximal to the distal extent of the osteotomy with a metal-cutting high-speed burr; as many of these stems are made of cobalt chrome, multiple tips are often required, particularly if the stem has a larger diameter (see Figs. 29 and 30). Once the stem has been cut, the proximal portion can be easily removed. The distal stem is removed with an appropriately sized trephine (see Figs. 31 and 32) placed around the cylindrical distal portion of the retained stem; ideally, the trephine should be 0.5 mm larger than the diameter of the stem to be removed. When using the trephine, irrigate it heavily to avoid thermal damage to the surrounding cortical bone. Definitive preoperative identification of the diameter of the component to be removed is helpful to ensure that an adequate number of appropriately sized trephines are available. In my experience, each trephine can

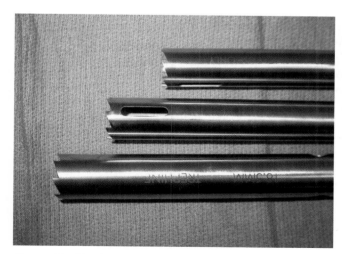

Figure 31. Trephines that are used to remove the distal stem segment once it has been cut.

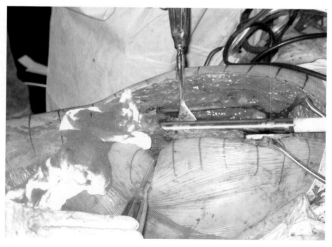

Figure 32. Using a trephine to remove the distal stem segment.

only be used for approximately 1 cm of cutting before if becomes dull if the stem is bone ingrown. Once the entire distal interface between the retained distal femoral stem segment and the host bone has been disrupted, the distal piece will become entrapped within the final trephine, and it comes out with the trephine when removed.

COMPLICATIONS

The most common complications relate to damaging native bone stock, which can compromise the subsequent reconstruction. During acetabular component removal, it is critical to ensure that the entire periphery of the component is exposed and free of overhanging soft tissue and bone to avoid difficulties during component extraction. Prior to attempting final component removal, the entire interface between the component and the surrounding host bone must be disrupted to avoid inadvert removal of host bone or the creation of a pelvic discontinuity. Contained cancellous bone defects can be managed by local grafting with fresh frozen cancellous bone grafts, whereas more severe damage may require structural grafting. If a pelvic discontinuity is created, plating of the posterior column should be performed to stabilize the pelvis.

The removal of femoral components can also lead to loss of host bone stock as well as fractures of the proximal femur and cortical perforations. As previously discussed, thorough clearing of soft tissue, bone cement, and overhanging bone from the lateral shoulder of the prosthesis is critical to assisting with component extraction and avoiding fractures of the greater trochanter. If a fracture of the trochanter occurs, rigid fixation with a claw or cable plate device is necessary. If during distal cement removal a cortical perforation is suspected, the area must be exposed to identify the extent of the perforation. A femoral component long enough to bypass the defect for at least two cortical diameters should be used to prevent the creation of a stress riser that can lead to late femoral fracture; alternatively, a strut allograft can be placed over the defect with cables. Similarly, more distal femoral fractures must be fully exposed with distal extension of the incision if needed and are treated by bypassing the fracture with a femoral component that extends past the fracture for a length of approximately two cortical diameters. Further fixation of the fracture can be obtained with the use of strut allografts fixed with cables along the fracture site. In any situation where a fracture is suspected, the liberal use of intraoperative x-rays is recommended to definitively identify and then fully define the extent of the fracture prior to films obtained in the recovery room.

RECOMMENDED READING

1. Glassman AH. The removal of cementless total hip femoral components. *Instr Course Lect* 51:93–101, 2002.
2. Meek RM, Garbuz DS, Masri BA, et al. Intraoperative fracture of the femur in revision total hip arthroplasty with a diaphyseal fitting stem. *J Bone Joint Surg Am* 86(3):480–485, 2004.
3. Mitchell PA, Masri BA, Garbuz DS, et al. Removal of well-fixed, cementless, acetabular components in revision hip arthroplasty. *J Bone Joint Surg Br* 85(7):949–952, 2003.
4. Paprosky WG, Weeden SH, Bowling JW Jr. Component removal in revision total hip arthroplasty. *Clin Orthop Relat Res* 393:181–193, 2001.

23

Cementing Long Stems

Donald W. Howie and Andrew D. MacDowell

INDICATIONS/CONTRAINDICATIONS

The indications for cemented long-stem revision total hip replacement are aseptic loosening, including osteolysis, in two thirds of our cases, and in the remaining one third, periprosthetic fractures, conversion of previous excision arthroplasties, recurrent dislocation, infection and, rarely, unexplained pain. This technique is used routinely in middle-aged and elderly patients. Femoral impaction grafting is used in young patients and in special circumstances, and cementless distal fixation is reserved for comminuted or difficult periprosthetic fractures and severe proximal cortical bone deficiency.

In general, cemented long-stem revision can be used for all deficiencies down to the lesser trochanter and in the older patient for deficiencies up to 2.5 cm below the lesser trochanter. Thus, this technique can be used for type 1 to 3 femurs as graded using the Gross classification of femoral deficiency, and some femurs with type 4 deficiencies (1).

Early experience with cemented femoral revisions was associated with an unacceptably high rate of complications and rerevision due to poor cementing, use of standard-length stems, acetabular component failure, and poor stem design. However, more recently, good results have been reported using improved cement techniques and long stems (2). Interestingly, similar problems of failure of the early designs of cementless revision stems were also seen.

Our results (3) and those of others (2,4) support the use of longer femoral components for cemented revisions. Bone strains can be reduced to near-normal levels if the revision stem passes beyond cortical diaphyseal defects by one and a half femoral canal diameters (5), and finite element analysis shows a significant improvement in the relative motion and cement-bone interface stresses (6). Given these findings, it has been our practice to bypass cortical defects by two canal diameters and to extend the femoral stem 5 cm past the areas of major endocortical damage.

Advantages of using cemented fixation of long stems at revision include immediate fixation allowing rapid full weight bearing and early rehabilitation. This is particularly valuable in middle-aged and elderly patients who do not cope well with partial weight bearing. An important advantage of cemented long-stem revision is that the procedure is simplified by using the stem and cement combination as a customized construct that fits the damaged femur exactly, while aiming for stem position that approximates the axial alignment of the femur without the need to be absolutely midline in both planes. Thus, this system is forgiving of femoral deformity and can be used to fit femoral deficiency and deformity without the need for aggressive bone removal or extended trochanteric or other corrective osteotomy.

Another advantage is that cemented fixation minimizes the risk of periprosthetic fracture because no impaction of the stem is necessary. Cement fixation also eliminates the need for reaming of bone to fit a stem. Furthermore, cement fixation is along the whole of the stem, so the construct can accommodate some proximal bone loss, provided there is still adequate proximal bone support for the stem.

The polished, collarless design and the continuous taper or the consecutive dual taper allow for stem removal from the cement in cases of rerevision for instability or infection. Leg length can be easily modified on the basis of the trial reduction. This may be achieved by seating the stem slightly proud or slightly recessed. There is minimal risk of stem fracture because a forged stem with inherent high strength is used. This stem design is also relatively low cost. A long cemented stem is approximately one third to one quarter the cost of a monobloc or modular cementless stem.

The rationale for using a polished cemented collarless double-taper femoral stem for long-stem revision is that the stem optimizes the transfer of compressive forces to the cement, the double taper wedging solidly in the bone cement mantle as the stem stabilizes. Thus, controlled subsidence in the first year following surgery is expected to occur, but after stabilization, further subsidence is minimal (7–11).

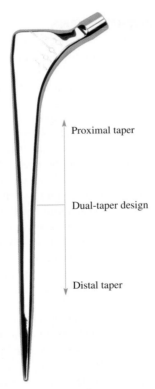

Proximal taper

Dual-taper design

Distal taper

Figure 1. Diagram showing a long, polished dual-taper stem with consecutive proximal to distal tapers, which optimizes the fit within the cement and optimally loads both cement and bone. (Courtesy of Zimmer, Inc., Warsaw, IN.)

Long cemented collarless double-taper stems are of two types. The shorter of the long stems has a continuous taper from proximal to distal and is suitable for some simple revisions. The longer stems have an intermediate segment in the midstem that is either another taper or, in some designs, a cylindrical portion. These longer stems are used for the more common revision scenario of proximal and/or more distal bone damage. Some stems have a distinctive dual-taper design in that they maintain the principle of the double-taper collarless tapered stem, but have two consecutive tapers from proximal to distal, with the proximal taper blending into the stem taper (see Fig. 1). The dual taper is designed to maximize the advantages of a tapered cemented stem.

PREOPERATIVE ASSESSMENT

Examination and Evaluation

The preoperative examination is thorough and in particular includes measurement of real leg length discrepancy, Trendelenberg test, assessment of power of hip abduction, and flexion and palpation of the glutei to ensure functioning muscle. Preoperative patient- and doctor-derived evaluation of pain and function is important for reporting outcomes.

Radiography

Preoperative radiographic evaluation of the femoral component and femur is undertaken using an anteroposterior (AP) pelvis radiograph centered on the pubis (see Fig. 2) and a long-leg anteroposterior hip (see Fig. 3) and lateral/oblique hip radiograph showing the femur down to the supracondylar region.

CEMENTED LONG-STEM REVISION

Preoperative Planning

Careful preoperative planning is vital to the success of revision hip arthroplasty. A general principle is to plan the most appropriate reconstruction for the individual patient needs but to have other choices available intraoperatively.

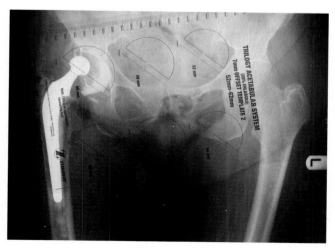

Figure 2. Preoperative AP pelvis radiograph. The AP pelvis radiograph is used to template the acetabular component and approximately determine the new center of hip rotation.

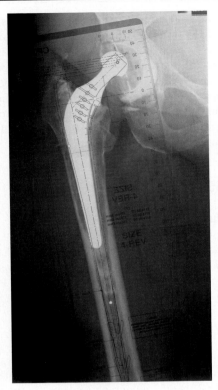

Figure 3. Preoperative AP radiograph with femoral template overlaid. Following templating of the femoral component on the preoperative pelvis radiograph to determine component depth of insertion and offset, the plug site, the extent of bone grafting, and the need for proximal reconstruction are planned. The presence of incongruities or an excessive bow or angulation in the AP or lateral planes is noted.

Templating should be carried out first for the acetabular component and then for the femoral component. The femur is templated to plan stem length, size, offset, depth of insertion, plug site, extent of bone grafting, and the need for proximal reconstruction. These may need to be modified according to intraoperative findings but provide a basis for planning. Areas of major osteolysis, stress risers, femoral perforations, and points of angulation or malrotation are clearly delineated, as all of these influence the size and length of stem required.

The template selected is one that best fits the proximal femur, leaving room for cement (Fig. 3). The femoral template is aligned so that it is centered in the diaphysis, and then the template is moved so that the center of the femoral head and shoulder of the stem are appropriately positioned to restore the planned amount of leg length. While aligning the femoral template in the canal, the presence of incongruities or an excessive bow or angulation in the AP or lateral planes will become evident. After indicating the planned center of rotation on the radiograph and the proper position of the femoral component, the optimal head position and stem offset are determined. In conjunction with clinical measurement and preoperative radiographs, limb length is predicted on the basis of the hip center and the height of the calcar and lesser trochanter. The appropriate relationship between the height of the tip of the trochanter, or other lateral landmark, and the center of femoral head rotation should be determined as well as potential difficulties in implant removal and insertion. If necessary, the level and type of femoral or trochanteric osteotomy and the bed for its reattachment is planned. The need for proximal reconstruction and the extent of bone graft required should also be determined. These may have to be modified intraoperatively but will provide a base for planning.

An important advantage of the collarless stem is that it can be adjusted proximally and distally as needed to the required leg length. Both when templating and intraoperatively, aim to achieve appropriate leg length without using the longer heads, which have a skirt. These are reserved for situations where an unplanned increase in leg length is required.

Surgery

Specifics of Positioning, Draping, and Organization of Operating Room.
Anesthesia by epidural catheter is routinely used for revisions and is often supplemented by a general anesthetic. Patients are placed in the lateral position, and anterior and posterior pelvic clamps are used to stabilize the pelvis. The pelvis is perpendicular to the operating table with the back parallel and the opposite hip flexed. A foam pad is placed between the knees and taped in place to allow knees and ankles to be palpated for leg length determination. Small foam pads are used to cushion the underlying fibula head and lateral malleolus.

Preparation and draping are along standard lines with aqueous povidone-iodine paint used to prepare the whole leg from the malleoli to nipple line and across the midline, the groin being painted last. A large drape is placed over the contralateral leg to the groin, and another is placed over the trunk above the iliac crest. A U-drape is used to drape off the perineum but permitting maximal posterior access and leaving the iliac crest exposed. The leg is bagged with crepe bandage to just above the knee. Large paper or plastic disposable hip drapes are placed over the leg and held to poles with clips. An iodized sterile, adherent, clear plastic incise drape is folded double under the thigh, and a large iodized drape is folded over the lateral thigh. Access should be available from the iliac crest and include the proximal two thirds of the femur. With the heels together, the positions of the flexed knees are compared as a guide to leg length.

Approach.
The hip joint is exposed using the approach of choice. More extensive exposure is generally required for revision surgery. An extensive exposure is recommended, especially in difficult revision cases. We would strongly recommend using a posterior approach, with or without a trochanteric slide, or an extended trochanteric (transfemoral) approach. A straight distal skin incision centered over the greater trochanter and curving slightly posterior proximally toward posterior superior iliac spine is used with the hip flexed 20 degrees and adducted across the contralateral thigh.

There are key points during the exposure to which we pay particular attention. First, as successful revision surgery is reliant on maintaining good abductor function, take time to clearly identify the gluteus medius muscle and tendon. The simplest way to do this is by finding the anterior aspect of the muscle and developing a plane between gluteus medius and gluteus maximus from anterior to posterior, eventually identifying clearly the plane between the main tendon posteriorly and the piriformis tendon. In this way, the abductors will always be protected, whereas simply dividing gluteus maximus in the line of its fibers can cause devastating and irreparable damage to medius in the common revision scenario where medius is adherent to maximus with scar tissue. We would always advise dividing the tendinous insertion of gluteus maximus from the femur during revision surgery to facilitate exposure. While doing this and while dividing the short external rotators, the foot is placed on a padded, draped Mayo table so that the femur drops into some internal rotation, allowing the sciatic nerve to fall away from the area of dissection. The sciatic nerve is identified in almost all cases, and having been visualized, its course is checked to make sure it is clear of the dissection. This does not require full exposure but at least palpation of the nerve course. In general, stay on bone during dissection. Cutting diathermy is used frequently throughout the procedure.

Determine Leg Length.
Prior to dislocating the hip, a baseline measurement of leg length is obtained. We recommend measuring from a pin in the ischium to a diathermy mark at the vastus ridge.

Remove Femoral Component.
The hip is carefully dislocated, and the femoral component is removed. We now routinely apply a cerclage wire to the proximal femur at this stage to protect the often fragile proximal femur. To protect the proximal femur during implantation of the acetabular component, any residual cement is left in the femur and removed following reconstruction of the socket.

Ideally, the femoral component is removed without an osteotomy because this unnecessarily converts a cavitory defect into an uncontained cortical defect, with increased risk of complications and which is a significant problem if union is not successful. Removal is simplified by aggressively clearing any overhanging medial bone at the greater trochanter. Sometimes further exposure is required for removal of the existing stem, especially if this is cementless with a fixation surface extending distally. We prefer to use the trochanteric slide, as it maintains the abductor-trochanter-vastus complex; however, if this is insufficient, such as in removing a well-fixed fully porous coated stem, the extended trochanteric osteotomy or transfemoral approach may be necessary and is reduced and fixed in place prior to preparing for a cemented long stem.

Revise Acetabular Component. Following removal of components to be revised, a new acetabular component is inserted, if necessary.

Femoral Canal Preparation. If there is residual cement left within the femur, this should be removed using a combination of hand tools, distal-controlled drills or burrs, and ultrasonic tools. A rasping and trial technique is used to prepare the femoral canal, ensuring sufficient bone removal at the greater trochanter to allow axial rasping. Rasps and provisional components are used to obtain the position of best fit of the stem. Before rasping, it is ensured that the bone is adequately removed from the trochanter by using a gouge, rongeurs, rasps, or a power burr. This will enhance axial alignment, preventing varus malpositioning, and is a key part of the preparation of the femur. While rasping laterally, the gluteus medius tendon is protected from damage using a curved retractor (see Fig. 4).

Rasping by hand alone is preferred. If a mallet is used, the rasp should advance with each moderate tap of the mallet. It is important to antevert the rasps by approximately 10 to 20 degrees, depending on the natural anteversion of the patient's femoral neck and the intraoperative plan. The rasp is gently seated to the appropriate depth mark indicator. When the final rasp is seated to the appropriate level, the rasp is left in place for a trial reduction, or the final rasp is removed and the appropriate provisional component is used for the trial reduction. Ideally, we aim to seat the rasp to the osteotomy level, thereby achieving a minimum 2 to 3 mm of cement mantle thickness throughout, although in revisions this may be compromised somewhat, depending on the shape of the damaged femur. The forgiving nature of the polished surface and tapered stem are ideal for these situations.

Trial Reduction. The ability to adjust leg length and offset at the time of the trial reduction is a distinctive feature of the trial reduction for this collarless polished taper system. With rasp in place, the cone provisional is applied, and a trial reduction is performed. If the rasps or provisionals are not stable, a trial locating pin is inserted through the depth indicator holes on the neck of the rasp or provisional, and lap pads or sponges are used as necessary to stabilize the rasp or provisional in the canal, preventing rotation.

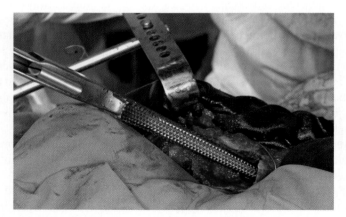

Figure 4. Diagram showing rasping of the femur. Rasps and provisional components are used to obtain the position of best fit of the stem, while ensuring that bone is adequately removed from the greater trochanter to enhance axial alignment.

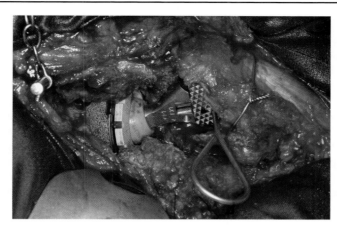

Figure 5. Diagram showing trial reduction with trial locating pin in situ. A trial reduction is undertaken by seating the final rasp or provisional to the appropriate level, and if necessary, the trial locating pin is used through the trial to maintain length.

The depth indicator holes correspond to the depth indicator markings on the final implant. Depth mark indicators below the osteotomy line indicate safe levels of stem seating under ideal circumstances of circumferential cement mantle and proximal bone support. If it is desired to seat the stem slightly proud, a trial locating pin is inserted into the appropriate hole to maintain the proud position during the trial reduction. The insertion depth is noted. Distal etch marks may be used to maintain stem alignment during insertion.

A trial reduction is performed, and if necessary, the provisional components are adjusted to optimize joint stability, leg length, and range of motion (see Fig. 5). Aim for a neutral head center trial to avoid the need for a skirted head. The relationship of the center of the femoral head to the top of the greater trochanter is noted to confirm the preoperative plan.

The sciatic nerve tension and range of motion are checked, and positions of potential instability are confirmed. Also, it is confirmed that the preoperative goal for leg length has been achieved by using the preferred method of measurement. After performing the trial reduction, the rasp and provisional components are removed.

The femoral canal is usually a mixture of predominantly sclerotic bone and some residual cancellous bone. However, on occasion, there may be an internal neocortex that can be removed with a burr or rongeur to expose underlying cancellous bone. In addition, the lesser and greater trochanters often have a neocortex that can be removed to aid cement interdigitation. To help cement interdigitation, horizontal grooves are made in thick areas of the endocortex (see Fig. 6). Distal cortical defects should be exposed and, after cementing the

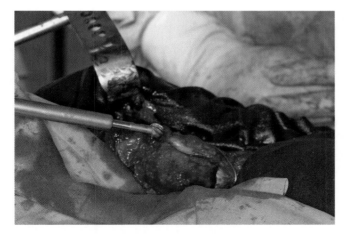

Figure 6. Burring the endocortex. To help cement interdigitation, horizontal grooves are made in thick areas of the endocortex, and sclerotic endocortex is removed, especially adjacent to the lesser and greater trochanters.

stem, the defect is bone grafted with mesh support. One technique is to first apply a temporary mesh with temporary wires over a dam made of a swab enclosed in a piece of glove and, when the cement has set, to graft this area and then apply the definitive mesh.

Cement Introduction. The distal canal is plugged, and cement is inserted in a retrograde manner, and cement is pressurized until the desired viscosity is achieved. Medullary canal sizers are used to determine the appropriate core size for the medullary bone plug (see Fig. 7). The bone plug is inserted to the mark on the inserter that corresponds to approximately 2.5 cm below the tip of the stem. The inserter is positioned laterally in the femur in the same orientation of the midline of the stem and level with the site of the neck cut normally made in primary arthroplasty. The plug is introduced with gentle hammering. If the site of the plug will be below the isthmus, a second plug is inserted over the initial plug if the initial plug is unstable. To do this, a larger plug, with some of its core having been removed with bone nibblers, is inserted. Otherwise, a small amount of cement is used or a temporary Steinmann pin is inserted through the femur at the site below the plug to support the plug.

Once the femoral canal is prepared, pulsatile lavage is used to remove any loose bone and to control bleeding. One technique for this is to use a femoral brush followed by pulsatile lavage, insertion of a thin plastic suction tube, and femoral packing (see Fig. 8). The pack may be presoaked in a variety of fluids to minimize bleeding. We use hydrogen peroxide.

Four packets of antibiotic polymethylmethacrylate (PMMA) bone cement, which contains tobramycin and to which is added 0.5 g of vancomycin powder for each 40-g packet of cement, are prepared. One large or two smaller cement cartridges are used (see Fig. 9). The bone cement is introduced in a relatively low viscosity state at approximately 2 to 3 minutes. The cement is injected into the canal in a retrograde fashion, and a femoral pressurizer seal is used to seal the cement proximally while pressurizing the cement for a few minutes (see Fig. 10).

Implantation. The stem is assembled to its inserter, and then the distal centralizer is attached. The stem is slowly advanced into the cement mantle, while maintaining appropriate anteversion and aiming for anatomical axial alignment. While inserting the stem, a valuable technique is for the surgeon to put his thumb posteromedially at the entry point to prevent varus alignment (see Fig. 11). The surgeon should aim for a minimum 4 mm of cement on the medial side of the stem but should be prepared to compromise the position somewhat so that the stem fits approximately down the middle of the cement column (see Fig. 12).

After inserting the stem to the final position, the stem is stabilized with one hand while removing the inserter with the other. It is recommended to gently push a small amount of cement over the lateral shoulder of the stem so that stem within cement subsidence may be evaluated on plain radiographs. This also helps prevent the remote possibility of the stem inadvertently backing out should a postoperative dislocation require reduction.

The aim is to have the stem reach its final position as the cement becomes quite viscous, thereby maintaining pressure on the cement. A horse collar cement seal is applied to maintain pressurization and stem position until the cement hardens (see Fig. 13). Once

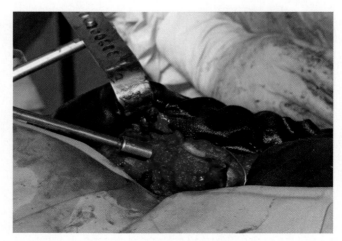

Figure 7. Sizing of the cement restrictor plug. Plug the distal canal, having used the medullary canal sizers to determine the appropriate core size for the medullary plug.

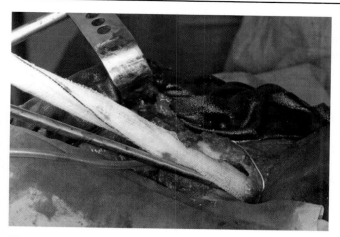

Figure 8. The femoral canal is being packed with gauze. Following pulsatile lavage and insertion of a thin plastic suction tube, the femoral canal is packed with peroxide-soaked ribbon gauze.

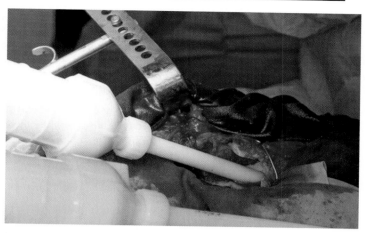

Figure 9. Two cement cartridges containing four packets of antibiotic containing PMMA bone cement. The canal is first filled in a retrograde fashion with relatively low viscosity cement.

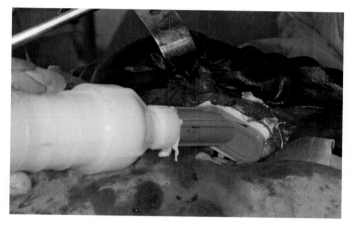

Figure 10. The use of the pressurizer seal. The cement cartridge is used with a femoral pressurizer seal to pressurize the cement for a few minutes.

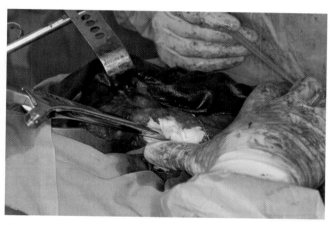

Figure 11. Stem introduction. The stem is slowly advanced into the cement mantle while maintaining appropriate anteversion. Axial alignment is assisted by placing a thumb medially and aiming to insert the stem approximately down the middle of the cement mantle.

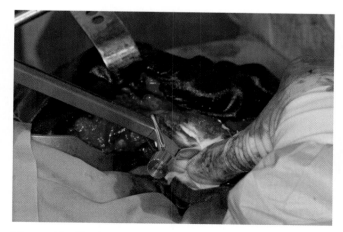

Figure 12. Final stem seating. The stem is introduced until the depth mark on the stem reaches the femoral neck reference point.

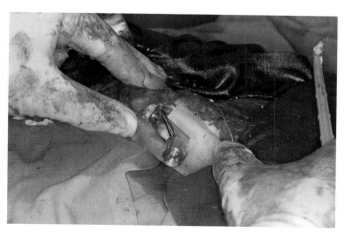

Figure 13. The use of the horse collar seal. The horse collar is applied to stabilize the stem and maintain a proximal seal while the cement polymerizes.

the cement has hardened, a further trial reduction is performed, and appropriate head size is selected. The neck taper is checked to ensure it is clean and dry. The femoral head is placed on the taper with a twisting motion until it locks on the taper. A pack or swab is placed over the femoral head to protect it, and then the femoral head is seated with one sharp blow using a femoral head impactor and mallet.

The femoral head is protected with a gauze pack, and it is held away from the acetabulum to avoid inadvertent impingement. The acetabulum is then cleaned and the joint is reduced, always while the operating surgeon's fingers protect the posterior structures containing the sciatic nerve. The gauze is removed from the femoral head as the head is reduced.

Wound Closure. After obtaining hemostasis, a wound drainage device is inserted, if desired. The wound is then closed in layers.

Postoperative Management

Excluding cases with structural weight-bearing graft, patients are mobilized with full weight bearing within 24 hours. If there is a calcar crack or other stable fracture, then partial weight bearing for 6 weeks is recommended. Patients are to sit out of bed on day 2 if cerebrally orientated and then are restricted to an elevated seat for 6 weeks. For revision, intravenous antibiotics are administered every 8 hours for 24 hours, followed by oral antibiotics until day 5 following surgery if the patient is at low risk for infection and the intraoperative gram stain and day 1 cultures are negative. Five-day cultures are reviewed, and treatment is altered appropriately if needed.

WHAT OUR EXPERIENCE HAS TAUGHT US AND EXPECTED RESULTS

Eighteen-year data are now available for this cemented long-stem femoral revision procedure. Aseptic loosening of the femoral stem is rare. In our experience, we have had only one stem loosen, and this was in a patient who had undergone three previous femoral revisions, including impaction grafting. When revision for aseptic loosening of the cemented collarless double-taper long stem is taken as the end point, the 5-year survival can be expected to be 100%, and the 8- and 10-year survival can be expected to be of at least 96% (95% confidence interval = 87% to 100%). Our intraoperative femoral fracture rate is approximately 6%, with femoral perforations occurring in about 6% of cases. Our

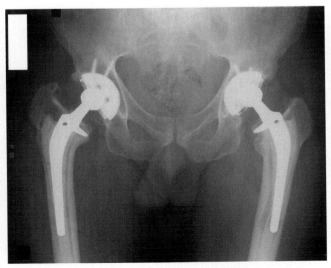

Figure 14. A: AP pelvis radiograph of bilateral loose precoated femoral components.

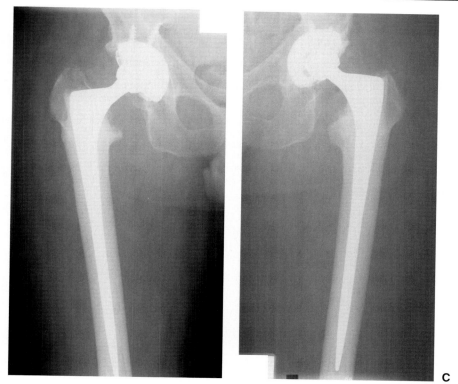

Figure 14. *(continued)* **B** and **C:** AP hip radiographs of bilateral cemented, polished, long dual-taper stems.

reoperation rate for infection is approximately 2%, and we feel that antibiotic-impregnated cement contributes to this low rate. The incidence of postoperative periprosthetic femoral fracture is approximately 2% to 3% in our series of patients but can often be successfully managed without reoperation of the femoral stem. While cement-bone radiolucencies are seen, evidence of definite femoral component radiographic loosening is not seen at long-term follow-up, and subsidence of the stem is not a problem. Radiographs of a patient who underwent bilateral femoral revision using polished dual-taper stems are presented in Figure 14. Second- or third-degree stress shielding is not present in these hips. Importantly, patients can expect on average to have minimal or no pain from the hip in the long term and for thigh pain not to be a problem.

ACKNOWLEDGMENTS

The authors thank Marg McGee, Tania Knight, and Kerry Costi for their assistance in the preparation of this chapter and Stephen Graves, Andrew Mintz, and joint replacement nursing staff of the Royal Adelaide Hospital for their clinical contributions.

RECOMMENDED READING

1. Saleh KJ, Holtzman J, Gafni A, et al. Reliability and intraoperative validity of preoperative assessment of standardized plain radiographs in predicting bone loss at revision hip surgery. *J Bone Joint Surg* 83:1040–1046, 2001.
2. Hultmark P, Karrholm, J, Stromberg C, et al. Cemented first-time revisions of the femoral component. Prospective 7 to 13 years' follow-up using second-generation and third-generation cementing technique. *J Arthroplasty* 15:551–561, 2000.
3. Howie DW, Wimhurst J, McGee MA, et al. Mid to long-term results of revision THR using cemented, collarless, double-tapered femoral stems. Presented at: 71st Annual Meeting of the American Academy of Orthopaedic Surgeons, March 10–14, 2004; San Francisco, Calif.

4. Gramkow J, Jensen TH, Varmarken JE, Repten JB. Long-term results after cemented revision of the femoral component in total hip arthroplasty. *J Arthroplasty* 16:777–783, 2001.
5. Panjabi MM, Trumble T, Hult JE, Southwick WO. Effect of femoral stem length on stress raisers associated with revision hip arthroplasty. *J Orthop Res* 3:447–455, 1985.
6. Mann KA, Ayers DC, Damron TA. Effects of stem length on mechanics of the femoral hip component after cemented revision. *J Orthop Res* 15:62–68, 1997.
7. Weidenhielm LRA, Mikhail WEM, Nelissen RGHH, Bauer TW. Cemented collarless (Exeter-C.P.T.) femoral components versus cementless collarless (P.C.A.) 2-14 year follow-up evaluation. *J Arthroplasty* 10:592–597, 1995.
8. Malchau H, Herberts P. Prognosis of total hip replacement. Presented at: 65th Annual Meeting of the American Academy of Orthopaedic Surgeons; March 19–23, 1998; New Orleans, La.
9. Fowler JL, Gie GA, Lee AJC, Ling RSM. Experience with the Exeter total hip replacement since 1970. *Orthop Clin North Am* 19:477–489, 1988.
10. Yates P, Gobel D, Bannister G. Collarless polished tapered stem. *J Arthroplasty* 17:189–195, 2002.
11. Williams HDW. The Exeter universal cemented femoral component at 8 to 12 years. a study of the first 325 hips. *J Bone Joint Surg Br* 84:324–334, 2002.

24

Modular Stems

Craig J. Della Valle

INDICATIONS/CONTRAINDICATIONS

Revision of a failed femoral component is a complex procedure with many potential technical pitfalls and problems that can adversely affect the patient's final outcome. There are multiple reconstructive options available for reconstructing the failed femur in revision total hip arthroplasty (THA), and a classification of femoral deficiency has been developed by W. G. Paprosky that assists the surgeon is selecting among these reconstructive options.

Classification of Femoral Deficiency

The radiographic classification system I use is based on the belief that a cylindrical, fully porous coated, diaphyseal-engaging femoral component can be utilized for the majority of femoral revisions. This type of component has been associated with excellent rates of stable fixation and a surgical technique that is straightforward and applicable to the majority of femoral reconstructions.

In this classification system, a type I femur is associated with minimal loss of metaphyseal cancellous bone and an intact diaphysis; it can be reconstructed with cemented or cementless fixation and is essentially equivalent to the situation encountered in primary THA (see Fig. 1). In a type II femur, there is extensive loss of metaphyseal bone; however, the diaphysis is intact (see Fig. 2). This type of defect either can be reconstructed with a proximally coated, cementless implant with diaphyseal stabilization or distal fixation can be achieved with an extensively coated implant.

A type III femur is associated with severe metaphyseal bone loss that precludes stable fixation with a proximally coated implant. Type III femurs are divided into IIIA (see Fig. 3) and IIIB (see Fig. 4) depending on the amount of intact diaphyseal bone available for fixation in the femoral isthmus; type IIIA femurs have more than 4 cm of isthmus available for distal fixation whereas type IIIB femurs have less than 4 cm available. This is a critical determination as femurs with more than 4 cm of femoral isthmus can be successfully reconstructed with a nonmodular, fully porous coated diaphyseal-fitting femoral component whereas femurs with less than 4 cm of intact femoral isthmus available for distal fixation have been associated with

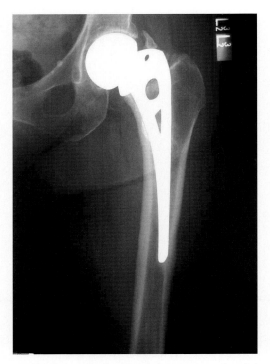

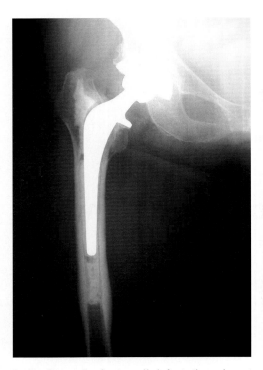

Figure 1. Radiograph of a type I defect; there is minimal loss of metaphyseal cancellous bone with an intact diaphysis. (Reprinted with permission from Della Valle CJ, Paprosky WG. The femur in revision total hip arthroplasty: evaluation and classification. *Clin Orthop Relat Res* 420:55–62, 2004.)

Figure 2. Radiograph of a type II defect; there is extensive loss of metaphyseal bone with an intact diaphysis. (Reprinted with permission from Della Valle CJ, Paprosky WG. The femur in revision total hip arthroplasty: evaluation and classification. *Clin Orthop Relat Res* 420:55–62, 2004.)

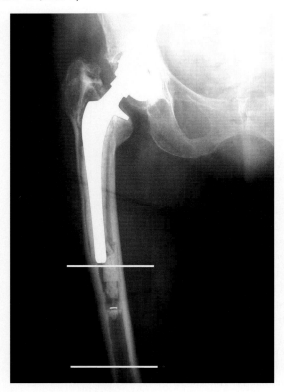

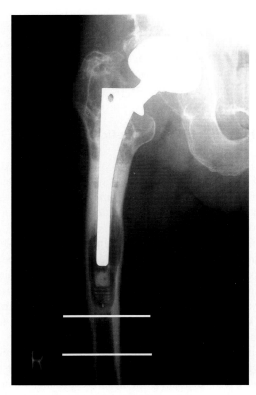

Figure 3. Radiograph of a type IIIA defect; the metaphysis is severely damaged and nonsupportive, and 4 cm of intact cortical bone is present in the femoral isthmus. The segment of usable bone in the femoral diaphysis is marked by the horizontal lines and is more than 4 cm. (Reprinted with permission from Della Valle CJ, Paprosky WG. The femur in revision total hip arthroplasty: evaluation and classification. *Clin Orthop Relat Res* 420:55–62, 2004.)

Figure 4. Radiograph of a type IIIB defect; the metaphysis is severely damaged with some intact cortical bone present distal to the isthmus (<4 cm). The segment of usable bone in the femoral diaphysis is marked by the horizontal lines and is less than 4 cm. (Reprinted with permission from Della Valle CJ, Paprosky WG. The femur in revision total hip arthroplasty: evaluation and classification. *Clin Orthop Relat Res* 420:55–62, 2004.)

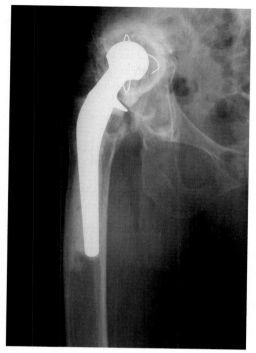

Figure 5. Radiograph of a type IV defect; there is extensive metadiaphyseal damage in conjunction with a widened femoral canal. (Reprinted with permission from Della Valle CJ, Paprosky WG. The femur in revision total hip arthroplasty: evaluation and classification. *Clin Orthop Relat Res* 420:55–62, 2004.)

higher rates of fibrous stable fixation and clinical failure when this type of implant is used. On the basis of these results, in the setting where 4 cm of diaphyseal interference fit cannot be obtained, a modular, cementless tapered implant is my choice for femoral reconstruction. An increasing number of cases with this type of femoral deficiency, associated with the failure of cemented femoral components that were inserted with second-generation cementing techniques that included longer femoral stems inserted with a correspondingly longer cement mantle and a distal cement restrictor, are currently encountered.

Type IV femoral deficiency (see Fig. 5) is associated with extensive metadiaphyseal damage and a widened femoral canal that precludes the use of a cementless femoral component. In these cases, impaction grafting can be employed if the femoral deficiency is contained and the cortical tube is intact. An allograft-prosthesis composite is used in younger, higher-demand patients whereas a proximal-femoral-replacing, modular oncology prosthesis is used in lower-demand, elderly patients.

Indications for the Use of Modular Femoral Revision Stems

The primary advantage of a modular femoral component is the ability to obtain maximal contact with the available host bone and to optimize initial implant stability required for successful osseointegration of the revision component. An additional advantage is the ability to accommodate proximal femoral remodeling with a proximal body segment that is placed independent of the distal segment. Further advantages relate primarily to the optimization of overall construct stability to prevent postoperative dislocations via intraoperative adjustment of the femoral anteversion employed and the ability to trial with different length and offset options to optimize stability. As instability is a common complication of revision THA, the benefit of these options cannot be underestimated. Modularity, however, is associated with the potential for additional sites for potential corrosion to occur, reports of breakage at the modular junctions, and a more complex surgical technique. On the basis of these limitations, I reserve the use of these components for the more complex femoral reconstructions that have been associated with higher rates of failure when a monobloc, fully porous coated stem is used.

Currently available modular revision femoral components can be categorized as belonging to one of three categories: components that rely primarily on proximal fixation that have a nonbioreactive distal stem segment, which adds secondary stabilization; components that rely primarily on diaphyseal fixation and have a porous coating present distally; and components that rely on distal fixation that is achieved with a straight, tapered component that has a bioreactive surface available for bone ongrowth. Modular stems that rely primarily on proximal fixation are commonly used in some centers but are beyond the scope of this contribution. Modular stems that use a fully porous coated distal segment are most useful for type IIIA femurs in which substantial proximal femoral remodeling into retroversion is encountered. If a monobloc, fully porous coated stem is used in these situations, proximal femoral fracture can occur, and in these cases the benefits of modularity outweigh the potential problems and drawbacks.

The main primary indication for the use of a modular revision femoral component is a type IIIB femur. In these situations, the femoral isthmus available for distal fixation is quite short (<4 cm), and poorer results have been associated with the use of a monobloc, fully porous coated, diaphyseal-engaging stem. A tapered distal segment allows the surgeon to gain axial stability by wedging into the available femoral isthmus; rotational stability is obtained by virtue of cutting flutes. These stems have been associated with excellent clinical and radiographic results; however, subsidence is a commonly noted problem as is leg length discrepancy, as it is difficult to predict accurately at what point axial stability will be obtained. In these situations, a modular stem allows the surgeon to fully impact the distal segment until adequate stability is obtained and then build up the proximal segment to recreate adequate leg length and achieve appropriate abductor tension to avoid prosthetic dislocation. Tapered stems are also often available in larger diameters (>20 mm) and thus may be appropriate for the failed femur with a larger-diameter femoral canal.

The final commonly encountered clinical scenario where the unique benefits of a modular stem outweigh the potential problems is in the management of periprosthetic femur fractures. In these cases, the available segment of diaphyseal bone available for distal fixation is often short (equivalent to a type IIIB femur), and thus reconstruction can be challenging. In addition, typically an extended trochanteric osteotomy to assist with the removal of retained cement and to optimize the achievement of stable fixation distally can be employed. As anatomic cues to femoral component rotation are often lost if this technique is employed, modular stems again afford the advantage of independent placement of the proximal body segment to adequately position the component to avoid dislocation.

PREOPERATIVE PLANNING

As discussed earlier in this volume, meticulous preoperative planning is critical to a successful outcome to ensure that appropriate revision components are available if needed. In planning for a femoral revision, high-quality plain x-rays are mandatory, including an anteroposterior (AP) view of the pelvis and AP and lateral views of the involved hip. The AP and lateral views of the hip should be of sufficient length to evaluate the integrity of the femoral isthmus and diaphysis, where component fixation is often achieved. It is my general practice to mark on the x-ray the most proximal and distal portions of the femoral isthmus that are available for distal fixation to determine if a tapered, modular stem is needed for stable fixation to be achieved (Figs. 3 and 4).

The diameter and length of the revision components to be implanted should be estimated using clear overlay templates (see Fig. 6). The implant selected also should have adequate femoral offset to optimize abductor function and prevent prosthetic impingement. Estimation of the implant diameter needed is critical, as in these situations, the femoral canal is often widened and larger-diameter components must be available to ensure that adequate implant stability can be achieved.

A critical and often overlooked portion of the radiographic review includes an assessment of femoral deformity. Loose femoral implants often undergo remodeling into varus and retroversion, and preoperative templating will assist in the identification of femoral re-

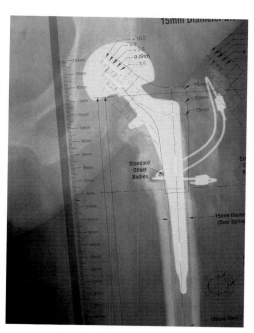

Figure 6. Clear overlay templates are used to estimate diameter and length of the distal segment as well as the size and configuration of the proximal body segment.

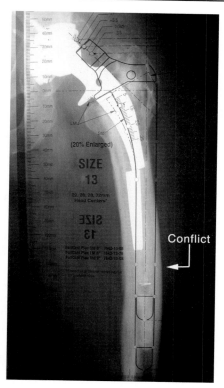

Figure 7. A clear overlay template is placed within the center of the femoral canal distally. The proximal portion lies outside the femur, indicating that varus femoral remodeling has occurred. An extended trochanteric osteotomy is required for appropriate reconstruction. (Reprinted with permission from Della Valle CJ, Paprosky WG. Revision total hip arthroplasty: extended trochanteric osteotomy. In: Grana WA, Fitzgerald RH, eds. *Orthopaedic Knowledge Online*. Rosemont, Ill: American Academy of Orthopaedic Surgeons; 2002. Available at www.aaos.org/oko. Accessed June 26, 2002.)

modeling (see Fig. 7). The distal portion of the stem to be implanted is centered in the femoral canal, and the relationship of the lateral border of the stem is compared with the orientation of the lateral femoral cortex. If the implant abuts or lies outside the lateral femoral cortex, femoral varus remodeling has occurred, and if an extended trochanteric osteotomy is not done, the surgeon is at risk for perforating the femoral canal while reaming, fracturing the femur during implant insertion, or placing an inadequately sized implant into the femoral canal.

SURGERY

Patient Positioning, Draping, Surgical Approach, and Organization of the Operating Room

Position the patient in the lateral decubitus position, taking care to rigidly secure the pelvis to the operating room table, perpendicular to the floor. Great care is taken to pad the down chest and the underside of the down leg, which is typically placed in a slightly flexed position. The lower extremity is prepped from the iliac crest proximally to just above the knee distally and draped free to ensure that adequate range of motion can be obtained to adequately test stability (see Fig. 8). Prior skin incisions are typically used to

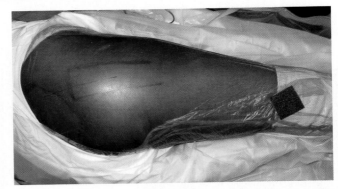

Figure 8. The extremity has been prepped and draped with the entire extremity free to allow for stability testing.

avoid wound-healing problems unless their position will inhibit appropriate exposure. My preference is to use a posterior approach to the hip, as it is extensile both proximally and distally, allows for access to the posterior column of the pelvis if needed, and is compatible with an extended trochanteric osteotomy if required. A wide exposure is necessary, and the femur must be sufficiently mobilized to allow for circumferential acetabular exposure when acetabular reconstruction is needed. An extended trochanteric osteotomy can be useful to assist with exposure, removal of retained implants, or deformity correction if deemed necessary as per the preoperative plan. A large operating room is generally used with adequate space for multiple tables given the large number of instruments and trials often required.

Details of Procedure

Once the failed femoral component has been removed, care is taken to ensure that any remaining soft tissue or overhanging bone on the medial side of the base of the greater trochanter is cleared to ensure that the femur is not reamed in varus (see Fig. 9); if substantial bone is present in this area, a high-speed burr is often required to adequately clear this area. Clear remaining debris from the femoral canal with crochet hooks to ensure that all retained cement and fibrous tissue have been removed that could potentially block or deflect the femoral reamers to be inserted (see Fig. 10). Next, gently ream

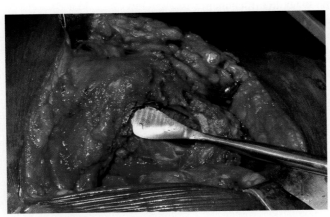

Figure 9. Soft tissue and bone are removed from the medial aspect of the base of the greater trochanter to ensure that the reamers and the implant are not placed in varus.

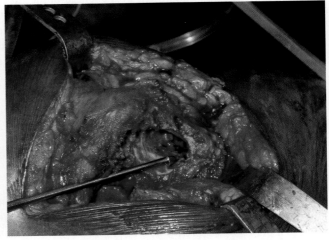

Figure 10. Crochet hooks are used to ensure that all cement and debris have been removed from the femoral canal to ensure that the reamers will follow a straight path.

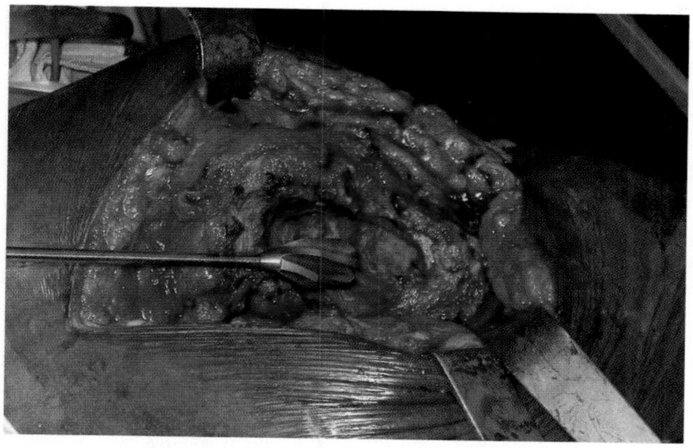

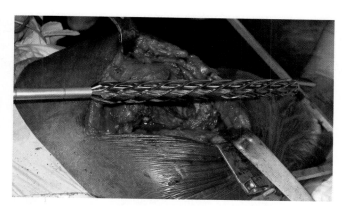

Figure 11. Flexible reamers are used to assist with de-bridement of the femoral canal.

Figure 12. The tapered reamers are inserted by hand.

the femoral canal with a flexible reamer (see Fig. 11); discontinue reaming as soon as cortical contact is made to avoid removing femoral isthmic bone, which will be used for distal fixation.

Progressively larger tapered reamers (see Fig. 12) are then inserted, and reaming is performed by hand until firm distal resistance is encountered and the reamer can no longer be advanced. It is critical that the reaming be performed by hand and that a large enough reamer be inserted so that even with firm axial pressure applied, the reamer cannot be inserted any deeper. Notched lines on the reamer handle (see Fig. 13) indicate the appropriate length of the distal femoral segment; in the system pictured, two different lengths are available in the selected diameter, and the relationship of the notches in the reamer when compared to the tip of the greater trochanter indicates the approximate length of the final construct when the shortest body segment is utilized. In the case pictured, the reamer has been advanced to just beyond the more distal line, indicating that the shorter of the two distal segments will be appropriate. If the surgeon is unsure if the appropriate diameter or length has been selected, an intraoperative radiograph with the reamer in place can be obtained to confirm appropriate fit and fill.

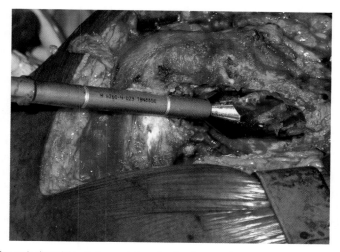

Figure 13. The relationship of the notches in the femoral reamer indicates the appropriate length of the distal segment; in this case the reamer has been advanced just beyond the more distal notch (when compared to the tip of the greater trochanter), indicating that the shorter distal segment will be of adequate length.

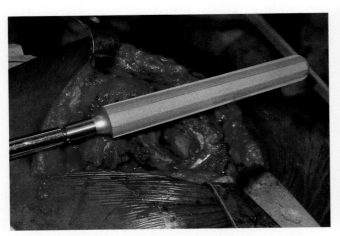

Figure 14. Distal segment of the revision femoral component. The tapered shape allows for the achievement of axial stability while the cutting flutes obtain rotational stability.

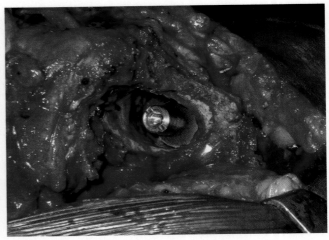

Figure 15. The distal femoral segment has been impacted into the femur.

Next, impact the selected distal body segment until axial and rotational stability have been achieved (see Figs. 14 and 15). If an extended trochanteric osteotomy has been used for the approach, place a cerclage wire distal to the osteotomy site to prevent a fracture during impaction of the distal segment. If the implant design includes a bow to accommodate the femoral bow, ensure that the implant is inserted in the appropriate alignment. The tapered distal segment gains stability by wedging into the femoral canal in the available femoral isthmus, and rotational stability is obtained via the cutting flutes. The principal advantage of modularity when applied to a tapered revision femoral component is the ability to fully impact the stem until stability has been obtained, thereby maximizing the chance for osseointegration and minimizing the risk of subsidence without concern about restoring leg length, which can be achieved by using a proximal body segment of appropriate length. The distal segment will often advance farther than the reamer advanced, and the surgeon should not be concerned if this occurs; however, impaction should continue until absolute stability has been achieved. Markings on the insertion handle will assist with choosing the appropriately sized proximal body length; for example, the most distal marking on the insertion handle corresponds to the shortest body length, and each subsequent marking denotes the next longer proximal body segment.

The next step includes trials with the proximal body segments. The majority of systems include the ability to use proximal bodies not only of differing lengths and offsets but also of different sizes and shapes to maximize proximal support and increase the amount of prosthesis in contact with host bone for osseointegration to occur (see Fig. 16). Initial trials are performed with the proximal body size indicated by the depth of insertion of the distal segment when referenced from the tip of the greater trochanter (see Fig. 17). Another advantage of modular systems is the ability to modify the amount of anteversion to maximize stability. Once the proximal body trial has been locked into place (see Fig. 18), perform an initial trial reduction. Larger-diameter (36 or 40 mm) femoral heads are used routinely in revision THA given the high risk of instability in this patient population.

Once restoration of leg lengths has been confirmed and stability has been optimized, the appropriate proximal body is brought onto the field. Once the desired anteversion has been selected, mark this position on the proximal femur with an electrosurgical pencil or a small notch with a burr to ensure that this position can be recreated when the final implant is inserted. The trunion of the already implanted distal femoral segment is cleaned and dried followed by impaction of the proximal body segment onto the Morse taper (see Fig. 19). Additional stability is obtained at this junction with a locking screw that is torqued into place to the appropriate tension (see Fig. 20). A final trial reduction is performed to confirm restoration of leg length and stability followed by impaction of the femoral head onto the

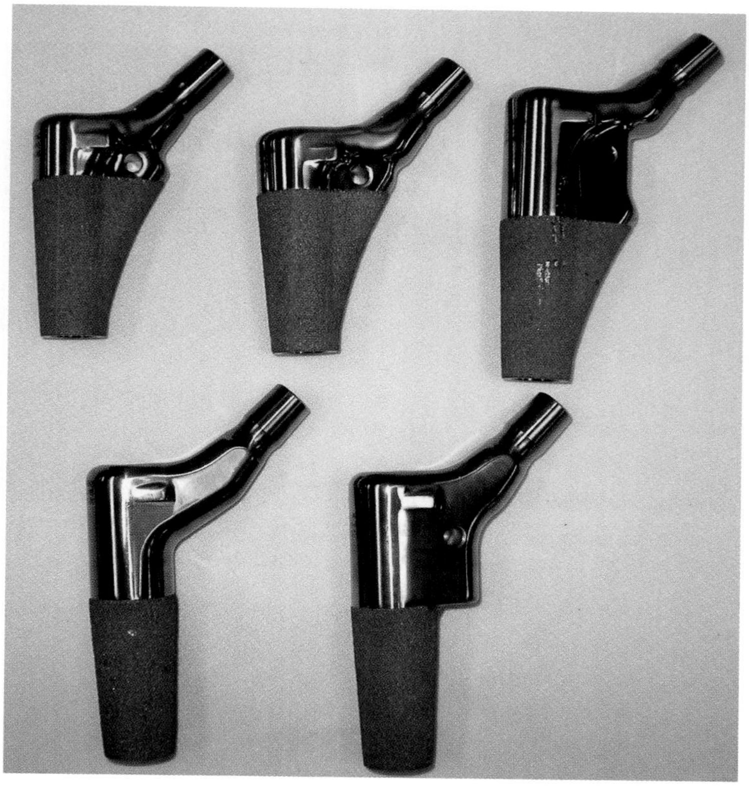

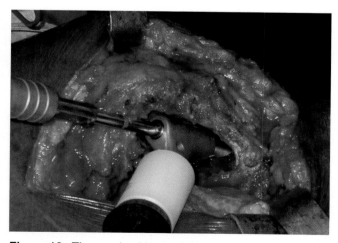

Figure 16. Multiple proximal body options are available in most modular femoral revision systems to maximize both proximal support and the area available for bone ingrowth.

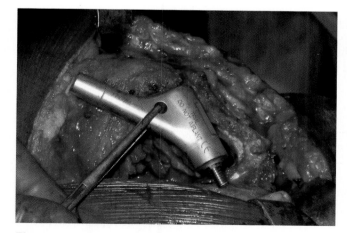

Figure 17. Trials are performed with different proximal body segments until the leg length has been restored and stability has been achieved.

Figure 18. The proximal body trial is locked into place; handles are often available to maintain the desired anteversion while tightening the set screw.

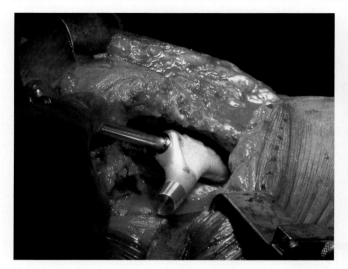

Figure 19. The proximal body implant has been engaged onto the Morse taper of the distal segment in the desired amount of anteversion.

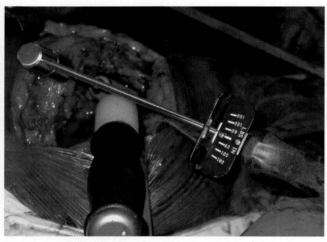

Figure 20. Final locking of the proximal body segment with a torque wrench.

Morse taper after if has been cleaned and dried (see Fig. 21). Closure is performed in a routine manner, including repair of the posterior soft tissue sleeve back to the posterior aspect of the greater trochanter (see Fig. 22) either at the insertion of the abductor musculature or through drill holes.

POSTOPERATIVE MANAGEMENT AND REHABILITATION

Final radiographs are obtained, and the patient is placed in a standard orthopaedic bed with an overhead trapeze. Prophylactic intravenous antibiotics may be continued until the final results of intraoperative cultures are known. Patients are anticoagulated with warfarin sodium (Coumadin) for a total of 3 weeks. They are mobilized from bed on the first postoperative day and instructed in touch-down weight bearing with a walker or two crutches. Touch-down weight bearing is continued for the first 6 weeks and then advanced to weight bearing as tolerated with two crutches or a walker for an additional 6 weeks. Abductor-strengthening exercises are initiated at 6 weeks postoperatively if an extended trochanteric osteotomy has been used and started immediately if not used. Patients are instructed in total

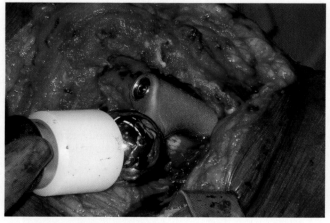

Figure 21. Impaction of the femoral head onto the Morse taper.

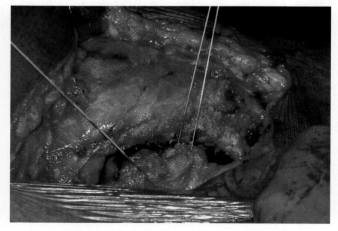

Figure 22. Repair of the posterior soft tissue sleeve.

hip precautions, and these are maintained for 3 months. An abduction orthosis is not necessary if a larger-diameter femoral head has been used for the reconstruction.

RESULTS

The majority of patients obtain good pain relief by 3 weeks postoperatively, and ambulatory capacity improves greatly by 3 months, at which point ambulatory aids can be discontinued. Serial radiographs will oftentimes show some restoration of bone stock as forces are transmitted over a longer segment of the femur than is often the case when a cylindrical, fully porous coated stem is used.

COMPLICATIONS

Although modularity has multiple benefits, as previously noted, there is concern that corrosion can occur at the junction between the proximal and distal body segments. In addition, breakages have been reported to occur at this junction.

The most common complication associated with a tapered revision femoral stem is subsidence of the femoral component. While the advent of modular systems decreases the risk of this complication, by virtue of its tapered geometry, subsidence can still occur; however, the majority of stems will gain stability. If subsidence occurs, patients are at increased risk for developing instability or a symptomatic leg length discrepancy. To avoid large amounts of subsidence, the distal femoral segment must be fully impacted until it no longer advances with firm blows of a mallet.

Dislocation is another common complication of revision THA in general, and particular attention should be given to intraoperative stability testing and adjustments in the femoral anteversion selected to decrease the risk of this complication. Great care is taken to debride anterior capsule and anterior prominences of the greater trochanter to remove sources of impingement. The routine use of larger-diameter femoral heads (36 or 40 mm) has dramatically decreased the incidence of instability at our center.

Periprosthetic fractures can also occur and most commonly are seen during impaction of the distal femoral segment. To avoid this complication, place a prophylactic cerclage cable just distal to an extended trochanteric osteotomy (if utilized for the approach), and impact the distal segment with firm mallet blows until the stem no longer advances with progressive blows of the mallet; further impaction beyond this point can lead to fracture. Late periprosthetic fractures can be avoided by bypassing cortical defects by at least two cortical diameters and placing strut allografts over areas of severely deficient femoral bony defects.

RECOMMENDED READING

1. Berry DJ. Treatment of Vancouver B3 periprosthetic femur fractures with a fluted tapered stem. *Clin Orthop Relat Res* 417:224–231, 2003.
2. Berry DJ. Femoral revision: distal fixation with fluted, tapered grit-blasted stems. *J Arthroplasty* 17(4 Suppl 1):142–146, 2002.
3. Bohm P, Bischel O. Femoral revision with the Wagner SL revision stem: evaluation of one hundred and twenty-nine revisions followed for a mean of 4.8 years. *J Bone Joint Surg Am* 83:1023–1031, 2001.
4. Christie MJ, DeBoer DK, Tingstad EM, et al. Clinical experience with a modular noncemented femoral component in revision total hip arthroplasty: 4- to 7-year results. *J Arthroplasty* 15:840–848, 2000.
5. Della Valle CJ, Paprosky WG. Classification and an algorithmic approach to the reconstruction of femoral deficiency in revision total hip arthroplasty. *J Bone Joint Surg Am* 85(Suppl 4):1–6, 2003.
6. Goldberg VM. Revision total hip arthroplasty using a cementless modular femoral hip design. *Am J Orthop* 31:202–204, 2002.
7. Kwong LM, Miller AJ, Lubinus P. A modular distal fixation option for proximal bone loss in revision total hip arthroplasty: a 2- to 6-year follow-up study. *J Arthroplasty* 18(3 Suppl 1):94–97, 2003.
8. Miner TM, Momberger NG, Chong D, Paprosky WL. The extended trochanteric osteotomy in revision hip arthroplasty: a critical review of 166 cases at mean 3-year, 9-month follow-up. *J Arthroplasty* 16(8 Suppl 1):188–194, 2001.
9. Sporer SM, Paprosky WG. Revision total hip arthroplasty: the limits of fully coated stems. *Clin Orthop Relat Res* 417:203–209, 2003.
10. Weeden SH, Paprosky WG. Minimal 11-year follow-up of extensively porous-coated stems in femoral revision total hip arthroplasty. *J Arthroplasty* 17(4 Suppl 1):134–137, 2002.

25

Cementless (Extensively Porous Coated) Stems

Mark Barba and Wayne G. Paprosky

INDICATIONS/CONTRAINDICATIONS

Fully coated stems can be used routinely for femoral stem revision. They are applicable in nearly all cases, with the exception of those requiring an allograft prosthetic composite because of massive proximal femoral bone loss or those with diaphyseal widening so great that an impaction bone-grafting technique would be considered, as in femurs with diaphyses wider than 22 mm.

The extended proximal femoral trochanteric osteotomy can aid in the four main objectives in revision surgery: exposure, implant removal, correction of deformity, and revision component implantation. Tissue quality can be poor in revision surgery. In certain cases of acetabular failure, revision of the femur may be indicated as an aid in soft tissue tensioning. Stability is paramount in revision surgery and should not be compromised in an effort to maintain equal leg lengths. It is important to counsel the patient regarding leg length issues. We have found that an additional benefit of the extended osteotomy is the ease with which it allows for soft tissue tensioning.

The following section describes the essential components of revision of a failed femoral stem with a fully porous coated straight stem designed to obtain distal ingrowth fixation.

PREOPERATIVE PLANNING

An anteroposterior (AP) view of the pelvis and AP and lateral views of the proximal two thirds of the femur are needed for planning.

Templates are used to choose the shortest stem possible that will be surrounded by a cylinder of cortical bone for 4 to 5 cm into the isthmus. This is the ultimate goal of the operation. The lateral view is used to determine whether a curved or straight stem is appropriate.

Templating the depth of implantation is now considered (see Figs. 1 and 2). First, the acetabular reconstruction is templated to determine the center of rotation. This is marked on the film. Next, femoral templates are applied by estimating the "anatomic position" of the

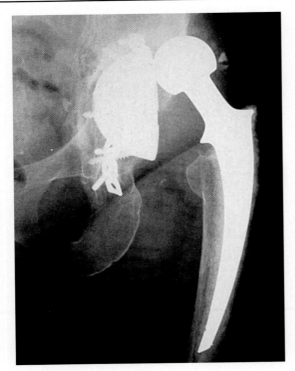

Figure 1. Preoperative view of a total hip reconstruction that failed secondary to instability. In this example, the socket is malpositioned and will require revision. The femoral component also demonstrates a significant radiolucency and will require concomitant revision.

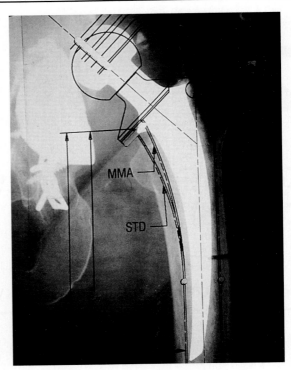

Figure 2. A templated radiograph using a 6-inch, fully coated stem. The template is aligned neutrally. Cement is some distance from the osteotomy site; however, note that the cement is poorly bonded and should pose no difficulty with removal.

component within the femoral canal. This is typically 1 cm proximal to the lesser trochanter. Using an intermediate neck length, the center of the head is then marked. By comparing the two marks, conclusions regarding tissue tension and leg lengths can be made. Typically, a combination of prosthetic height and neck length that increases offset and length is chosen, as this is often needed to achieve stability.

The distalmost level of the extended trochanteric osteotomy is determined by the following factors. First, the osteotomy should not jeopardize fixation. The transverse limb of the osteotomy should be at a level that will preserve approximately 4 to 6 cm of tight isthmic fit of the distal portion of the ingrowth stem cement. If the cement plug is more substantial than that seen in Figure 2, a more distal osteotomy can be selected, but attention must be paid to the planned location of the distal 4 to 6 cm of the implanted stem. This section should not be compromised by the osteotomy. Fortunately, the osteotomy provides unimpeded access to the isthmus. We have noted that a significant number of revision femurs have a preoperative varus deformity. This places the femur at risk for a varus and undersized implantation. Use of the osteotomy helps to avoid this consequence.

The distal osteotomy level is measured from an easily identified landmark such as the vastus tubercle for use as an intraoperative reference.

SURGICAL TECHNIQUE

Exposure

We use a posterior approach. The pseudocapsule and external rotators are raised in a single flap. The gluteus maximus tendon is released. When the hip is encountered, we dislocate the joint, if possible. However, with severe protrusio or heterotopic ossification, dislocation may be difficult to achieve. If the joint cannot be dislocated, we perform the extended osteotomy and remove heterotopic ossification.

Extraction

After thoroughly clearing the introitus of the femur of granuloma, scar, and bone, a loose prosthesis has a chance of being pulled free. Be aware of any impingement of the prosthesis shoulder and the greater trochanter, as this can fracture the trochanter. Use of a barrel-shaped high-speed burr can help open this area. If the prosthesis pulls out readily, we then proceed to the osteotomy. If it does not, we will perform the osteotomy with the prosthesis in situ. It is technically easier if the prosthesis is removed prior to osteotomy.

Osteotomy

The hip is extended and internally rotated 15 to 20 degrees to allow for proper positioning of the femur. The vastus lateralis is separated from the posterolateral femur along the linea aspera down to the level of the distal extent of the osteotomy. This is determined from the preoperative templating and can be measured either from the tip of the greater trochanter or by using the removed stem as a guide. The vastus is then elevated anteriorly off the femur only at the distal site of the osteotomy, and a retractor is placed at this site to protect the tissue during completion of the distal osteotomy cut. The osteotomy site is marked along the posterolateral femur just anterior to the linea aspera (see Fig. 3).

When the incision is viewed posteriorly (see Fig. 4), the sucker is on the tip of the greater trochanter, and the gluteus medius muscle is to the right. In this case, the prosthesis was easily removed after clearing the shoulder area of bone and soft tissue and using a tamp on the collar to facilitate extraction. An oscillating saw is then used to section the proximal femur in half distally to the area where the Hohman retractor is located in the bottom right corner. The transverse limb of the osteotomy is made with a

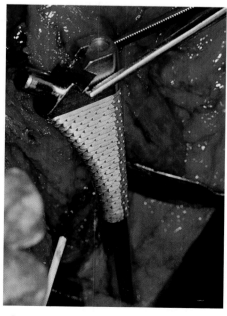

Figure 3. Cautery is used to mark the distal extent of the osteotomy at a level that will provide adequate coverage of the cylindrical distal portion of the fully coated stem.

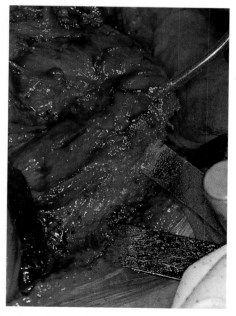

Figure 4. Viewed posteriorly, the sucker is on the tip of the greater trochanter, and gluteus medius muscle is to the right.

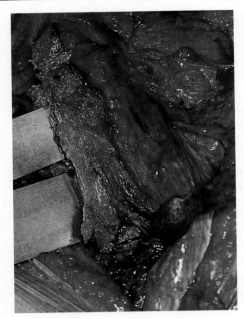

Figure 5. Wide Lambotte osteotomes are passed from posterior to anterior and used to lever open the osteotomy in a controlled fashion.

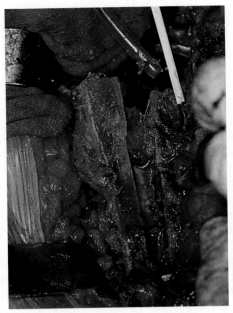

Figure 6. The release of anterior scar tissue with the cautery device is shown.

thin high-speed burr at the level of the Hohman retractor, which corresponds to the tip of the removed prosthesis.

Wide Lambotte osteotomes are then passed from posterior to anterior (see Fig. 5); the multiple osteotomes are used to lever open the osteotomy in a controlled fashion, protecting both the osteotomy fragment and the anterior soft tissue attachments. The gluteus medius, gluteus minimus, and vastus lateralis remain attached to the osteotomized portion of bone.

Release of anterior tissue must be performed carefully prior to reflecting the osteotomized fragment anteriorly. This maneuver prevents fracture of the medial posterior femur or the osteotomized fragment (see Fig. 6). The assistant initially holds the trochanteric fragment by hand as the tissue is released. After the fragment is mobilized anteriorly, a Hohman retractor can be inserted to facilitate exposure.

Pedestal

Often, a distal cement plug or bony pedestal remains. Burring the visible area of the canal and making a perforation with a drill or pencil burr will allow the passing of a crochet hook. The bone or cement can then be pulled out. Care must be taken to avoid a perforation, and it is prudent to advance cautiously with the drills or burrs. An alternate style is to drill the distal cement 1 to 2 cm with cement drills and tap the cement plug with cement taps. This is repeated as needed.

Reaming

After all the cement, neocortex, and distal pedestal have been removed, reaming is undertaken. A clear canal will help keep the reamer centered and neutrally aligned in the femoral canal. With straight stems, solid reamers are utilized, whereas for curved stems, flexible reamers are used.

The length of reaming is determined from the length of stem necessary to achieve fixation. Only the length necessary for fixation is reamed. In general, this is 4 to 6 cm distal to the osteotomy. Reaming is performed in neutral alignment with special attention to avoid varus. Varus orientation of the reamers occurs if the proximal trochanteric region is not osteotomized and the reamer obtains three-point contact with the diaphysis distally and the trochanter proximally. If the proximal trochanteric region is left intact, reaming must be started laterally enough while avoiding impingement from the greater trochanter. As mentioned, this can be impossible in cases with a preoperative varus deformity and is a specific indication to perform an osteotomy. A Charnley T-handled awl must insert freely into the diaphysis without proximal obstruction to assure neutral reamer positioning.

Sequential reaming is then performed, increasing reamer diameter until good endosteal cortical contact is obtained (see Fig. 7). Reaming is stopped 0.5 mm below the size of the prosthesis to be implanted. This point is one of the most crucial in cementless femoral revisions.

Templating is a helpful, albeit inexact, way to size the canal with respect to final reamed diameters. The template is probably accurate to plus or minus one size, but bone quality and magnification must be considered. A patient with healthy cortices will give good feedback during reaming. The reamer will labor through the strong bone, and there is little question when to stop. This is not as pronounced in patients with diminished bone quality.

To facilitate the decision of when to stop reaming, we insert a T-handled reamer the same size as the prosthesis to be implanted into the prepared channel. If rotational stability is achieved with 4 to 5 cm of reamer remaining proud, this is the diameter prosthesis chosen. If rotational stability is not obtained, the femur is reamed up. If more than 5 cm of reamer are showing, then the introitus is reamed line to line to prevent fracture on insertion. Underreaming insures a tight fit, but at the risk of fracturing. In our experience, a 4- to 5-cm distance of 0.5 mm underreamed canal is safe. In addition, a prophylactic Luque wire placed 1 cm distal to the osteotomy is a wise precaution.

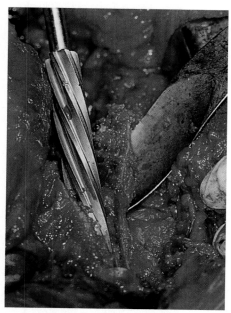

Figure 7. The hash mark on the reamer corresponds to the level of the collar and should be referenced to the templated implantation level. In the case shown, the canal was ultimately reamed up to 16.0 mm, and a 16.5-mm component was implanted. Reaming was begun at 10 mm and increased until there was minimal bite at 13.5 mm. The 15.0/13.5 broach fit line to line and could be used as a trial, but reaming to 14.0 mm provided an extra measure of safety and adjustment. The canal was thus reamed to 14.0 mm, and a 15.0/13.5 broach was placed and trial reduced until a stable height and neck length were determined.

Broaching

Next, the appropriate broach is inserted. Usually, broaching is unnecessary for proximal preparation due to the loss of proximal bone. However, it is useful for trial reduction. The cylindrical distal portion of the broaches is 1.5 mm in diameter less than the actual prosthesis. For example, a 15.0-mm broach has a stem diameter of 13.5 mm (referred to as 15.0/13.5). Solution prostheses are manufactured in 1.5-mm increments, beginning at 10.5 mm and ending at 22.5 mm.

Broaching is undertaken chiefly to determine stem version and neck length, since there is usually adequate space in the proximal femur to accommodate a prosthesis without the broaching procedure (see Fig. 8). Additionally, one may select a prosthesis with a more narrow proximal profile. These stems have utility, especially when the surgeon is working without an osteotomy and when a tight proximal femur can limit anteversion in the standard body prosthesis.

With a broach implanted, a midrange neck length is chosen, and the hip is reduced. If the hip remains reduced in the 90–90 position (90 degrees flexion–90 degrees internal rotation) (see Fig. 9), adequate soft tissue tension has been obtained. We also test the limb in the "sleeping position" lateral decubitus with the operated leg crossed over the non-operative one.

Trial reduction is one of the most important steps in revision and total hip arthroplasty. It is through the trial reduction that the component positions can be altered to achieve stability. This is accomplished by modifying neck length, height, and version. The most important consideration is stability. If the hip is unstable, the cause may be simply poor tensioning. In that case, either add neck length or implant the stem proudly while maintaining good fixation.

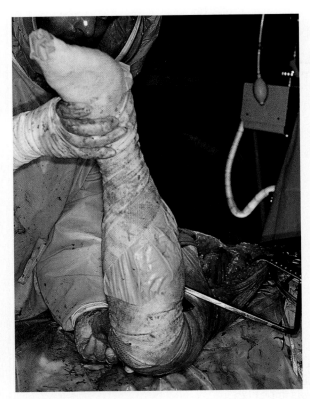

Figure 8. With a trial broach in place, the hip is checked in the 90–90-degree revision. In this example, the hip is placed in 90 degrees of internal rotation and flexed to the limit of the soft tissue. In reality, this is often somewhat short of 90 degrees.

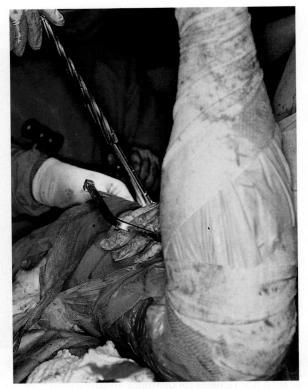

Figure 9. Implantation of the component is shown with a reamer placed to control rotation. The degree of anteversion can be seen clearly by observing the angle of the reamer to the leg.

Management of Impingement

When ranging the hip, attention must be paid to impingement. This can be due to contact of the trunion with the perimeter of the cup. This is easily recognized and can be managed by modifying the component position. However, occasionally the anterior femur at the level of the calcar can act as a fulcrum against the anterior soft tissues, remaining pseudocapsule, and pelvis. Thinning the anterior trochanteric bone with an oscillating saw can manage this problem. Less commonly, the hip can be tight in external rotation, and a limited anterior capsulectomy is done until proper tension is achieved.

Implantation

The component is implanted using a reamer placed in the extraction hole to help control rotation (see Fig. 10). On average, the angle of the inserted reamer to the leg is 25 degrees and is the femoral anteversion. Initial insertion of the stem may require little force and can usually be accomplished by hand until the stem engages the region of the canal that is relatively undersized by 0.5 mm. Insertion of the femoral stem past this point should require repeated blows from a heavy mallet on the stem impactor. Once the stem begins to engage the underreamed segment of femur in which fixation will be achieved, it becomes more difficult to alter the anteversion. Thus, the anteversion must be closely monitored during the initial 2 to 3 cm of prosthetic seating into the segment of the canal that will provide fixation.

As the stem engages, the surgeon must determine the depth of insertion based on the trial insertion and reductions and landmarks chosen to measure the depth of implant insertion. This is most commonly the relationship of the inferior border of calcar with remaining medial bone stock. If the stem stops advancing, a shorter neck length may be employed,

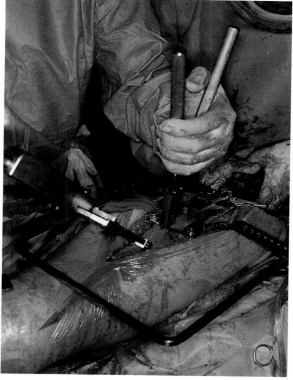

Figure 10. Following cable tightening and prior to crimping, the hip can be tested for shuck and stability. Problems of insufficient abductor tension can be managed by removing bone from the distal segment of the osteotomy fragment and advancing the segment distally on the femur.

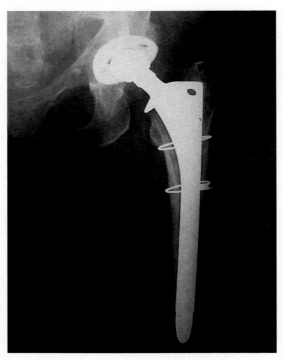

Figure 11. Postoperative view of a 6-inch, fully coated stem with osteotomy fixed with two cables. Note that the stem is implanted in neutral alignment and there are greater than 4 cm of canal-filling fit. The stem is placed with a collar in anatomic purchase and gains stability from distal purchase.

and if a more distal insertion is required to obtain good fixation, either a longer neck or advancement of the trochanteric fragment may be needed.

Once the stem has been inserted, trial heads may be used to perform a final trial reduction to assess hip stability and length.

Once the revision prosthesis has been inserted, the osteotomy fragment is shaped with a high-speed burr to shape the fragment to fit over the lateral shoulder of the prosthesis. Multiple wires or cables are then used to secure the fragment to the shaft. Abductor laxity can be addressed by shortening the fragment and advancing it distally (see Fig. 11). The limb can be put through a range of motion before the cables are crimped so that the trochanteric fragment position can be fine-tuned.

In cases where the proximal femur is very thin, atrophic, patulous, or porotic, the cables used to hold the osteotomy segment in place may be used to "collapse" the proximal medial bone sleeve to the implant. As all stem stability has been gained from the distal "scratch fit," this maneuver only serves to bring the healthy proximal bone closer to the ingrowth surface of the proximal stem.

POSTOPERATIVE MANAGEMENT

All revision patients are placed in an off-the-shelf abduction orthosis. It is set at 30 degrees of abduction with a flexion stop at 70 degrees. This brace is continued for 8 weeks. For 6 weeks, the patients are kept at 30% weight bearing with a walker. They are then advanced to full weight bearing by 8 weeks and protected as needed with a cane. We use fully coated ingrowth stems widely in our revision practice. We have noted a loosening rate of 2.4% of 311 hip revisions at an average of 8.2 years.

While thigh pain is uncommon and rarely clinically bothersome, it may occur. Patients with thin, osteopenic femurs and large stems seem to be at greater risk. Fortunately, there is clinical evidence that stiffening the femur by placement of allograft bone plates may be useful in managing this complication.

COMPLICATIONS

Specific complications referable to this technique relate specifically to component implantation, and in this regard, two alternate complications are worth discussing. Fracture of the femur may occur on insertion of a stem into a canal that has been inadequately prepared for the implant. Alternatively, an undersized stem may fail to obtain rotational and axial stability so that micromotion is present with loading, leading to ingrowth failure.

For the experienced surgeon, implantation of the appropriately sized stem is guided by several clues, including visual, auditory, and tactile feedback that can be gained only with experience. These clues are obtained by paying careful attention to parameters such as "cortical chatter" during reaming, the quality of bone encountered at various depths of reaming, and the appearance of bone in the reamer flutes from those depths. The feel of reamers on a hand chuck at the final reaming size, rather than a power reamer, can give the surgeon a good sense of the actual quality of the bone at the reamed size chosen. Fracture may be avoided in particularly hard bone by reaming a short transition zone (1 cm) between the open intramedullary cavity above and the interference fit segment below. If there is any question of difficulty at the initial insertion into this zone, a cerclage wire placed at this region may decrease the incidence of fracture at the time of stem insertion. Unfortunately, a stem that is implanted and found to be loose—either by virtue of rotational instability or insufficient resistance encountered during component insertion—should be removed, and the femur should be prepared to accept a larger component.

26

Grafting: Impaction and Strut

John Charity, Anthony D. Lamberton, Graham A. Gie,
and Andrew John Timperley

INDICATIONS/CONTRAINDICATIONS

Femoral impaction grafting is indicated in any patient where revision of the femoral stem is required during revision total hip arthroplasty and where, after removal of the femoral component, there remains a smooth endosteal surface of the femur with little cancellous bone remaining to provide adequate fixation for a cemented femoral component. The technique is also indicated in any revision situation where it is desirable to restore bone stock and also where the intramedullary canal diameter is equal to or greater than 18 mm, as the use of an uncemented stem in this situation has a high incidence of thigh pain. It is further indicated, even in the hands of surgeons dedicated to uncemented stems, where the required length of "scratch" fit cannot be achieved, as in situations where there is significant bone loss to below the isthmus of the femur.

The technique is applicable to patients of any age but is most useful in the younger patient where it is desirable to restore bone stock.

There are no contraindications, and although we advise that the procedure be performed in two stages in the presence of infection, there are surgeons using this technique as a one-stage procedure in infected cases. Where complete loss of the proximal femur exceeds 10 cm, reconstruction with femoral impaction grafting becomes extremely complex, and other methods of stem fixation are recommended.

Although the technique works in all ages, it may not be indicated in the very old or in medically unfit patients where bone stock recovery is not necessary, where a relatively short revision operation is desirable, and where distal fixation is achievable with an uncemented stem.

PREOPERATIVE PLANNING

Exclusion of Infection

Screening of patients for infection is carried out along conventional lines. Where there is a clinical suspicion of infection or where anti-inflammatory markers are raised, aspiration of the joint is carried out prior to the definitive revision procedure. Antibiotic powder is added to the graft at the subsequent impaction-grafting procedure (1).

Analysis of Bone Deficiencies

Prerevision radiographs are analyzed in detail. Anteroposterior (AP) pelvis, AP femur, extending to well below the tip of the existing implant, and lateral radiographs are taken to detect endosteal and cortical femoral bone deficiencies. Donor allograft femoral heads or condyles and strut grafts, if necessary, are ordered from a bone bank. Femoral reconstruction metal meshes (see Fig. 1) must be available to reconstruct the femoral tube where preoperative x-rays indicate cortical deficiencies or where there is loss of medial femoral neck.

Templating

Femoral Component. From the radiographs, the size, length, and offset of the stem required for revision are determined with the appropriate translucent templates (see Fig. 2). The stem must bypass the most distal significant femoral defect, i.e., a cortical defect or an endosteolytic lesion involving 50% or more of the cortex seen on two views, by at least one, and preferably two, cortical diameters. The femoral impaction grafting system of X-Change Revision Instruments (Stryker Corp., Rutherford, NJ) allows for implantation of all Exeter stems from 30- to 50-mm offset (see Fig. 3) and from 125 to 260 mm in length (see Figs. 3 and 4).

Canal Plug. The threaded femoral plug (see Fig. 5) must be templated to lie at least 2 cm beyond the tip of the stem to be used at the revision operation. If there is significant limb shortening, the plug should be placed a little more distal in the femur in case trial reduction is too tight and the femoral component needs to be inserted deeper than expected.

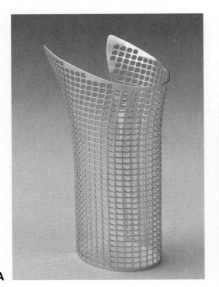

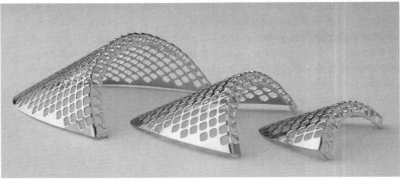

A   B

Figure 1. Femoral reconstruction metal meshes.

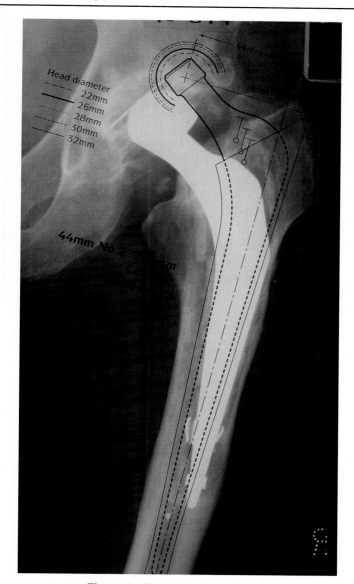

Figure 2. Templating of the stem.

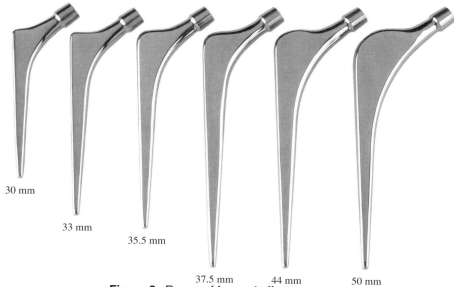

Figure 3. Range of femoral offsets.

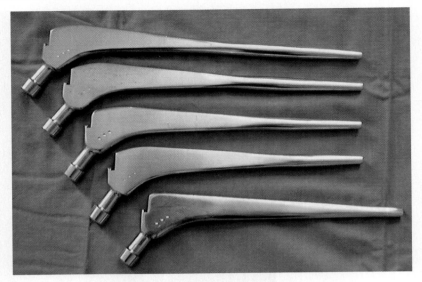

Figure 4. Long stem range 200 to 260 mm.

If a well-fixed cement plug lies at least 2 cm distal to the most distal bony defect and the tip of the stem to be used, it can be left in situ.

SURGERY

Patient Positioning

The patient is positioned securely by the operating surgeon personally on his/her side in the lateral decubitus position. The lower limb is free-draped, giving exposure from the iliac crest to the knee.

Surgical Approach

Incision. We use a posterior approach exclusively for its versatility and extensibility, and we are not concerned about previous approaches to the hip. A posterolateral incision is made, incorporating or excising the previous scar if possible. There is no place for

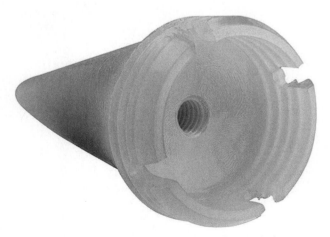

Figure 5. Threaded polyethylene femoral plug.

minimally invasive surgery when bone quality is such that femoral impaction is required. Limited clearing of subcutaneous fat from the fascia lata is made in the line of the incision to facilitate closure. The fascial incision follows the line of the skin incision with the gluteus maximus muscle being split in the line of its fibers.

Identification of the Sciatic Nerve. The sciatic nerve is identified by palpation and blunt dissection. It is not formally exposed unless the posterior column of the pelvis is deficient and requires augmentation. When incising the external rotator muscles and hip capsule, cautery is used, giving due warning should the dissection approach the sciatic nerve.

Aspiration of the Hip. The hip is aspirated prior to opening the joint capsule. The fluid obtained is sent for immediate microscopy and for routine and enrichment culture. If microscopy reveals greater than 100 neutrophils per high-powered field or if organisms are identified, the revision is abandoned, the hip is carefully debrided, and a temporary hip spacer is inserted. This involves the appropriate metal and polyethylene components with 4 g of vancomycin and 1 g of gentamicin added to each mix of cement. Frozen section of multiple tissue samples may be useful if there remains any doubt about the possibility of the joint being infected (2).

Exposure of the Joint. With the hip positioned in slight flexion, adduction and internal rotation and the vastus medialis muscle retracted anteriorly, the tendinous insertion of gluteus maximus is released from its femoral insertion. Gluteus minimus is lifted off the capsule and is retracted anteriorly.

If a previous posterior exposure has been used, the external rotators and capsule are raised as a single layer, incising them with cautery close to the posterior aspect of the greater trochanter and obtaining as much length as possible to facilitate closure at the end of the procedure. This is best achieved by the limb being held in 45 degrees of flexion and internal rotation during capsular incision. If previous surgery involved an anterior approach, the external rotators and capsule are raised as separate flaps. A single, straight longitudinal incision is made in the capsule to the upper border of the acetabulum with no posterior curve or T-shaped incision. This helps create a large, sturdy posterior flap for later bony repair and reduction of dislocation risk. Stay sutures are placed in the flap and used to reflect it posteriorly, protecting the sciatic nerve.

Dissection of the tissues off the bone is carried distally to the level of the lesser trochanter. To further facilitate exposure and to help deliver the femur out of the wound, particularly in obese patients or muscular men, the psoas tendon is released from the lesser trochanter and the anterior capsule is released from the anterior aspect of the femur. It is important to carry out this release before the leg is significantly flexed and internally rotated since the anterior wall of the femur is often flimsy from osteolysis and may fracture or avulse during dislocation of the joint. The hip is then dislocated with as little force as possible, aided by a bone hook around the prosthetic neck and a gentle lift.

Explantation, Debridement, and Graft Preparation

Removal of the Femoral Component. Once the proximal femur is adequately displayed with the aid of a femoral elevating retractor, cement is removed from over the shoulder of the prosthesis using a high-speed burr. The femoral component is then extracted with gentle persuasion, care being taken to ensure that impingement on the greater trochanter does not occur. An instrument is applied to the neck of the prosthesis to control rotational forces, which may fracture the femur during component removal.

If an uncemented component is being removed, a single longitudinal femoral split or an extended trochanteric osteotomy may be required (3). This does not preclude the technique of impaction grafting and indeed has been used in our center in more than 20 cases without any aseptic loosenings or trochanteric nonunions to date. The osteotomy must be soundly repaired with cables.

Further Femoral Exposure. The proximal part of the greater trochanter must be exposed sufficiently to allow insertion of the guide wire down the medullary canal in the midline axis, so that the neomedullary canal that is subsequently formed is in neutral

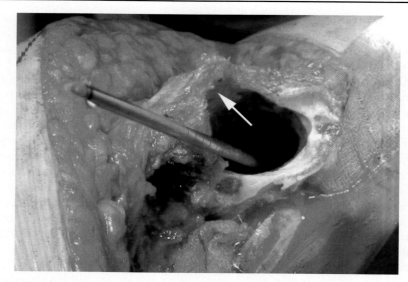

Figure 6. The neomedullary canal must be in neutral alignment. Arrow indicates opening of trochanteric overhang.

alignment, avoiding either varus or valgus. This often requires opening of the trochanteric overhang laterally by around 1 cm to accommodate the introduction of instruments in the correct alignment, without risking fracture of the trochanter (see Fig. 6).

Cement and Membrane Removal. Cement and membrane removal must be complete in the area for impaction grafting. However, if the distal cement plug is greater than 2 cm beyond the tip of the stem to be used, it may be left in position and used to occlude the distal canal during reconstruction.

Several separate specimens of tissue and membrane from the interfaces are routinely sent for microbiological examination.

Preparation of the Graft. We use almost exclusively allograft from fresh-frozen femoral heads, sourced from our own bone bank, which complies with the standards and procedures laid down by the UK Tissue Banking Standards Authority. ABO compatibility between graft donor and recipient is not necessary. Rhesus compatibility is only important when the patient is a rhesus-negative woman of child-bearing age.

Graft preparation is critical to the success of the procedure. All soft tissue and cartilage must be removed from the bone. Two sizes of bone chips are required: 3- to 4-mm chips for packing the distal three quarters of the canal above the plug and 8- to 10-mm chips for the proximal quarter. Even in a nonectatic femur, never fewer than two femoral heads are required. Note that neither very fine milled bone nor bone slurry is suitable for impaction grafting. These do not have the mechanical properties required for adequate impaction, and their usage will lead to failure.

Femoral Preparation for Impaction

In essence, the technique of femoral impaction grafting restores the femur to a state equivalent to that at the time of primary arthroplasty. The first step, if required, is cortical tube restoration with mesh, followed by cancellous restoration with impaction grafting. The success of impaction grafting is dependent upon adequate physical constraint of the graft material. The surgeon should therefore have a low threshold for prophylactic cerclage wiring, and any defects in the femoral diaphysis must be repaired prior to impaction grafting.

Malleable stainless steel meshes (Stryker Corp., Rutherford, NJ) are secured with monofilament cerclage wires or cables to contain any cortical defects or perforations. Periprosthetic fractures are addressed in a similar fashion. These meshes are placed with as little soft tissue dissection as possible. Cortical strut allografts may additionally be required to augment the diaphysis in certain situations. (Uncontained defects of the proximal femur in the calcar region are reconstructed later in the procedure.)

Distal Occlusion of the Femur

Prior to grafting, the medullary canal must be occluded distally in order to contain the graft. The canal size is determined with canal sounds (see Fig. 7). An appropriately sized threaded polyethylene plug (see Fig. 5) is screwed onto an intramedullary guide rod and inserted into the medullary canal with a cannulated introducer sleeve coupled to a slap hammer (see Fig. 8). The plug is advanced to the templated level, and the introducer is removed. Calibrations on the introducer sleeve ensure placement at the correct depth. If the plug must be placed beyond the isthmus, then the largest plug that passes through the isthmus to the correct depth is used and secured by passing a Kirschner wire percutaneously into, or immediately below the level of, the plug.

The guide wire remains in situ for cannulated instruments to pass over for the impaction grafting (see Fig. 9).

If a retained cement plug is to be used, then the largest-diameter distal impactor that will pass down the canal is introduced to the level of the plug to act as a drill centralizer. The intramedullary drill is passed through the impactor, and the cement is drilled to a depth of 6 mm. The threaded guide rod can then be passed through the impactor and screwed into the predrilled hole in the cement plug.

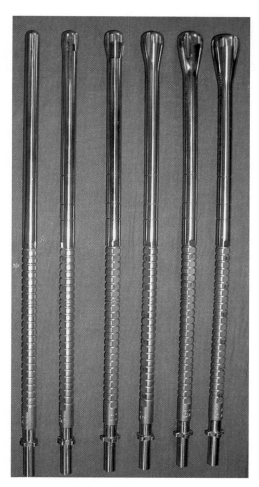

Figure 7. Canal sounds used to determine canal size.

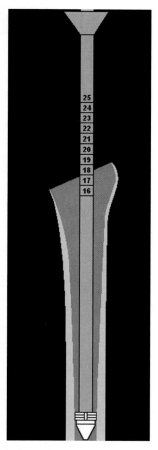

Figure 8. Polyethylene plug screwed onto an intramedullary guide rod and inserted into the medullary canal.

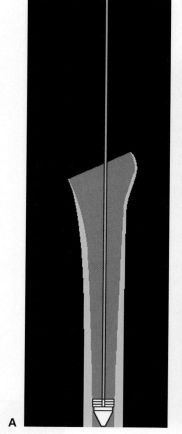

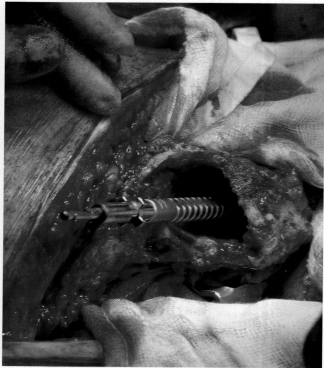

A   B

Figure 9. Guide wire in situ.

Impaction of the Graft

Alignment and Size Check. Cannulated instruments are used to pack the graft in the distal and proximal femur by passing over the guide wire (see Fig. 10). First, the largest impactor stem, or "phantom," of the appropriate offset is passed over the guide rod into the canal and, working progressively smaller, the first "phantom" to pass easily into the canal without obstruction to the required depth is the correct size for impaction.

Care should be taken that the rod is not driven into varus as the impactor is inserted. If this occurs, further development of the posterolateral slot in the trochanter is necessary until neutral alignment of the proximal impactor can be achieved. The guide wire should lie freely in the canal proximally and align with the midpoint of the popliteal fossa when viewed from its proximal end.

Distal Impaction. Before using the distal impactors to impact the bone chips, it is important to establish the distance down the canal that each size of impactor can be passed without jamming in the canal and potentially causing a fracture.

Select a distal impactor one size smaller in diameter than the intramedullary plug diameter. This should pass easily over the guide wire down to the plug without obstruction. Withdraw this impactor 2 cm and attach a marker clip to grooves on the impactor at the level of the greater trochanter to mark the intended depth of insertion (see Fig. 11). Bearing in mind that the impactor will be carrying bone graft ahead of it, impaction is stopped 2 cm above the plug to avoid driving the plug further distally. Larger-diameter impactors are in turn introduced as far down the canal as they will pass and similarly marked with a clip (see Fig. 12). When subsequently impacting the bone chips, do not drive the impactor beyond this depth, or a femoral blowout fracture will occur.

The smaller-diameter allograft chips are introduced into the medullary canal around the guide rod using an open-ended 10- or 20-mL syringe (see Fig. 13). The chips are then

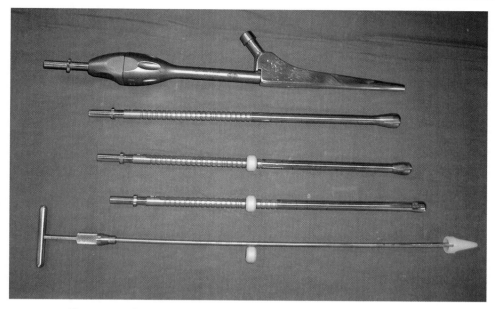

Figure 10. Cannulated instruments are passed over the guide wire.

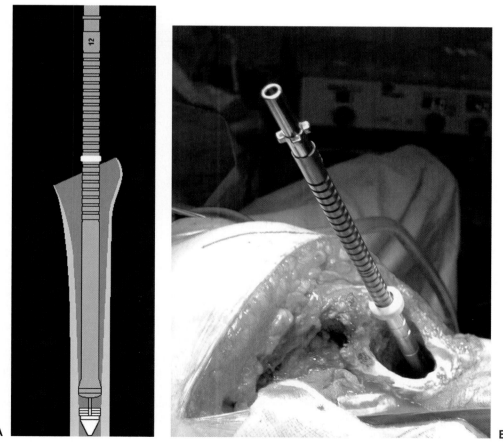

Figure 11. A marker clip is attached to the grooves of the impactor at the level of the greater trochanter to mark the depth of insertion.

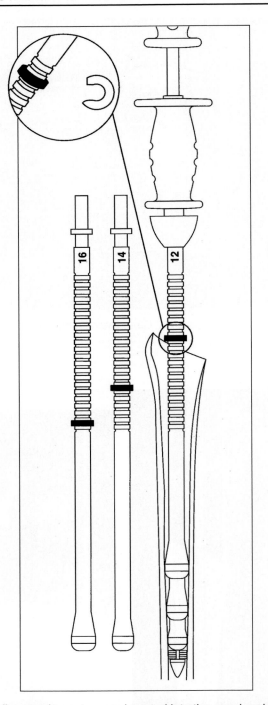

Figure 12. Larger-diameter impactors are inserted into the canal and marked with a clip.

manually pushed down the canal using one of the larger impactors. Using the first impactor (the one that passes right down to the plug), bone chips are firmly compacted to the marked depth using the slap hammer.

The impaction process is continued by introducing and impacting more chips and using progressively larger impactors (see Fig. 14) to their marked depth. An eye should be kept on the calibrations on the guide rod to ensure that the plug is not migrating distally, and if it is, it should then be temporarily skewered with a 2-mm Kirschner wire.

Impaction is continued until the distal impactors cannot be introduced beyond the distal impaction line. This is indicated by the most distal groove on the distal impactors (see Fig. 15) or as an extra line on the long-stem impactors. Once this point has been reached, the

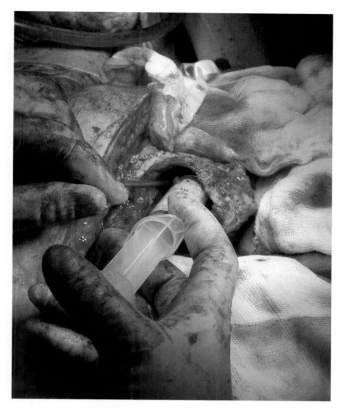

Figure 13. A syringe is used to introduce allograft chips into the intramedullary canal.

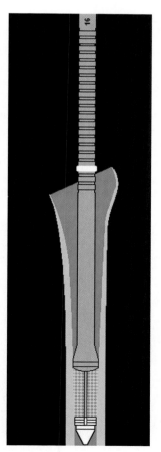

Figure 14. The impaction process involved adding and impacting more chips and introducing progressively larger impactors.

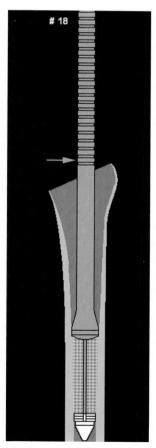

Figure 15. Impaction is continued until the distal impactors cannot be introduced beyond the distal impaction line.

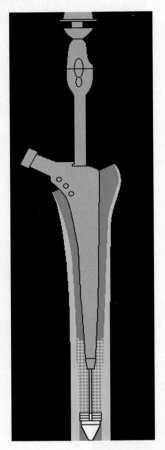

Figure 16. A slap hammer is used to drive the phantom into the distal bone plug.

"phantoms" should be used. If the canal is filled beyond this point, then it will be impossible to introduce the phantom to the required level.

Midstem Impaction. The previously determined "phantom" is mounted on the slap hammer assembly and passed over the guide rod. Using the slap hammer, the phantom is driven into the distal bone plug (see Fig. 16). It is then removed, and more chips are inserted. The phantom is reintroduced. A trial reduction is performed as soon as there is enough stability to do so. The slap hammer is removed, a trial head is placed onto the neck of the phantom, and the hip is reduced with the guide wire remaining in situ (see Fig. 17).

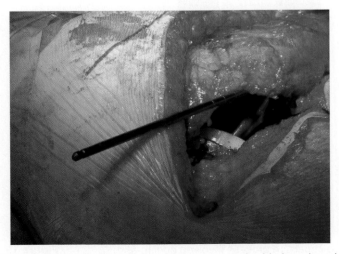

Figure 17. The guide wire remains in situ as the hip is reduced.

Hip stability and leg length are checked. The level to which the phantom is inserted is marked on the proximal femur with methylene blue for later reference (see Fig. 18). At this time, any calcar or proximal femoral deficiency can be assessed and reconstructed using the appropriate metal meshes, keeping the phantom in situ while this is done (see Fig. 19). Reconstruction must be performed to a level that at least reaches the most distal of the three ring marks on the phantom. The higher the reconstruction, the better the rotational stability that will be achieved.

Once the position of the phantom is marked in relation to the bone or mesh, it is removed, and more graft is introduced into the canal, approximately 10 cm³ at a time, and initially advanced by using a distal impactor by hand (see Fig. 20). The phantom is then repetitively driven into the graft using the slap hammer (see Fig. 21).

The slap hammer handle is used to control rotation of the phantom to ensure that the neomedullary canal that is formed is in the correct amount of anteversion, usually 10 to 15 degrees.

Graft is sequentially added and vigorously impacted until the canal has been filled to within a few centimeters of the calcar. Impaction is only tight enough when the phantom barely reaches the required depth with vigorous slap hammer blows.

Proximal Graft Packing. At this stage, change to the larger-diameter bone chips for final proximal packing. The proximal tamping instruments are used to introduce these chips around the seated phantom, first by hand and then impacted with a mallet (see Fig. 22). This is continued until no further chips can be introduced.

When it seems that the femur is fully grafted, one final maneuver is performed. The phantom is withdrawn by 2 cm using the slap hammer, and a last introduction of the large allograft chips is made. These are hammered around the phantom with the proximal tamps. The phantom is then driven into this bone, resulting in impressive final graft impaction.

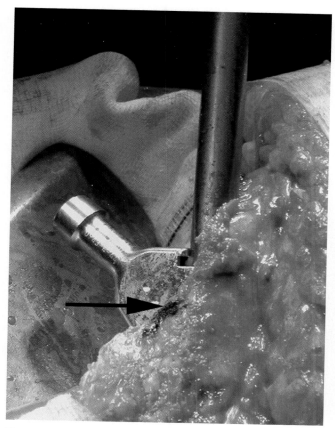

Figure 18. Methylene blue is used to mark the level to which the phantom is inserted.

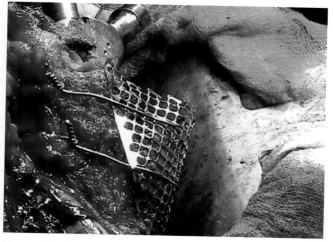

Figure 19. Metal mesh is used to reconstruct calcar or proximal femoral deficiency.

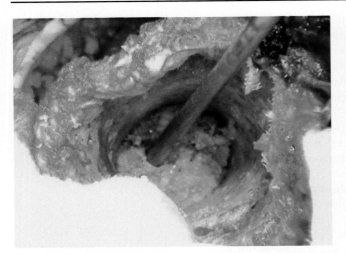

Figure 20. More graft is introduced to the medullary canal and advanced by hand with a distal impactor.

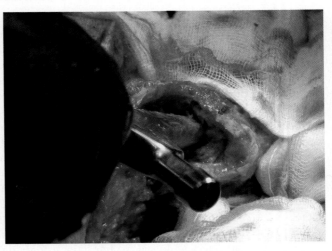

Figure 21. A slap hammer is used to drive the phantom into the graft.

Absolute axial and torsional stability of the phantom should be evident at the conclusion of impaction. Several blows with the slap hammer should result in minimal axial advancement of the phantom (<1 mm), and withdrawal should be extremely difficult or impossible without the use of the slap hammer. A second trial reduction can be performed at this time, if desired.

Cancellous restoration is now complete, with the formation of a neomedullary canal ready to accept the prosthesis (see Fig. 23). The definitive stem chosen for implantation has

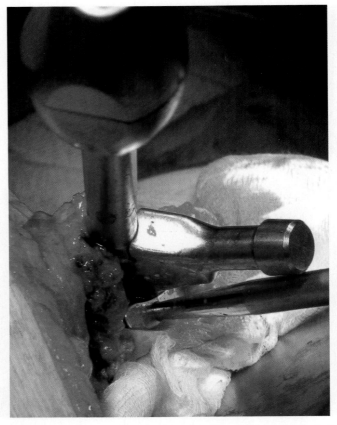

Figure 22. Larger-diameter bone chips are introduced around the seated phantom with proximal tamping instruments and are then impacted with a mallet.

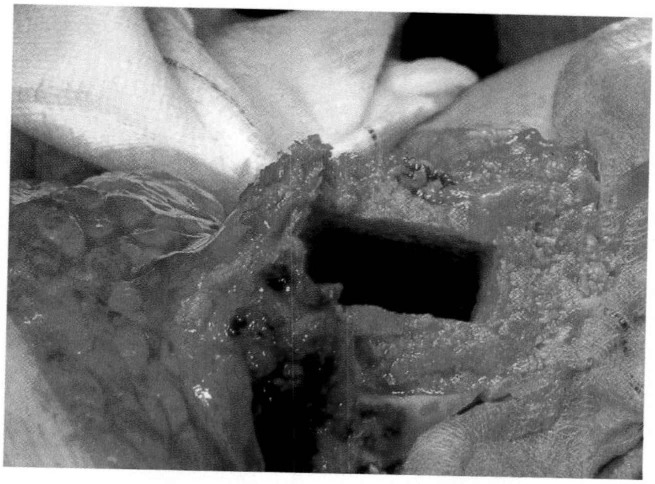

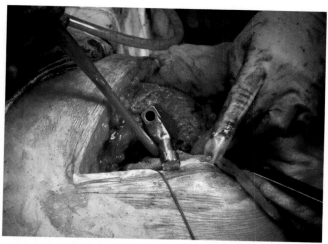

Figure 23. The neomedullary canal is ready to receive the prosthesis.

Figure 24. The phantom is left in place to keep the graft under compression until cement insertion.

the same number as the phantom impactor used for the impaction, the phantom being oversized to allow for cement mantle and the distal centralizer.

Cementation, Stem Insertion, and Closure

The slap hammer is removed, followed by the guide wire. The phantom is left in position until just before cement insertion, keeping the graft under compression (see Fig. 24). The canal can be kept dry by placing a no. 14 French-gauge suction catheter down the lumen of the phantom (see Fig. 25).

Cementation is performed with an identical technique as used for an Exeter primary total hip replacement. Simplex bone cement (Stryker Corp., Rutherford, NJ) is used, introduced retrograde after removal of the phantom at about 2 min from mixing, using a revision cement gun with a tapered or narrow nozzle to ensure that the graft is not disrupted (see Fig. 26).

Once the canal has been filled, a flexible femoral seal is placed over the nozzle, which is then cut off flush with the seal. The cement gun is reapplied to the proximal femur, and cement is then pressurized into the graft (see Fig. 27). Pressurization is maintained, with

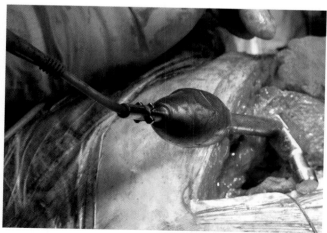

Figure 25. A no. 14 French suction catheter placed down the lumen of the phantom keeps the canal dry.

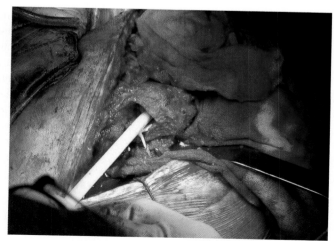

Figure 26. Simplex bone cement is introduced retrograde with a revision cement gun.

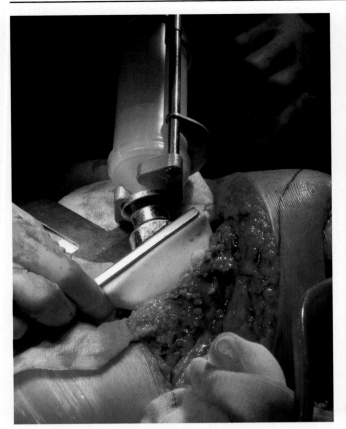

Figure 27. A cement gun with a flexible femoral seal placed over the nozzle is used to pressurize cement into the graft at the proximal femur.

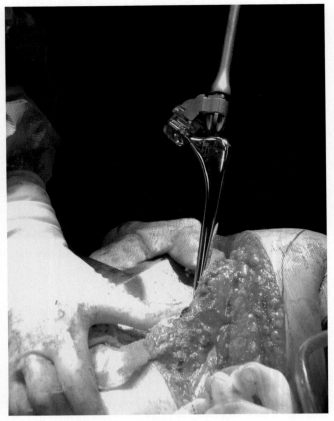

Figure 28. The surgeon's thumb maintains pressurization of the cement.

the continuous injection of cement, until the viscosity of the cement is appropriate for stem insertion: normally around 6 min after mixing if the room temperature is 20°C. At least two 40-g cement mixes are required.

The definitive component with the wingless centralizer applied is inserted to its predetermined position, as indicated by the previously placed methylene blue mark. The surgeon's thumb is applied to the medial aspect of the femoral neck throughout insertion to occlude cement extrusion from the medullary canal and thus maintain pressurization of the cement (see Fig. 28).

When the desired position of the prosthesis is reached, the stem introducer is removed, and a seal is applied around the proximal femur in order to maintain pressure on the cement and graft while the cement polymerizes (see Fig. 29).

A final trial reduction is carried out (see Fig. 30), the head with the appropriate neck length is then applied, and the hip is reduced.

The posterior capsule is reattached via drill holes to the posterior aspect of the femur with no. 2 nonabsorbable braided sutures. Routine wound closure is completed. Although drainage is no longer used in primary hip surgery, where there has been significant soft tissue release in revision surgery, a single deep suction drain is used.

Strut Grafts

Since the introduction of long stems, the use of strut grafts has significantly decreased. They are seldom used proximally, where metal meshes are preferred to build up and reinforce the proximal femur. They are easier to mold to fit and also allow for easy access of a blood supply through the mesh holes to the impacted bone graft within.

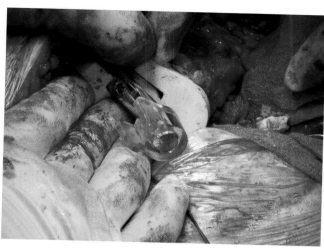

Figure 29. To maintain pressure on the cement and graft while the cement polymerizes, a seal is applied around the proximal femur.

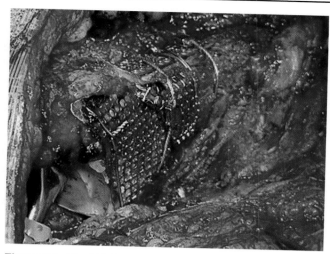

Figure 30. Final trial reduction.

Strut grafts, however, still have a very definite place, namely:

1. Where the femoral diaphysis is so flimsy that application of wires or cables will simply crush or slice through the cortex.
2. Where, despite the use of a long stem, a significant stress riser is present within two cortical diameters of the stem tip, at the stem tip, or beyond the stem tip.
3. Where a long stem is required but the femur is too small to accept the smallest long cemented stem and a short stem has to be used. A strut graft is used to overlap the tip of the stem by two cortical diameters and to bypass the most distal lytic lesion by a similar amount.

Application. Minimal stripping of tissues from the femoral cortex should be performed. Only tissues the width of the strut graft need to be elevated from the femur. The graft is usually placed laterally.

The appropriate length graft is applied to the host cortex and assessed for fit. A high-speed burr is then used to shape it appropriately to achieve maximum possible contact between the strut and host cortex. Cables or wires are then passed around the femur from posterior to anterior (less chance of snaring the sciatic nerve) at the levels where the strut makes direct contact with host bone. If wires or cables are tightened where there is no contact, the strut may fracture acutely or fatigue in due course. Drill holes should not be made in the strut.

Immediately prior to application of the strut, milled autograft or allograft is placed within its concave surface. The strut is then wired or cabled firmly to the host cortex. The strut should not be applied onto underlying mesh.

POSTOPERATIVE MANAGEMENT

The patient is nursed supine with an abduction pillow between the legs.

The drain is removed on day one, and AP pelvis and full-length femoral radiographs are obtained prior to mobilization of the patient, which takes place as soon as the patient is comfortable enough to do so. If an epidural anesthetic has been used, the epidural catheter is removed on the second postoperative day, and the patient is then mobilized. Touch to partial weight bearing on crutches is advised for the first 6 weeks when major reconstruction has been performed. When impaction grafting is performed for lack of cancellous bone only and when the cortex is of good quality, full weight bearing is allowed as comfortable.

Clinical and radiographic surveillance is carried out at 6 weeks, 6 months, 2 years, and then every 2 years indefinitely.

RESULTS

In revision total hip surgery, the technique of impaction grafting has the advantage over other forms of femoral reconstruction in that it offers restoration of bone stock in deficient femora as the impacted allograft chips incorporate and subsequently remodel in the host skeleton.

The results of impaction grafting at our center have generally been very good (4) with regard to the clinical outcome scores for patients, the survivorship of the implants, and the radiological evidence of bone stock restoration. Survivorship for all indications with multiple surgeons is greater than 90% at an average 6.7 years in over 540 cases with minimum 2-year follow-up (5).

Potential problems associated with the technique are now well known—principally, femoral fracture and massive subsidence. Prophylactic wiring, strut allograft reinforcement of type 4 femurs, and long-stem implants have dramatically reduced the fracture rate. The incidence of significant subsidence has now been reduced by the use of larger bone chips proximally and in capacious canals, a better distribution of particle size, tighter impaction of these chips within the femoral canal, and—in the case of severe bone stock loss—the use of longer stems (5–11).

Most of the complications reported from centers that have used this technique, including our own, have resulted from inappropriate surgical technique (5,12–16). Application of the methods described in this chapter should further improve the results possible using the impaction-grafting method.

RECOMMENDED READING

1. English H, Timperley A, Dunlop D, Gie G. Impaction grafting of the femur in two-stage revision for infected total hip replacement. *J Bone Joint Surg Br* 84:700–705, 2002.
2. Athanasou NA, Pandey R, de Steiger R, et al. Diagnosis of infection by frozen section during revision arthroplasty. *J Bone Joint Surg Br* 77(1):28–33, 1995.
3. Younger TI, Bradford MS, Magnus RE, Paprosky WG. Extended proximal femoral osteotomy. A new technique for femoral revision arthroplasty. *J Arthroplasty* 10(3):329–338, 1995.
4. Gie GA, Linder L, Ling RS, et al. Impacted cancellous allografts and cement for revision total hip arthroplasty. *J Bone Joint Surg Br* 75(1):14–21, 1993.
5. Lamberton TD, Charity JA, Kenny PJ, et al. Impaction grafting in revision total hip joint replacement results of 540 cases with 2–15 year follow up. Presented at: Stryker Hip Symposium; May 2002; Gold Coast, Queensland, Australia.
6. Brewster NT, Gillespie WJ, Howie CR, et al. Mechanical considerations in impaction bone grafting. *J Bone Joint Surg Br* 81(1):118–124, 1999.
7. Ullmark G, Nilsson O. Impacted corticocancellous allografts: recoil and strength. *J Arthroplasty* 14(8):1019–1023, 1999.
8. Karrholm J, Hultmark P, Carlsson L, Malchau H. Subsidence of a non-polished stem in revisions of the hip using impaction allograft. Evaluation with radiostereometry and dual-energy x-ray absorptiometry. *J Bone Joint Surg Br* 81(1):135–142, 1999.
9. Giesen EB, Lamerigts NM, Verdonschot N, et al. Mechanical characteristics of impacted morsellised bone grafts used in revision of total hip arthroplasty. *J Bone Joint Surg Br* 81(6):1052–1057, 1999.
10. Malkani AL, Voor MJ, Fee KA, Bates CS. Femoral component revision using impacted morsellised cancellous graft. A biomechanical study of implant stability. *J Bone Joint Surg Br* 78(6):973–978, 1996.
11. Hostner J, Hultmark P, Karrholm J, et al. Impaction technique and graft treatment in revisions of the femoral component: laboratory studies and clinical validation. *J Arthroplasty* 16(1):76–82, 2001.
12. Eldridge JD, Smith EJ, Hubble MJ, et al. Massive early subsidence following femoral impaction grafting. *J Arthroplasty* 12(5):535–540, 1997.
13. Masterson EL, Masri BA, Duncan CP. The cement mantle in the Exeter impaction allografting technique. A cause for concern. *J Arthroplasty* 12(7):759–764, 1997.
14. Jazrawi LM, Della Valle CJ, Kummer FJ, et al. Catastrophic failure of a cemented, collarless, polished, tapered cobalt-chromium femoral stem used with impaction bone-grafting. A report of two cases. *J Bone Joint Surg Am* 81(6):844–847, 1999.
15. Meding JB, Ritter MA, Keating EM, Faris PM. Impaction bone-grafting before insertion of a femoral stem with cement in revision total hip arthroplasty. A minimum two-year follow-up study. *J Bone Joint Surg Am* 79(12):1834–1841, 1997.
16. Pekkarinen J, Alho A, Lepisto J, et al. Impaction bone grafting in revision hip surgery. A high incidence of complications. *J Bone Joint Surg Br* 82(1):103–107, 2000.

27

Allograft Prosthetic Composite

Allan E. Gross

The most important parameter that determines the complexity and prognosis of revision arthroplasty of the hip is bone stock (1). Several classification systems are used to evaluate femoral bone loss (1–3). The system that we use has five types (1). A type 1 has no significant loss of bone stock and can be managed by conventional cemented or uncemented components. A type 2 has contained loss of bone stock and can be managed by one of several methods: long, full, porous coated implants for ingrowth; long, roughened, titanium implants for ongrowth; impaction-grafting, modular implants for proximal or extensive ingrowth or ongrowth, or long-stemmed cemented implants. A type 3 has segmental (full circumferential) bone loss from the proximal femur that is less than 5 cm in length and involves the calcar and lesser trochanter but does not extend into the diaphysis. These defects can be managed by any implant system as described above that also offers calcar buildup. A defect is of type 4 when segmental (full circumferential) bone loss of greater than 5 cm in length extends into the diaphysis (see Fig. 1). This type of defect can be managed by tumor prosthesis or an allograft prosthetic composite. A type 5 is the same as a type 4 with the addition of a periprosthetic fracture and can also be managed by an allograft prosthetic composite or tumor prosthesis (1) (see Fig. 2).

The tumor or megaprosthesis has the advantages of being modular, is available off the shelf, and carries no possibility of disease transmission. Its disadvantages are that host bone or muscle cannot be effectively reattached, it does not restore bone stock, and it violates the distal host canal with cement or a porous coated stem, making further revisions difficult. A proximal femoral allograft, on the other hand, allows bone and muscle attachment and, using appropriate technique, does not violate the distal canal, which may facilitate further revision surgery. Its disadvantages are the potential for disease transmission and the possibility of a poor result from biological complications including resorption, fracture, and host-graft nonunion. Patients with malignancies may be better off with tumor implants because of the detrimental effects of chemotherapy and radiation on allograft-host healing. Also, extensive resection of muscle and bone, including the greater trochanter, makes reattachment of muscle and bone irrelevant. In addition, patients with a guarded prognosis benefit from an operation that does not require an extended period of non–weight bearing. Surgery in the revision population, on the other hand, does require a method for reattachment of the greater trochanter and soft tissues and benefits from a procedure that facilitates further revision surgery.

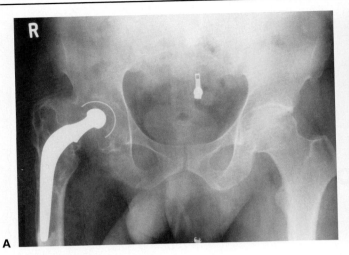

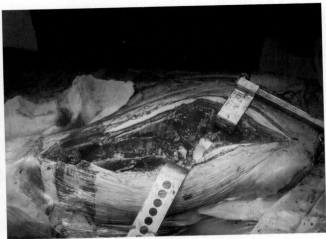

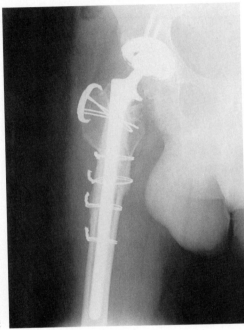

Figure 1. A: Preoperative x-ray of 45-year-old man several years after cemented total hip replacement. The femoral component is loose, and there is segmental bone loss extending into the diaphyses. **B:** Intraoperative photograph illustrating segmental loss of proximal femoral bone stock. **C:** Postoperative x-ray 8 years after reconstruction with proximal femoral allograft.

SURGICAL TECHNIQUE

Preoperative Planning

Routine x-rays are used to determine the approximate level of deficient proximal femur and the length of allograft required. Also, the length and extent of remaining bone of the deficient proximal femur can be estimated. It is prudent to order an allograft that is longer than estimated. The diameter of the host femur and allograft should be approximately the same. It is best not to have an allograft that has a diameter that is significantly wider than the host femur. It is common for the allograft diameter to be smaller than the host femur because of lysis and cavitation, and this is not disadvantageous because under these circumstances the allograft can be telescoped into the host femur for 1 or 2 cm, and this enhances union. It is important that the allograft canal will accommodate the implant to be used. X-rays of the allograft are therefore important for preoperative planning, as is a template of the proposed femoral implant.

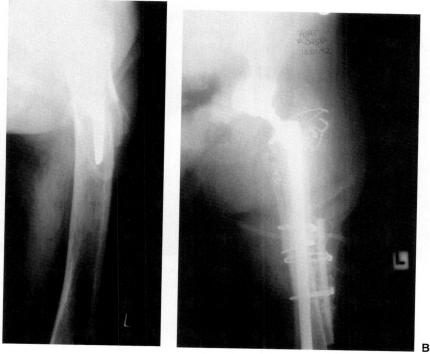

A   B

Figure 2. A: X-ray illustrating periprosthetic femoral fracture with loose femoral component and loss of bone stock extending into the diaphysis. **B:** Five years after reconstruction with proximal femoral allograft.

Preparation of the Allograft

We prefer to use fresh frozen allograft from an American Association of Tissue Banks–accredited tissue bank. The larger banks process the bone in bactericidal and virocidal solutions before the bone is deep-frozen. Some banks provide irradiated bone, which can be 10% to 20% weaker, depending on the radiation dose (4). The author has had no experience with freeze-dried structural grafts, but they are weaker and more brittle than deep-frozen grafts (5). To replace a proximal femur, we prefer to use a proximal femoral allograft; however, a distal femur will accept a larger implant, and this is recommended by some surgeons. The allograft is thawed in 50% Betadine solution after cultures have been taken. To save time during the procedure, one of the surgical assistants can work on the graft on a separate "back" table while the rest of the surgical team prepares the patient. After the bone has thawed and been stripped of soft tissue it is prepared for the femoral implant. The femoral head is excised about 1 cm above the lesser trochanter or even at the base of the lesser trochanter, facilitating insertion of the implant and allowing room for adjusting the version. Lengthening of the leg is not carried out via the neck cut but rather by the length of the allograft below the lesser trochanter. If the patient does not have a greater trochanter, then the allograft greater trochanter should be left in place with a cuff of abductor muscle insertion for attachment of the patient's abductors. If the host trochanter is present, the greater trochanter is excised, allowing for reattachment of the host trochanter.

Reaming is then carried out (see Fig. 3) with straight, rigid reamers for a straight implant or with flexible reamers for a bowed implant. We ream to the cortex but try not to ream the cortex itself in order to allow placement of a larger-diameter implant. It is important not to ream excessively in order to allow insertion of a larger-diameter implant in an attempt to obtain a press fit for the implant into host bone distally. However, if the allograft is excessively reamed, it may be weakened. We ream only enough cortex to allow insertion of the implant. The reason for this is because the host canal is almost always larger than the allograft canal, and if the surgeon attempts to use an implant large enough to obtain a press fit distally, then the allograft will have to be excessively reamed and weakened.

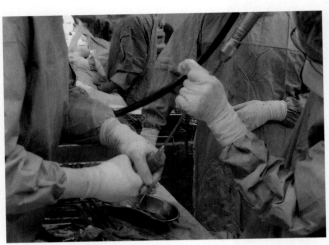

Figure 3. Intraoperative picture of reaming of proximal femoral allograft on a separate table.

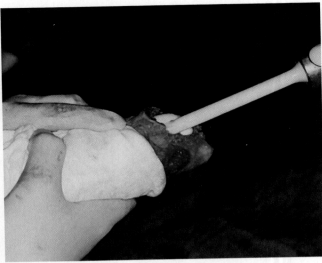

Figure 4. Cement is introduced into the allograft medullary canal. It may be pressurized by occluding the canal distally with a fingertip.

Preparation of the Allograft Prosthetic Composite

The implant that we are presently using is a monobloc type with increasing diameters and two lengths (250 and 300 mm). The stem is not bowed. We most commonly use a 13.5-mm diameter stem, which does not usually give us a press fit distally. Since the implant is cemented into the allograft but not the host, we are dependent on the stability of the graft-host junction to stabilize the construct. Usually, the implant does not obtain a press fit distally because of the relatively large host canal relative to the allograft. To obtain a press fit distally, it would be necessary to use a large-diameter implant, which would necessitate excessive reaming and subsequent weakening of the allograft. This is because, in most situations, the femoral canal of the host revision femur is cavitated and dilated by previous surgery whereas the allograft is normal healthy bone.

Another approach would be to cement the stem both proximally in the allograft and distally into the host. This technique interferes with graft-host union by destressing the graft-host junction and also may lead to graft resorption by destressing the graft (6). Also, by cementing distally, future revision surgery is compromised. A modular femoral implant that has different length bodies that could be cemented into the allograft and large-diameter stems to obtain a press fit in the host would be ideal but is not yet available.

Our technique has been to cement the femoral component into the allograft but not into the host (see Fig. 4). This spares the distal canal for future revisions if necessary. The monobloc stem that we use is smooth with no coating and is small proximally so that the allograft does not have to be broached and weakened. We use straight, rigid reamers to ream the allograft canal and mill the calcar region until the implant can be seated. The host canal only requires gentle reaming since a press fit is not being attempted.

It is necessary to have a stable graft-host junction. We use either a step cut or oblique graft-host osteotomy to obtain stability (see Figs. 5 and 6). An oblique osteotomy is easier and allows adjusting the version without having to make major changes to the osteotomy. The osteotomy should be at least 2 cm in length. Sixteen-gauge stainless steel cerclage wires are used to secure the osteotomy. Any available residual host femur with its soft tissue attachments is also cerclaged around the junction as a vascularized autograft to enhance union (see Figs. 7 and 8). Any autograft bone that is available from reamings, etc., is placed around the junction. If the stability of the junction is not optimal, then a cortical strut allograft is used as a biological plate (see Fig 9). It is stabilized with cerclage wires. A short,

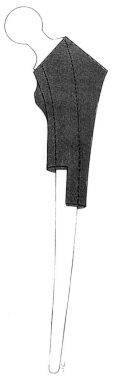

Figure 5. Drawing illustrates femoral implant and proximal femoral allograft. A step cut is used at the junction with host.

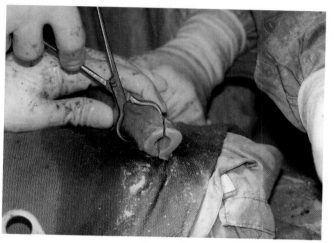

Figure 6. Intraoperative picture to demonstrate cutting an oblique osteotomy in the allograft to stabilize the graft-host junction.

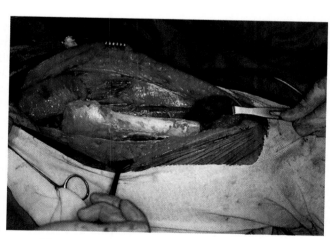

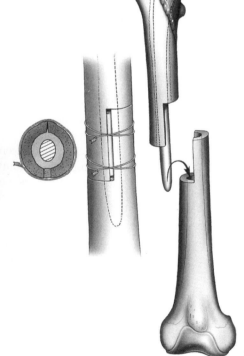

A   B

Figure 7. A: The allograft prosthetic composite (APC) stem is inserted into the host canal but not cemented. **B:** The step cut is stabilized by cerclage wires.

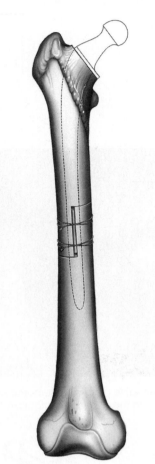

Figure 8. APC after attachment of host greater trochanter and cerclage of graft host junction.

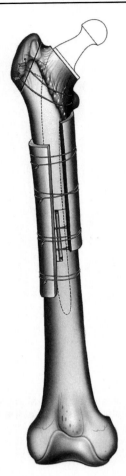

Figure 9. APC after insertion with stabilization by cortical strut allograft.

four- or six-holed plate is another option, but this weakens the allograft with screw holes. If possible, we do not violate the graft with any holes, even for trochanteric attachment. Occasionally, there is enough discrepancy of canal diameter between the graft and the host so that the graft can be telescoped into the host canal for several centimeters, making a step cut or oblique osteotomy unnecessary.

The final determination of the length of the allograft, the fashioning of the step cut or oblique osteotomy, and cementation cannot be done until the acetabular reconstruction has been done and a trial reduction has been performed. This is done initially with the femoral component without the graft (see Fig. 10) and then with the implant in the graft but not cemented. Before cementing the implant into the allograft, the graft is triple washed in half-strength Betadine solution followed by 1% hydrogen peroxide and Bacitracin (50,000 units per liter of saline). We then use the hydrogen peroxide again because it is a drying agent. The graft is then dried with sponges passed through the canal. A cement gun is used, and the cement is pressurized by plugging the canal distally with a finger. The implant is then inserted in the correct version, which has been determined along with the length by a trial reduction. After the implant is seated, the cement is cleaned off the part of the stem that is distal to the allograft using damp sponges and also off the surface of the osteotomy. The graft implant composite is then ready for insertion into the host (see Fig. 11). Additional fine-tuning of length of the graft and version of the osteotomy may be necessary depending on the final trial reductions.

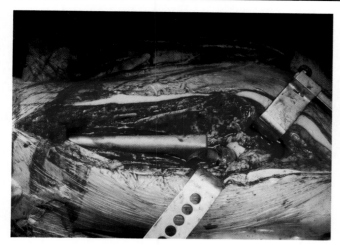

Figure 10. Intraoperative picture showing femoral implant inserted into host femur in order to estimate approximate length of allograft required. The acetabular reconstruction has been completed at this point.

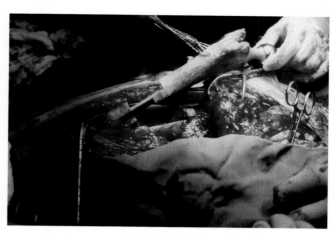

Figure 11. Intraoperative picture of allograft prosthetic composite ready for insertion into host. This was prepared on a separate table.

THE REVISION

The revision is carried out with the patient positioned on their nonoperative side. A straight lateral incision is used, incorporating old scars if possible. We prefer to use a trochanteric slide for exposure (7) (see Fig. 12). Often, the proximal femur is so deficient that the trochanteric fragment is very thin, but it is important to keep it in continuity with the abductors and vastus lateralis. We have modified the trochanteric slide to reduce the incidence of posterior dislocation (8). We leave the posterior capsule and external rotators intact by leaving about 1 cm of posterior greater trochanter attached to the femur.

Site of step cut
or oblique osteotomy

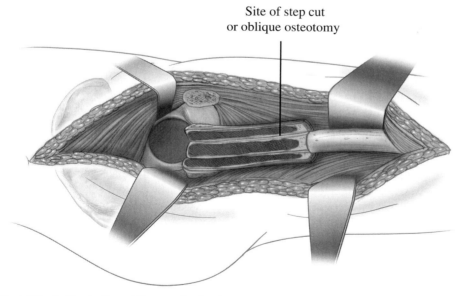

A

Figure 12. A: Illustration of the greater trochanter retracted anteriorly (still attached to the abductors and the vastus) and the femur split in the coronal plane to remove the prosthesis. *(continues)*

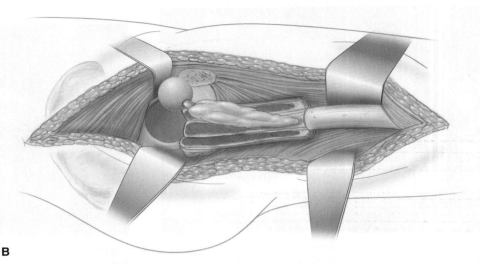

B

Figure 12. *(continued)* **B:** Illustration of how the femoral split is carried down to the level of good host bone. The horizontal cuts extending anteriorly and posteriorly allow the femur to be pried open.

After the trochanteric osteotomy has been completed, the vastus lateralis is reflected off the septum down to the level to which the coronal femoral split is to be carried out. This is determined by preoperative planning and intraoperative visualization of the junction of the deficient femur and healthy host femur. The vastus is only reflected anteriorly enough to do the split, about 1 or 2 cm. The trochanter is retracted anteriorly, and the femur is then split in the coronal plane down to the level of femur that is considered healthy enough to not require replacing by allograft (Fig. 12). The femoral split is easily done by a saw or osteotomes because the proximal femur is so deficient. At the level of healthy femur, transverse cuts are made anteriorly and posteriorly, each extending about a quarter of the way around the femur, leaving the medial half of the femur intact. The deficient femur is then pried open using multiple osteotomes. At the level of the horizontal cut, the medial half of the femur stays intact and can be used as the step cut or oblique osteotomy (Fig. 12). Before the femoral implant is removed, a pin is inserted into the iliac crest, and a fixed point on the host femur is identified and marked with a drill hole. This point must be in the healthy host femur distal to the allograft because it is a reference point for measuring the leg length (see Fig. 13). The deficient femur is then cleaned of residual cement and granulation tissue. Any residual bone in the deficient proximal femur is left with its soft tissue attachments so it can be used as a vascularized bone graft to wrap around the allograft, particularly at the graft-host junction, where it enhances union. The residual host bone proximal to the junction does not replace the allograft, but it may reinforce it by uniting to it. This, however, does not really determine the success of the allograft, and there is usually very little host bone to wrap around the allograft. The host bone that is wrapped around the junction is more important because it enhances union between host and allograft. The host femur distal to the split is gently reamed (see Fig. 14). It is not usually necessary to ream cortex because, using this technique, a press fit for the femoral implant is not attempted or necessary. Any cement or granulation tissue distal to the split is removed, but most often, the split is down to the level beyond which the previous implant did not extend.

At this point, the acetabular revision is performed. Once the acetabular reconstruction is completed and a trial cup is in situ, the length of the allograft can be determined. The femoral implant that best fits the allograft and extends at least 6 cm beyond the host allograft junction is inserted without the allograft into the host canal and reduced into the trial cup (Fig. 10). Using the pin in the crest and the previously placed drill hole in the distal healthy host

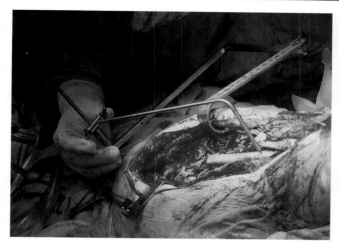

Figure 13. Intraoperative picture showing leg length and offset reference guide. A pin has been inserted into the iliac crest, and there is a mark on the host femur.

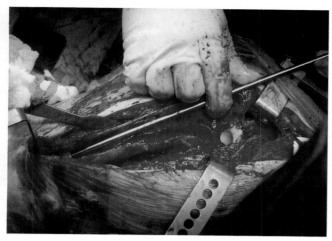

Figure 14. Intraoperative picture showing reaming of distal femur. Note the deficient proximal femur where allograft is to be inserted.

femur, the leg length is estimated, and the length of allograft is determined (Fig. 13). The allograft is then trimmed slightly longer than this length including the step cut or oblique osteotomy, and a trial reduction is performed. Final adjustments of length version and step cut or oblique osteotomy are done, and this usually requires multiple trial reductions (see Fig. 15). When final adjustments are completed, the implant is cemented into the allograft as described above (see Fig. 16). With the implant now cemented into the allograft, fine-tuning, stability adjustment, and length adjustment can still be carried out with regard to version and the osteotomy. When all parameters have been satisfied, the allograft prosthetic composite is inserted and fixed to the host at the junction by cerclage wires (see Fig. 17). All residual host femur is cerclaged to the allograft, particularly at the junction. If the junction is not perfectly stable, a cortical strut is cerclaged to the junction as a biological plate. We prefer a cortical strut because a plate and screws weakens the allograft, but if necessary, a plate is acceptable. Any residual autograft bone (reamings, etc.) is placed around the graft-host junc-

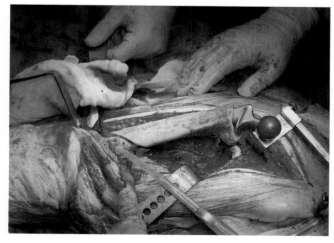

Figure 15. Intraoperative photograph showing trial with femoral implant and allograft before cementing implant into allograft. Final adjustments for length and version are made. Note the oblique cut osteotomy.

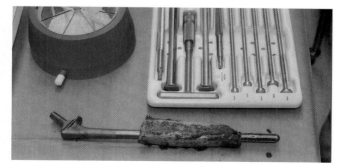

Figure 16. Intraoperative picture showing that the allograft and implant are ready for cementing on a separate table.

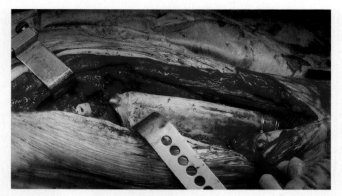

Figure 17. Intraoperative picture showing allograft now in situ with oblique osteotomy fixed with cerclage wires.

tion. The greater trochanter is attached to the allograft with two 16-mm stainless steel cerclage wires. Drill holes in the allograft are avoided if possible by placing the wires distal to the lesser trochanter so they will not migrate proximally. The vastus lateralis is reattached to the septum, and the posterior border of the gluteus medius is reattached to the capsule and external rotators. The rest of the closure is routine.

POSTOPERATIVE CARE

Intravenous antibiotics are started intraoperatively after cultures are taken and continued for 5 days. If the patient is not allergic to penicillin, cefazolin sodium (Ancef) 1 g q8h is given, and if the patient is allergic to penicillin, clindamycin 300 mg IV q6h is used. After the course of intravenous antibiotics 5 days of oral antibiotics are given, cephalexin hydrochloride (Keflex) 500 mg q6h or clindamycin 150 mg q8h. If the patient is catheterized, one dose of 80 mg of gentamycin is administered intravenously, and then trimethoprim and sulfamethoxazole (Septra) double-strength once per day until the catheter is removed. Prophylactic anticoagulation with warfarin sodium (Coumadin) is continued for 3 weeks. The patient is kept on complete bed rest for 3 days and then is kept non–weight bearing until there is radiographic evidence of union of the graft-host junction, usually at between 6 and 10 weeks. No resisted abduction is allowed for 6 weeks (see Fig. 18).

RESULTS

Between April 1984 and December 1989, the author performed 63 proximal femoral allografts in 60 patients for proximal segmental femoral deficiencies of over 5 cm in length (9) (Gross type IV, Paprofsky type IV, and American Academy of Orthopaedic Surgeons type 3) (1–3). The minimum length of allograft was 10 cm. There were 20 men and 40 women with an average age of 62.5 (30.2 to 81.6). An average of 3.8 previous arthroplasties had been performed. The average length of the allograft was 15 cm (10 to 22 cm).

A modified Harris hip score was used for clinical evaluation (10). Clinical success was defined as a postoperative increase in the hip score of greater than 20 points, a radiographically stable implant, and no need for additional surgery related to the allograft.

Radiographs were examined for trochanteric union, allograft-host union, allograft resorption, component loosening, and fracture. Implant stability was evaluated by lucent lines and migration. Definite loosening was defined as migration of the implant of greater than 3 mm or fracture of the cement. Resorption of the allograft was graded as mild (partial thickness <1 cm in length), moderate (partial thickness >1 cm in length), and severe (full thickness of any length). Kaplan-Meier survivorship analysis was performed (11). Failure

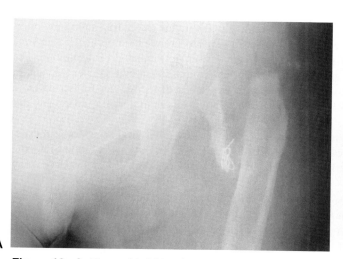
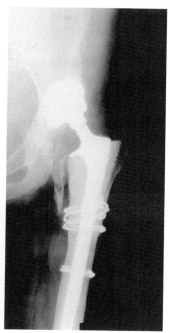

Figure 18. **A:** X-ray of left hip of 50-year-old woman who had undergone an excisional arthroplasty for infection 2 years previously. **B:** X-ray 10 years after reconstruction with a proximal femoral allograft.

was defined as planned or actual removal of the allograft prosthetic construct or severe radiographic resorption.

According to our definition of clinical success (increase in point score of 20 points, stable implant, and no need for additional surgery related to the implant), 14 hips were considered failures (22%). There were five infections, four nonunions, two dislocations requiring a reoperation, and three cases of late aseptic loosening. The success rate of the entire series (including 15 patients who died) was 78% (49 of 63 hips), at an average follow-up of 9 years (2.4 to 15 years). The success rate of those patients still alive at the time of follow-up was 77% (37 of 48 hips), at an average follow-up of 11 years. Of the clinical failures, three nonunions and both dislocations were treated successfully with retention of the allograft. Four of the five infections and two aseptic failures were treated successfully with a new proximal femoral allograft. According to the Kaplan-Meier survivorship analysis, the probability of the construct surviving for 5 years was 90% (95% confidence limits, 80% to 95%), and the probability of the construct surviving for 10 years was 86% (95% confidence limits, 74% to 93%).

Radiographic analysis revealed four nonunions (6%). Three required surgery consisting of cortical struts and autografting, and all eventually united. The fourth nonunion was treated nonoperatively because the patient was elderly and asymptomatic. Trochanteric escape of greater than 1 cm was seen in 14 hips (22%). Many of the hips in this series were done with a transverse trochanteric osteotomy, and we now prefer to do a trochanteric slide to avoid this complication.

In the living patients, allograft resorption was seen in 13 of 48 hips (27%). The resorption was mild in 10 hips (21%), moderate in 2 hips (4%), and severe in 1 hip (2%). The resorption occurred on the periosteal side and in 9 of 13 hips was associated with cerclage wires. There was no endosteal resorption, and there were no cement fractures. No revisions were carried out for graft resorption.

There were three aseptic loosenings, all at the interface of cement and implant. The time to loosening was 9 years, 10 years, and 11 years, and all required revision for symptoms.

CONCLUSIONS

The multiply revised femur with significant segmental bone loss extending into the diaphysis is a challenging problem. The allograft prosthetic composite is a viable solution that provides pain relief, function, and a stable implant and does not compromise the distal host canal, facilitating further revision surgery.

Allograft prosthesis composite is an alternative to the tumor prosthesis, and in my opinion is more appropriate for the revision population. This technique requires access to a bone bank and an experienced surgical team. There are advantages in using this technique. The allograft unites to host bone and allows reattachment of muscle and the greater trochanter. The host medullary canal distal to the allograft is preserved, facilitating further revision surgery if necessary. The host canal is not violated with cement or a porous coat using our technique.

As with any allograft tissue there is always the concern about viral transmission, especially human immunodeficiency virus. Adherence to the American Association of Tissue Banks' standards (12,13) reduces the risk of transmission of human immunodeficiency virus to 1 in 1,667,600.

The proximal femoral allograft has to be of sufficient size to accommodate the implant and the cement mantle without excessive reaming. The implant must be long enough to reach the distal diaphyseal-metaphyseal junction, but a distal press fit is not essential, and distal cementing is not advisable. As distal press fit is not usually obtained, rigid stability of the graft-host junction must be obtained intraoperatively to stabilize the construct. Failure to do so results in nonunion and necessitates more fixation (usually cortical struts) and autografting. We are increasingly using more cortical struts at the initial procedure to enhance stabilization. Long-term stability is obtained when the graft-host junction unites. In this regard, it is also very important to wrap any available vascularized bone around the junction as well as placing any autograft reamings at the host-graft interface.

REFERENCES

1. Saleh KJ, Holtzman J, Gafni A, et al. Reliability and intraoperative validity of preoperative assessment of standardized plain radiographs in predicting bone loss at revision hip surgery. *J Bone Joint Surg Am* 83:1040–1046, 2001.
2. Krishnamurthy AB, MacDonald SJ, Paprosky WG. 5-to-13 year follow-up study on cementless femoral components in revision surgery. *J Arthroplasty* 12(8):839–847, 1997.
3. D'Antonio J, McCarthy JC, Bargar WL, et al. Classification of femoral abnormalities in total hip arthroplasty. *Clin Orthop Relat Res* 296:133–139, 1993.
4. Tomford WM. Disease transmission, sterilization and the clinical use of musculoskeletal tissue allografts. In: WM Tomford. *Musculoskeletal Tissue Banking*. New York, NY: Raven Press, 1993: 209–230.
5. Strong MD, Mackenzie AP. Freeze-drying of tissues. In: WM Tomford. *Musculoskeletal Tissue Banking*. New York, NY: Raven Press, 1993: 181–208.
6. Haddad FS, Garbuz DS, Masri BA, et al. Femoral bone loss in patients managed with revision hip replacement: results of circumferential allograft replacement. *J Bone Joint Surg Am* 81:420–436, 1999.
7. Glassman AH, Engh CA, Bobyn JD. A technique of extensile exposure for total hip arthroplasty. *J Arthroplasty* 2:11–21, 1987.
8. Goodman S, Pressman A, Saastamoinen H, Gross AE. Modified sliding trochanteric osteotomy in revision total hip arthroplasty. *J Arthroplasty* 19(8):1039–1041.
9. Blackley HR, Davis AM, Hutchison CR, Gross AE. Proximal femoral allografts for reconstruction of bone stock in revision arthroplasty of the hip. *J Bone Joint Surg Am* 83(3):346–354, 2001.
10. Gross AE, Hutchison CR, Alexeeff M, et al. Proximal femoral allografts for reconstruction of bone stock in revision arthroplasty of the hip. *Clin Orthop Relat Res* 319:151–158, 1995.
11. Kaplan EL, Meier P. Nonparametric estimation from incomplete observations. *J Am Stat Assoc* 53:457–481, 1958.
12. Jacobs NJ. Establishing a surgical bone bank. In: Fawcett KJ, Barr HR, eds. *Tissue Banking*. Arlington, Va: American Association of Blood Banks, 1987: 67–96.
13. Buck BE, Resnick L, Shah SM, Malinin TI. Human immunodeficiency virus cultured from bone. Implications for transplantation. *Clin Orthop Relat Res* 251:249–253, 1990.

28

Megaprosthesis: Proximal Femoral and Total Femoral Replacement

Javad Parvizi and Franklin H. Sim

During the past decade, remarkable advances in the field of revision hip reconstruction have been made. One such improvement has been the introduction of second-generation modular prosthetic components (see Fig. 1A) that allow better ability to restore limb length and achieve optimal soft-tissue tension, which may reduce the incidence of instability that frequently occurs following insertion of a monolithic megaprosthesis (Fig. 1B). The new generation of megaprosthesis also provides a better environment for soft tissue reattachment and the ability to reapproximate the retained host bone to the prosthesis. However, with current improvements in alternative reconstruction methods and increased use of cortical strut grafts to augment host bone, the indications for the use of the megaprosthesis have narrowed.

INDICATIONS

We currently reserve the use of the megaprosthesis (proximal femoral replacement and total femur replacement) to expedite recovery for elderly or sedentary patients with massive bone loss that may have occurred after failed total hip arthroplasty (see Fig. 2), deep infection, periprosthetic fracture (see Fig. 3), fracture nonunion with failed multiple attempts at osteosynthesis, and hip salvage after a failed resection arthroplasty. In younger patients in whom bone loss of high magnitude is encountered that cannot be reconstructed by conventional means, an allograft prosthetic composite would be preferred over femoral prosthetic replacement. An important prerequisite for the use of prosthetic femoral replacement and allograft prosthetic composite is the availability of sufficient distal femoral length (>10 cm) for secure fixation of the cemented or uncemented femoral stem. When distal bone is severely deficient, consideration may be given to total femoral replacement.

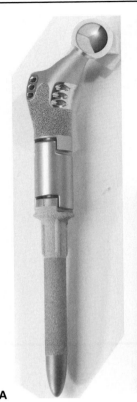

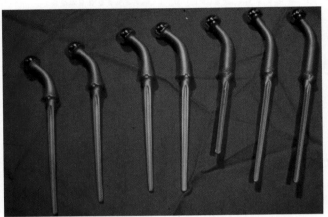

Figure 1. A: New generation of modular proximal femoral replacement prostheses. **B:** First-generation segmental replacement prostheses in various sizes.

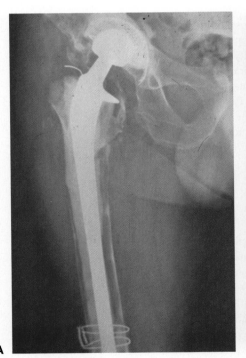

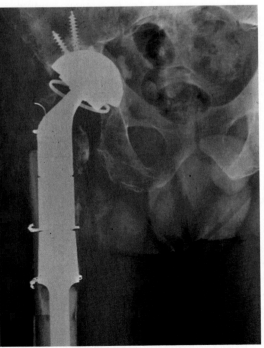

Figure 2. Anteroposterior radiograph of a patient with multiple previous surgeries for deep infection that had resulted in massive proximal femoral bone loss **(A)** that necessitated the use of a megaprosthesis for reconstruction **(B)**.

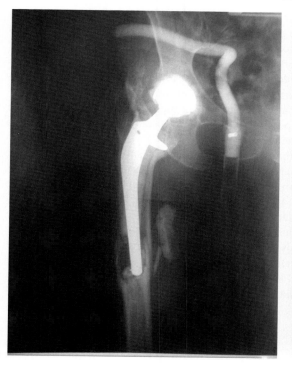
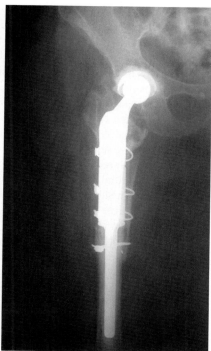

Figure 3. A: Seventy-two-year-old patient presenting with periprosthetic fracture. **B:** Because of severe bone loss, reconstruction with a megaprosthesis was carried out.

CONTRAINDICATIONS

The presence of superficial or deep infection around the hip is considered an absolute contraindication for insertion of a megaprosthesis. In addition, an uncooperative patient, vascular insufficiency that may prevent healing, and the presence of significant medical comorbidities precluding administration of anesthesia also are considered additional contraindications.

PREOPERATIVE PLANNING

The importance of preoperative planning in hip arthroplasty in general and in megaprosthesis reconstruction in particular cannot be overstated. These cases can be technically demanding, requiring meticulous attention to detail to achieve success.

Most patients undergoing megaprosthesis reconstruction have had multiple previous procedures. Therefore, it is imperative to examine the incision site carefully for the presence of skin lesions that may predispose to infection and to determine the appropriate previous scar to be used. A new incision may occasionally have to be used if the previous scars are inappropriately placed to access the hip. On occasion, involvement of plastic surgeons may be necessary to evaluate the status of the soft tissue in case local or free flap may be required for reconstruction. Thorough examination of the hip with particular attention to the status of the abductors and the limb length should be carried out. Preoperative clinical and radiographic (standing films) assessment of the limb length is carried out and recorded. Patients should be counseled about the possibility of limb length discrepancy that may result from surgery. In our opinion, lengthening of the limb up to 4 cm can be carried out safely. Any lengthening beyond this point is likely to place the neurovascular structures at risk. Intraoperative monitoring of the sciatic and femoral nerves may need to be performed in patients in whom extensive (>4 cm) limb lengthening is anticipated.

All patients (other than those undergoing tumor resection) needing a megaprosthesis have undergone multiple previous surgeries of the hip. We always order a white blood cell count with differential, C-reactive protein, and erythrocyte sedimentation rate to rule out infection. On the basis of clinical and radiographic examinations and the result of serology, hips with a high index of suspicion are also preoperatively aspirated to rule out deep infection. All patients should also receive a thorough medical examination with appropriate laboratory investigation. Revision hip arthroplasty with a megaprosthesis with extensive soft-tissue dissection, usually long operative time, and large volume of blood loss places immense physiological demand on the patient.

Preoperative templating to select the appropriate stem length and diameter is essential. Problems with removal of existing hardware, specific needs for acetabular reconstruction and the potential need for insertion of constrained liners, and ensuring the absence of prior infection should be anticipated and addressed appropriately. Despite the most accurate preoperative measurements, a variety of prosthesis sizes should be available in the operating room as intraoperative adjustments with change in anticipated size of prosthesis are common. The megaprosthesis manufacturing company representative should be contacted to be present in the operating room. Experienced operating room personnel, particularly the scrub person, should assist with this procedure. An experienced anesthesia team should administer anesthesia, as invasive monitoring in these often elderly and frail patients is warranted.

SURGICAL TECHNIQUE

Anesthesia and Patient Positioning

Regional anesthesia is preferred in these patients. Intraoperative blood salvage (cell saver) should be used in these patients. The anesthesia team should be warned about possible large volume loss and encouraged to monitor this closely. Invasive monitoring with the use of arterial lines or pulmonary catheters may be necessary in some patients. We place the patient in lateral decubitus position and use hip rests to secure the patient (see Fig. 4). Nonpermeable U-drapes are used to isolate the groin. The distal one third of the extremity is also isolated from the field using impermeable drapes. It is very important to include the knee in the operative field on all of these patients—even in those undergoing proximal femoral replacement. Extension of the incision and arthrotomy of the knee to address intraoperative problems such as fractures extending distally is not uncommon.

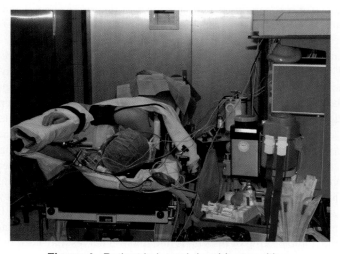

Figure 4. Patient in lateral decubitus position.

The skin is scrubbed with Betadine solution for at least 10 min, and Duraprep is applied prior to application of Ioband to the skin.

Surgical Approach

We use the direct lateral approach (Hardinge) or the posterolateral approach with trochanteric slide to gain access to the hip and maintain a low threshold to extend the incision as needed (see Fig. 5). When extensile exposure of the femur is needed, a vastus slide as described by Head et al. (1) mobilizes the anterior abductors, vastus lateralis, and vastus intermedius muscles anteriorly in unison and exposes the anterior and lateral aspects of the femur (see Fig. 6). Meticulous soft-tissue handling helps the tissues to heal and minimizes postoperative complications. Deep tissue specimens for frozen section and culture are obtained in all cases. Meticulous debridement of the hip is carried out to remove previous metal debris and hardware around the femur, if present.

Femoral Reconstruction

Proximal Femoral Replacement. If intact, an osteotomy to split the proximal femur may be required in order to facilitate the removal of the previous prosthesis and/or hardware. A transverse osteotomy is first made in the host bone at the most proximal area of circumferential adequate quality bone. Because the outcome of this procedure is influenced directly by the length of the remaining femur, maximum length of the native femur is maintained at all costs (2). We then prefer a longitudinal Wagner type of coronal plane osteotomy to split the proximal femur with poor bone quality. Soft-tissue attachments to the proximal femur, particularly the abductor mechanism, if present, should be retained if at all possible. Once the femur is exposed, the distal portion of the canal is prepared by successive broaching. Preserve the cancellous bone, when present, for better cement interdigitation. After completion of femoral preparation and determination of the size of best fit broach, trial components are inserted, and the stability of the hip is examined. A distal cement restrictor is used whenever possible. The restrictor is introduced and advanced distally to allow for at least 2 cm of bone cement at the tip of the stem. The cement is pressurized, and the final component is implanted, ensuring that the porous coated portion of the stem is placed directly and firmly against diaphyseal bone with no interpositioning cement. Either the prosthesis can be assembled and then cemented distally or the stem can be cemented and then the body can be assembled onto it. In any case, extreme care needs to be exercised to prevent rotational malpositioning (see Fig. 7). To mark the rotation, we use a sharp osteotome to scratch the distal femoral cortex once the trial component is appropriately positioned. The rotation of the component cannot be changed once the distal stem is cemented in place.

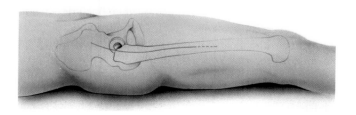

Figure 5. Diagram showing the placement of incision.

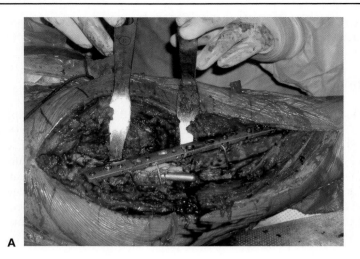

A

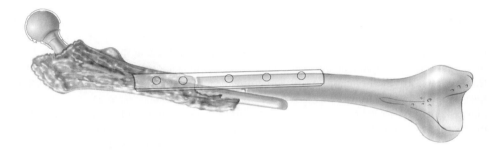

B

Figure 6. A: Intraoperative picture showing exposure of femur in a patient who has sustained periprosthetic fracture. **B:** Diagram of the same picture.

Total Femur Replacement. The indication for total femoral replacement is rare and generally includes inadequate length (<10 cm) or poor quality of distal femoral bone for fixation of a femoral stem (see Fig. 8). In the majority of cases, adequate length and quality of distal femur can be retained to allow secure fixation. Total femoral replacement includes an arthrotomy of the knee to allow prosthetic replacement of the knee. Once exposure of the femur using a lateral vastus reflecting approach is completed (Fig. 8), then the entire femur is split longitudinally in the coronal plain. Again, despite what may be extremely poor quality, as much of the bone with its soft-tissue attachment is retained as possible. The subvastus approach is extended to include a lateral or a medial arthrotomy of the knee and eversion of the patella. The amount of tibial bone resected is kept to a minimum but should be of adequate thickness to allow implantation of the components and insertion of polyethylene without elevating the joint line. Preparation of the tibia is carried out in the same manner as for total knee arthroplasty. Once the appropriate tibial component size is determined, preparation of the tibia followed by insertion of the trial component is carried out. A full-length trial femur is assembled, ensuring that appropriate limb length is restored. Unless constrained liners are to be used, we prefer to use a large femoral head size to improve arc of motion and minimize instability. The thickness of the tibial

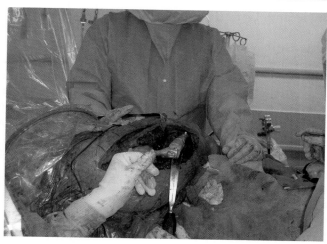

Figure 7. Intraoperative picture demonstrating how the rotational positioning/version of the femoral component is determined. The version of the femoral stem is judged by appropriate positioning of the knee.

polyethylene is usually between 15 and 20 mm but may have to be adjusted to obtain appropriate length of the extremity and restore the joint line.

A linked, articulated knee design is necessary because of loss of the stabilizing ligamentous structures. Once the prosthesis is assembled, a trial reduction is carried out and tested for stability. We usually do not resurface the patella unless severe wear of the articular cartilage is noted.

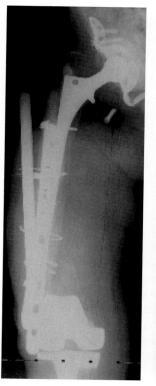
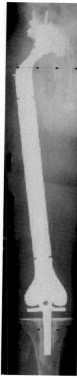
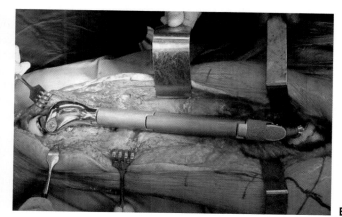

B

A,C

Figure 8. A: Preoperative radiograph of a 78-year-old patient with failed hip arthroplasty who has a knee arthroplasty in place. **B:** Distal femoral bone length and quality were deemed too poor for femoral stem fixation. **C:** Total femoral replacement was performed in this patient.

Determination of Limb Length

The length of the femoral component is determined through careful preoperative planning and intraoperative assessment. Two methods may be used for proper leg length determination. The first method is to apply traction to the limb with measurement from the cup to the host bone osteotomy site (for the proximal femoral replacement cases). The second and preferred method is to place a Steinmann pin in the iliac crest to measure a fixed point on the femur before dislocation. With the long-stem trial prosthesis in place, proper leg length can be accurately restored. For patients with total femur replacement, radiographs of the opposite and normal femur may be obtained preoperatively and used for accurate templating for length. The length of the prosthesis usually equals the length of the bone being resected, although in many of these patients, the integrity of the bone has been breached and the anatomy has been markedly altered. Ultimately, the femoral prosthesis length depends on the soft-tissue tension about the hip. Balancing tension, restoring limb length, and avoiding excessive tension on the sciatic nerve are of utmost importance if complications are to be avoided.

Acetabular Reconstruction

The acetabulum is exposed at the beginning of the operation and examined carefully. If a previous acetabular component is in place, the stability and positioning of the component is scrutinized. If the component is appropriately placed and stable, it is left in place, and the liner is exchanged. If a previous acetabular component is not in place, a new component is inserted in a press-fit manner with screw fixation. More complex acetabular reconstruction such as the use of an antiprotrusio cage occasionally may be needed. The type of acetabular liner is determined after completion of reconstruction of the femur, because constrained liners may have to be utilized in patients with poor soft-tissue tension and a high probability of instability. If instability is of concern, a constrained liner is used. The constrained liner may be cemented into a well-fixed acetabular shell. In these cases, the shell should be scored with a burr, grooves should be made on the back of the liner, and a liner that is sufficiently small as to allow for 1 to 2 mm of cement mantle should be selected.

The constrained liners can be inserted either snap-fit or cemented into the shell, depending on the type of the acetabular component implanted. In our experience, constrained liners are required in approximately one half of patients receiving a megaprosthesis. Our absolute indication for the use of a constrained liner is for patients with properly positioned components and equal or near-equal leg length who have intraoperative instability secondary to soft-tissue deficiency.

Closure

The femur, however poor in quality, is maintained and wrapped around the megaprosthesis at the conclusion of implantation. The muscle-tendon attachments are preserved whenever possible. The soft tissues and, in particular, the abductors, if present, are meticulously secured to the prosthesis (see Fig. 9). Multiple loops of nonabsorbable sutures are passed around the trochanter remnant and the attached soft tissue. The leg is brought to abduction, and the trochanter is firmly fixed onto the proximal portion of the prosthesis by passing the sutures through the holes in the prosthesis or around the proximal body and the deep tissues. We occasionally suture the abductors to the vastus lateralis, the tensor fascia lata, or the host greater trochanter, if available (Fig. 6). Two surgical drains are inserted before closure of the wound in layers using interrupted resorbable sutures. Meticulous skin closure, with excision of hypertrophic prior scar, if necessary, is carried out to minimize postoperative wound drainage.

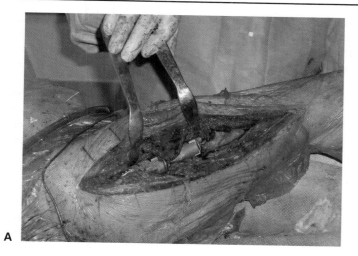

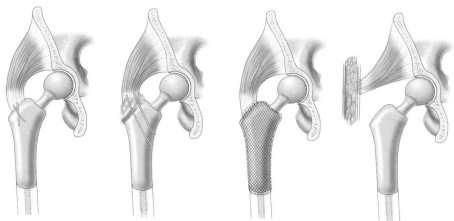

Figure 9. A: Intraoperative picture demonstrating soft-tissue closure around the femoral stem. Proximal bone and soft tissue, however poor in quality, need to be reapproximated to the stem as meticulously as possible. **B:** Various methods of soft-tissue reapproximation to the femoral stem.

POSTOPERATIVE MANAGEMENT

Intravenous prophylactic antibiotics are given and maintained until final cultures are obtained. Thromboembolic prophylaxis for 6 weeks is also administered. Patients are allowed to commence protective weight bearing on postoperative day 1. We recommend the use of abduction orthosis for all patients and protective weight bearing for 12 weeks until adequate soft-tissue healing occurs. Patients are usually able to ambulate with the use of a walking aid during this time. Patients receiving total femur replacement may require continuous passive motion machines for rehabilitation of the knee replacement. Daily physical therapy for assistance with ambulation and range of motion exercise for the knee are recommended.

RESULTS

Our early experience with the use of a megaprosthesis after tumor resection was encouraging. Therefore, we began using prosthetic femoral replacement in patients with failed hip prosthesis and severe bone loss for whom the only viable option was resection arthroplasty. Our initial review revealed that the mode of failure of the megaprosthesis is similar in patients with or without neoplastic conditions. We were unable to detect any significant difference in the outcome of the megaprosthesis with respect to failure, incidence of radiographic lucency, limp, pain relief, or the use of walking aids in these two groups.

The initial use of a megaprosthesis for reconstruction of the proximal femur in nonneoplastic conditions at our institution first was reported in 1981 (3). Although all 21 patients had significant pain relief, there were two failures. One patient required acetabular component revision, and the second patient needed revision of the femoral component for recurrent instability.

Another retrospective study reported the outcome of 50 revision hip arthroplasties using prosthetic femoral replacement in 49 patients with nonneoplastic conditions (2). All patients had massive proximal bone loss, and some patients had multiple failed attempts with other reconstructive procedures. The mean follow-up was 11 years. The mean preoperative Harris hip scores of 43 ± 13 points improved significantly to 80 ± 10 points at 1 year and improved to 76 ± 16 points at the latest follow-up. Before surgery, 86% of the patients had moderate to severe pain. Pain relief was achieved in 88% of patients at 1 year and 73% of patients at the latest follow-up. There was significant improvement in gait and the ability to ambulate. However, there was some deterioration in all parameters with time.

Detailed radiographic analysis revealed an increase in the incidence of progressive radiolucent lines on the femoral and acetabular sides. Progressive radiolucency was seen around 37% of the acetabular components and 30% of the femoral components. Aseptic loosening constituted the main reason for revision surgery. Using revision as an end point, overall survivorship in the aforementioned series was 64% at 12 years. The most common complication was dislocation, with an overall rate of 22%.

The results of 11 patients undergoing total femur replacement at Mayo Clinic were recently evaluated. Six of these patients had total femur reconstructions performed for multiple failed ipsilateral total knee arthroplasty and total hip arthroplasty. Five patients underwent total femur replacement as limb salvage for musculoskeletal malignancy, four of whom had pathologic fractures. Of the six patients who had total femoral replacement for failed arthroplasties, hip instability in two necessitated conversion to a constrained acetabular liner. Of two patients with prior infections, one developed recurrent infection despite staged total femoral reimplantation, and one has an elevated sedimentation rate on chronic antibiotic suppression but no evidence of clinical infection. All patients ambulated with either a walker or a cane. Of the five patients who had total femoral replacement for treatment of tumor, one developed hip and knee pain within 3 years, had wear of the knee hinge bushings, and is seeking disability. One patient developed wound dehiscence and sepsis in the postoperative period and expired. Two patients ambulate with a cane, and three ambulate without the routine use of any gait aids.

COMPLICATIONS

The major complications encountered following the use of a megaprosthesis are early dislocation and aseptic loosening. The etiology of instability in this group of patients is multifactorial. First, these patients often have had multiple previous reconstructive procedures that have led to compromised abductors around the hip. Furthermore, the inability to achieve a secure repair of the residual soft tissues to the metal prosthesis predisposes these patients to instability (4). The problem is additionally exacerbated in patients in whom the proper leg length and appropriate soft-tissue tension are not achieved.

We have implemented changes in our practice to minimize instability. These include the use of constrained cups in selective cases, routine use of a postoperative abduction brace, and augmentation of the proximal bone with the use of a strut allograft that imparts more rigidity for soft-tissue attachment. It is conceivable that the problem of soft tissue to metal attachment may be better addressed in the future with the use of trabecular metals such as tantalum, with its excellent potential for soft-tissue ongrowth.

The other common complication of megaprosthesis reconstruction is the relatively high incidence of acetabular and femoral radiolucency in most reported studies. The reason for this complication lies in the biomechanical aspect of this reconstructive procedure. The diaphyseal cement fixation predisposes the bone-cement prosthesis to high torsional and compressive stresses, leading to early loosening. Cemented long-stem revision implants are known to have limited success and currently are recommended for elderly and sedentary patients (5). As would be expected, the incidence of radiolucency after the use of press-fit or proximally or extensively coated ingrowth stems is, in comparison with megaprosthesis, markedly less (6,7).

The incidence of radiolucency after megaprosthesis reconstruction at our institution has declined somewhat in latter years. This may be caused by using improved cementing techniques, namely using pulse lavage and plugging of the canal for better cement interdigitation. However, the more likely reason for the reduction in the incidence of radiolucency is that we have narrowed the indications for the use of megaprosthesis to elderly and sedentary patients who place lower demands on the prosthesis.

Conclusions

Despite all of the aforementioned concerns, the megaprosthesis is valuable in the armamentarium of the reconstructive hip surgeon who treats patients with extensive bone loss, for whom other available reconstructive procedures cannot be utilized. This prosthesis will have an unacceptably high failure rate in the younger patients, and other reconstructive options should be exploited.

SURGICAL PEARLS

- Examine patients thoroughly. Note various previous scars, status of abductors, and limb length.
- Communicate with the patient, and help make their expectations realistic.
- Perform detailed preoperative templating. Have the company representative available to review your templating and to ensure that correct components, and neighboring sizes, are available on the day of surgery.
- Ensure that thorough medical optimization of the patient has been carried out.
- Ask for an experienced scrub and anesthetic team.
- Minimize soft-tissue dissection off the native bone, and retain as much of the host bone as possible.
- Restore appropriate leg length and soft-tissue tension.
- Have a low threshold for the use of constrained liners.
- Ensure good hemostasis, and perform a meticulous wound closure.

RECOMMENDED READING

1. Head WC, Mallory TH, Berklacich FM, et al. Extensile exposure of the hip for revision arthroplasty. *J Arthroplasty* 2:265–273, 1987.
2. Malkani A, Settecerri JJ, Sim FH, et al. Long-term results of proximal femoral replacement for non-neoplastic disorders. *J Bone Joint Surg Br* 77:351–356, 1995.
3. Sim FH, Chao EYS. Segmental prosthetic replacement of the hip and knee. In: Chao EYS, Ivins JC, eds. *Tumor Prostheses for Bone and Joint Reconstruction: The Design and Application.* New York: Thieme Medical Publishers, 1983: 247–266.
4. Gottasauner-Wolf F, Egger EL, Schultz FM, et al. Tendons attached to prostheses by tendon-bone block fixation: an experimental study in dogs. *J Orthop Res* 12:814–821, 1994.
5. Mulroy WF, Harris WH. Revision total hip arthroplasty with the use of so-called second-generation cementing techniques for aseptic loosening of the femoral component: a fifteen-year average follow-up study. *J Bone Joint Surg Am* 78:325–330, 1996.
6. Berry DJ, Harmsen WS, Ilstrup D, et al. Survivorship of uncemented proximally porous-coated femoral components. *Clin Orthop Relat Res* 319:168–177, 1995.
7. Paprosky WG. Distal fixation with fully coated stems in femoral revision: a 16-year follow-up. *Orthopedics* 21:993–995, 1998.

8. Berry DL, Chandler HP, Reilly DT. The use of bone allografts in two-stage reconstruction of failed hip replacements due to infection. *J Bone Joint Surg Am* 73:1460–1468, 1991.

9. Callahan JJ, Salvati EA, Pellici PM, et al. Result of revision for mechanical failure after cemented total hip replacement, 1979 to 1982. *J Bone Joint Surg Am* 67:1074–1085, 1985.

10. Chandler HP, Clark J, Murphy S, et al. Reconstruction of major segmental loss of the proximal femur in revision total hip arthroplasty. *Clin Orthop Relat Res* 298:67–74, 1994.

11. Donati D, Zavatta M, Gozzi E, et al. Modular prosthetic replacement of the proximal femur resection of a bone tumor. *J Bone Joint Surg Br* 83:1156–1160, 2001.

12. Emerson RH, Malinin TI, Cuellar AD, et al. Cortical strut allografts in the reconstruction of the femur in revision total hip arthroplasty: a basic science and clinical study. *Clin Orthop Relat Res* 285:35–44, 1992.

13. Gie GA, Linder L, Ling RS, et al. Impacted cancellous allografts and cement for revision total hip arthroplasty. *J Bone Joint Surg Br* 75:14–21, 1993.

14. Giurea A, Paternostro T, Heinz-Peer G, et al. Function of reinserted abductor muscles after femoral replacement. *J Bone Joint Surg Br* 80:284–287, 1998.

15. Gross AE, Hutchinson CR. Proximal femoral allografts for reconstruction of bone stock in revision arthroplasty of the hip. *Orthop Clin North Am* 29:313–317, 1998.

16. Haentjens P, De Boeck H, Opdecam P. Proximal femoral replacement prosthesis for salvage of failed hip arthroplasty: complications in 2–11 year follow-up study in 19 elderly patients. *Acta Orthop Scand* 67:37–42, 1996.

17. Johnsson R, Carlsson A, Kisch K, et al. Function following mega total hip arthroplasty compared with conventional total hip arthroplasty and healthy matched controls. *Clin Orthop Relat Res* 192:159–167, 1985.

18. Kantor GS, Osterkamp JA, Dorr LD, et al. Resection arthroplasty following infected total hip replacement arthroplasty. *J Arthroplasty* 1:83–89, 1986.

19. Morrey BF. Bone deficiency in reconstruction surgery of the joints. In: Morrey BF, ed. *Joint Replacement Arthroplasty*. 2nd ed. New York: Churchill Livingstone, 1996: 1569–1586.

20. Morris HG, Capanna R, Del Ben M, Campanacci D. Prosthetic reconstruction of the proximal femur after resection for bone tumors. *J Arthroplasty* 10:293–299, 1995.

21. Roberson JR. Proximal femoral bone loss after total hip arthroplasty. *Orthop Clin North Am* 23:291–302, 1992.

22. Ross AC, Tuite JD, Kemp HBS, Scales JT. Massive prosthetic replacement for non-neoplastic disorders. *J Bone Joint Surg Br* 77:351–356, 1995.

23. Rubash HE, Sinha RK, Shanbhag AS, Kim S. Pathogenesis of bone loss after total hip arthroplasty. *Orthop Clin North Am* 29:173–186, 1998.

24. Sim FH, Chao EYS. Hip salvage by proximal femoral replacement. *J Bone Joint Surg Am* 63:1228–1239, 1981.

25. Xenos JS, Hopkinson WJ, Callahan JJ, et al. Osteolysis around an uncemented cobalt chrome total hip arthroplasty. *Clin Orthop Relat Res* 317:29–36, 1995.

26. Zehr RJ, Enneking WF, Scarborough MT. Allograft-prosthesis composite versus megaprosthesis in proximal femoral reconstruction. *Clin Orthop Relat Res* 322:207–223, 1996.

29

Cementless Acetabular Revision

R. Michael Meneghini, David G. Lewallen,
and Arlen D. Hanssen

INDICATIONS/CONTRAINDICATIONS

Acetabular revision is often challenging because of the extreme variation in bone quality and magnitude of bone deficiency. Uncemented hemispherical cups are extremely versatile and may be used for the vast majority (>90% to 95%) of acetabular revisions with a high success rate.

The primary indications for acetabular revision include aseptic mechanical loosening, hip instability due to component malposition, and periprosthetic osteolysis associated with wear debris. An additional indication for revision total hip arthroplasty, albeit in a staged manner, is periprosthetic infection necessitating removal and reimplantation of implants. *Relative* contraindications to acetabular revision with a hemispherical revision shell include acetabular osteonecrosis due to radiation exposure, pelvic discontinuity, and severe global acetabular bone loss precluding adequate apposition of the hemispherical implant to viable host bone. However, it should be emphasized that these contraindications are relative, and many clinical situations exist, such as in pelvic discontinuity, where a hemispherical implant may be used with success. Clinical success is achieved in conjunction with modalities to augment component stability, such as plating the posterior column in pelvic discontinuity.

Inherent in these indications and contraindications are the requisites for success with a cementless hemispherical acetabular implant in the revision setting. These requirements include an adequate amount of viable host bone contact to provide sufficient mechanical stability and the appropriate biological conditions to allow bone ingrowth and long-term clinical success.

PREOPERATIVE PLANNING

Serial radiographs are helpful to assess component migration and osteolysis progression. The anteroposterior (AP) hip radiograph is used to more closely evaluate the periacetabular bone for osteolysis, as well as critically assess the femoral component for radiographic signs of aseptic loosening or osteolysis. The cross-table lateral radiograph provides valuable information on the degree of posterior osteolysis in the ischium, as well as an approximation of acetabular component version. In addition, the AP dimension of the remaining acetabular bone stock can be assessed if a jumbo cup is considered. Finally, if pelvic discontinuity is suspected, because of acetabular component position medial to Kohler's line or excessive teardrop osteolysis, Judet views are warranted and provide valuable information regarding the integrity of the posterior column. A computed tomography scan is rarely needed unless adequate plain film radiographs are unobtainable or questions persist regarding the integrity and location of the remaining host periacetabular bone.

The assessment of mechanical integrity by radiographic evaluation of the ischium, teardrop, medial wall, Kohler's line, and superior bone for osteolysis and bone loss is critical. Medial wall and teardrop osteolysis is indicative of medial wall and anterior column deficiency. Radiographic ischial lysis represents a potential deficiency in the posterior column, which may necessitate adjunctive means of fixation to support a cementless hemispherical cup. Superior migration and osteolysis, if directly superior, suggest a contained defect with an intact supporting rim. In contrast, superior and lateral migration may represent a segmental defect requiring structural support in conjunction with a hemispherical cup. An accurate assessment and knowledge of the patterns of bone deficiency combined with a familiarity with the appropriate methods of acetabular reconstruction are essential in preoperative planning to enact clinical success in the revision acetabulum.

Once the decision to perform acetabular revision surgery is made, a surgical plan is developed on the basis of the details of the clinical and radiographic pathology. The appropriate surgical approach is chosen on the basis of issues such as access to particular acetabular regions, abductor muscle integrity, any preexisting instability, and surgeon preference. If the acetabular component is being removed for malposition or infection and is deemed well fixed, the explant instrumentation should be available in the operating room to facilitate component removal with preservation of acetabular bone stock. If large cavitary or segmental defects are anticipated, bulk and particulate allograft, as well as newly available modular acetabular wedges and cages, should be available to the operating surgeon. The femoral implant is evaluated for any signs of loosening and, if deemed well fixed, should be assessed for neck length and taper to obtain modular femoral heads of various sizes with matching tapers. Whenever possible, the hemispherical cup should be the first implant of choice, with use of alternatives reserved for situations where a hemispherical cup is deemed unsatisfactory.

SURGERY

Surgical Approach and Exposure

The surgical exposure for acetabular component revision is determined by a combination of surgeon preference and the particular surgical demands imparted by the specific anatomical and functional circumstances encountered in the surgery. The majority of hip revision surgery can be accomplished successfully through a posterior, anterolateral, or direct lateral approach. If an isolated acetabular revision is anticipated, with retention of a well-fixed femoral component, a more extensile approach may be necessary to facilitate exposure of the acetabulum. A thorough capsular debridement is performed, emphasizing the creation of a capsular rent or pocket, which allows the neck of the retained femoral component to be retracted posteriorly or anteriorly, depending on the selected surgical approach. If both components are to be revised, acetabular exposure can be facilitated by one of the extensile techniques, such as an extended trochanteric or transfemoral osteotomy, utilized in the setting of complex femoral revision. In addition, a transtrochanteric approach may be beneficial in the setting of hip instability due to inadequate soft tissue tension, as it allows trochanteric advancement and subsequent tensioning of the abductor mechanism.

Regardless of the surgical approach utilized, it is critical to have unobstructed access to the entire acetabular rim. In addition, the posterior and anterior columns should be readily accessible, as well as the origins of the ilium, ischium, and pubis. Failure to adequately visualize the anatomic deficiencies and accurately ascertain the location and quality of viable host bone could result in inadequate implant stability and subsequent clinical failure. Finally, intraoperative evaluation for infection is essential and entails tissue sent for frozen section pathological evaluation, as well as culture and sensitivities.

Procedure

Removal of loose acetabular components (see Fig. 1) is relatively straightforward once adequate acetabular exposure has been obtained. The surgeon should clearly identify the interface between implant and bone and utilize a variety of curved osteotomes to facilitate complete separation of the implant from surrounding bone. However, the surgeon should be extremely careful when removing the acetabular component to protect the surrounding bone and soft tissues to prevent further inadvertent bone loss or destruction, especially in the setting of osteolysis, where bone quality is typically less than optimal.

Removal of well-fixed cementless acetabular components (for instability or infection) has been greatly facilitated by the Explant system (Zimmer, Warsaw, IN), a system of curved osteotomes attached to a central femoral head that inserts into the native polyethylene liner or trial liner. The femoral head is located a distance from the osteotome blade that corresponds to the outer shell diameter. As the osteotome is rotated circumferentially around the centered femoral head within the acetabular liner, the bone-implant interface is separated in a manner that preserves the majority of surrounding bone. This system facilitates removal of well-fixed acetabular components with minimal bone loss (1).

Once the acetabular component has been safely removed, a meticulous debridement of the acetabulum is performed, removing all fibrous membrane and interposed soft tissue (see Figs. 2 and 3). The acetabular bone deficiency is now classified. An assessment of the quality and location of viable host bone that will support an acetabular component is performed, which will ultimately determine the type of acetabular reconstruction that is chosen. The acetabular rim is examined for segmental loss and structural integrity. The location and severity of cavitary lesions are noted, and the integrity of the anterior and

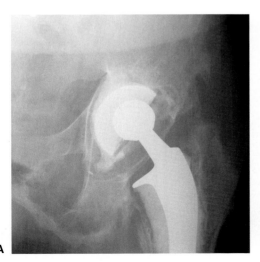 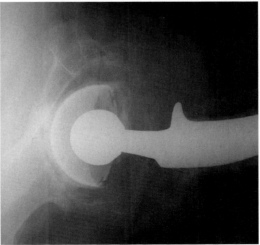

A   B

Figure 1. (A) AP and **(B)** lateral radiographs of a loose, cemented acetabular component.

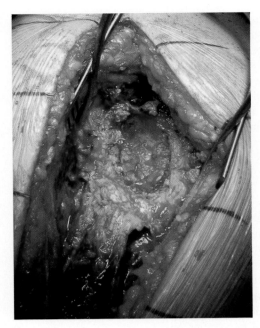

Figure 2. Complete exposure of the acetabulum depicted in Figure 1 through a transfemoral approach.

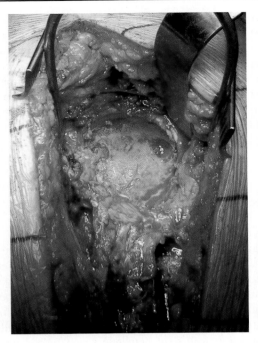

Figure 3. Exposure of acetabulum after thorough debridement of fibrous tissue, demonstrating an intact peripheral rim and only small cavitary medial defects.

posterior columns is carefully assessed. The medial wall is carefully palpated to ascertain any deficiency and subsequent need for particulate graft. This thorough acetabular exposure and careful evaluation provides the surgeon with an overall assessment of the ability to insert a hemispherical acetabular component with the required host bone apposition necessary for mechanical stability. The majority of acetabular component revisions are successfully performed using an uncemented hemispherical acetabular component with cancellous bone grafting of residual defects. The two most commonly used uncemented, hemispherical acetabular revision cups are a titanium, porous coated implant and a recently developed, acetabular implant of porous tantalum material, termed Trabecular Metal (Zimmer, Warsaw, IN) (see Fig. 4).

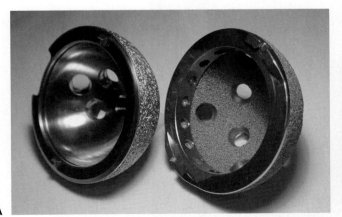

A

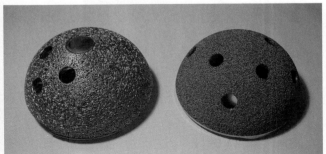

B

Figure 4. Porous coated titanium (left) and porous tantalum (right) hemispherical acetabular components used in cementless revision acetabular reconstruction as viewed from the **(A)** concave and **(B)** outer convex surfaces.

Regardless of the type of hemispherical acetabular implant chosen for reconstruction, the preparation of the acetabulum is the same. The acetabulum is exposed, debrided, and well visualized, and then it is progressively reamed until a viable hemispherical bed of bleeding host bone is present. The surgeon must be careful not to eccentrically ream away any anterior or posterior column that could potentially compromise the ability to obtain rigid implant fixation to host bone. In addition, as progressively larger reamers are used, the reamer is directed inferiorly to prevent inadvertent superior reaming and subsequent superior migration of the hip center.

Small- and medium-sized cavitary defects are filled with particulate allograft and can be combined with any autograft that is obtained from the reamings taken from acetabular preparation. The graft is packed into the acetabulum by hand and contoured to fill the cavitary defects in a hemispherical geometry by utilizing the reamers in the reverse direction (see Figs. 5A,B). This facilitates pressurized packing of the graft into the cavitary defects

Figure 5. (A) Cancellous allograft placed in the acetabular cavity and **(B)** impacted using an acetabular reamer on reverse. **C:** This technique effectively fills small cavitary defects.

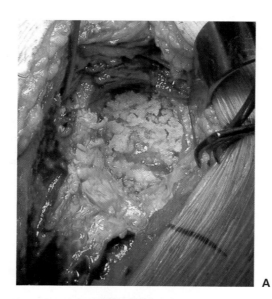

A

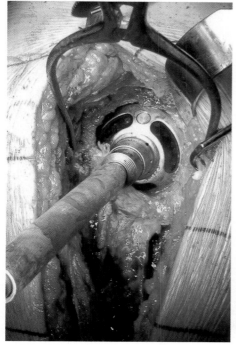

B

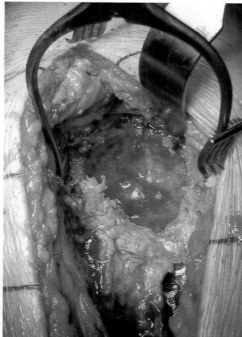

C

while preserving the exposed surface of the viable host bone for contact with the acetabular component (Fig. 5C). This technique is particularly appropriate for medial wall deficiencies with an intact acetabular periphery, in order to reconstitute medial wall integrity. A hemispherical, uncemented acetabular implant, sized approximately 2 mm larger than the last reamer used, is impacted into the acetabulum to obtain interference fit and mechanical stability against viable host bone (see Fig. 6).

In the overwhelming majority of revision cases, socket fixation is augmented with multiple screws placed through the socket into the pelvic bone. Obtaining screw fixation in the revision setting can be difficult and tenuous, depending on the location and quality of host pelvic bone remaining. At a minimum, multiple screws should be placed into the superior iliac bone, angling slightly posteriorly to avoid neurovascular injury. In addition, screw fixation into the intact posterior column is advantageous and should be strongly considered, especially if marginal fixation is obtained with the superior screws. Finally, ischial screws are very important and are frequently necessary in the complex revision setting to optimize component stability. Biomechanical studies demonstrate that forces across the hip during weight bearing cause distraction forces on the acetabular implant away from the ischial bone, highlighting the importance of ischial screw fixation in the revision setting.

If a modular titanium implant is utilized, the manufactured screw holes should be aligned in the proper position in anticipation of the adjuvant screw fixation. The authors currently employ the recently developed revision acetabular component made of porous tantalum (Figs. 4 and 6). A distinct advantage of this material is the ability to create screw holes in the implant material with a high-speed burr, allowing the surgeon the flexibility to place screws in the direction and location of maximal bone quality. This flexibility is not afforded with modular, titanium implants, as the surgeon is relegated to screw placement as dictated by screw hole locations created by the manufacturer.

If a modular acetabular component is used, the liner is inserted once screw fixation has been obtained. The porous, tantalum revision acetabular component relies on cementation of a polyethylene liner into the Trabecular Metal implant. All screw heads are sealed with bone wax to facilitate removal, should that be required. The outer surface of the polyethylene liner is roughened with a high-speed burr to facilitate mechanical interlock with ce-

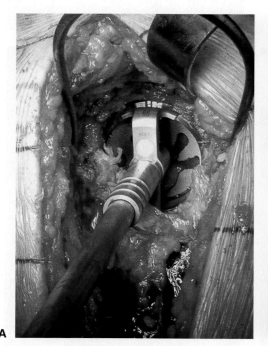
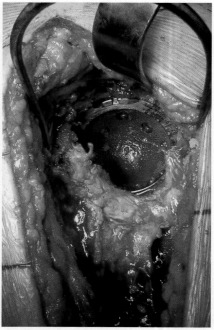

A   B

Figure 6. (A) Porous tantalum revision acetabular component is properly positioned using the specialized inserter and impacted into the acetabulum, **(B)** gaining excellent interference fit and mechanical stability.

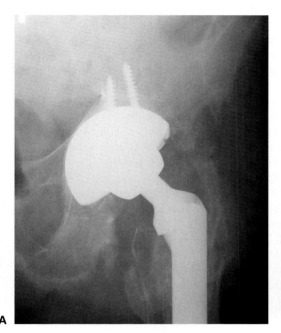

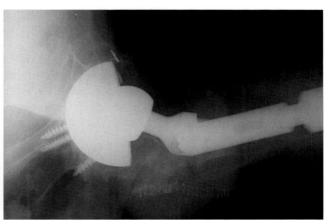

A   B

Figure 7. (A) AP and **(B)** lateral postoperative radiograph of the revision acetabular reconstruction depicted in Figures 2 to 6.

ment, and the liner is cemented into the acetabular shell (see Fig. 7). Once the femoral head is reduced into the liner, the hip is taken through a range of motion to assess stability and evaluate potential sources of impingement.

Large Acetabular Defects

Accurate intraoperative assessment of the acetabular defects and remaining viable host bone is essential in establishing the correct classification and the ability to gain sufficient mechanical stability for cementless fixation with a hemispherical component. It is generally agreed upon that hemispherical components will obtain sufficient mechanical stability and bone ingrowth if a minimum of 50% host bone contact exists with the surface of the implant. Large defects may necessitate the use of alternative methods of acetabular reconstruction such as an extralarge cementless hemispherical socket, high hip center, or adjunctive techniques of mechanical fixation such as bulk allograft or reconstruction cages.

Small to moderate segmental bone deficiencies can be successfully treated with hemispherical, uncemented porous coated or porous metal sockets. Medial segmental deficiencies can be treated with morselized cancellous bone if sufficient peripheral rim remains intact to provide mechanical stability to the implant. Small to moderate peripheral segmental deficiencies can be managed with bone grafting to reconstitute bone stock, provided sufficient acetabular rim is intact for cup stability. Moderately sized segmental peripheral defects, frequently located superolaterally, may be treated successfully by accepting a higher hip center and placing the acetabular component against viable host bone for mechanical support. Large peripheral segmental defects typically require the use of structural allograft or newly developed porous metal augments, with or without the use of reconstruction cages, to provide the required mechanical support for osseointegration of the hemispherical cementless socket. The majority of cavitary deficiencies can be successfully treated with hemispherical uncemented sockets, with varying amounts of bone grafting and socket sizes depending on the severity of the defect. A requisite for successful treatment of cavitary defects is that they remain contained with an intact rim for mechanical support of the socket. Mild to moderate combined segmental and cavitary defects can be treated with extralarge uncemented hemispherical sockets, sequentially reaming through defects and expanding the acetabulum to optimize mechanical support against viable host bone. However, this technique is limited by the anteroposterior dimension of the acetabulum, which is difficult to assess by standard preoperative imaging. A slightly elevated or medialized cup position may be accepted in order to obtain maximal contact with viable host bone, and offset acetabular liners are available to facilitate correction of the hip center in this difficult setting.

Large acetabular defects are a challenging problem, frequently requiring additional reconstruction methods such as corticocancellous allograft or antiprotrusio cages to gain mechanical stability. However, because of the relatively high failure rates of complex acetabular reconstructions with bulk allograft (2), a novel method of reconstruction utilizing modular porous metal augments has been developed for this challenging problem (3). The rationale for developing this modular system was to provide the potential for biological fixation, in addition to mechanical fixation, to avoid the use of structural allograft, to obviate the need for custom fabrication of implants, and to extend the feasibility of uncemented hemispherical acetabular components by using these modular augments to address the wide variety of bone deficiencies frequently encountered in acetabular revision. Multiple sizes and shapes accommodate the various acetabular defects encountered and the various sizes of hemispherical acetabular components (see Fig. 8). In addition, the augments are fenestrated to allow supplementation with morselized autograft or allograft.

Classification

Accurate radiographic and intraoperative classification of acetabular defects and identification of viable host bone are essential to enacting the appropriate treatment algorithm using this modular system. The authors favor the Paprosky classification (4) of acetabular defects, as it has proven beneficial in ascertaining appropriate treatment plans in acetabular revision and correlates well with the classification system developed by the authors to describe and facilitate the appropriate modular acetabular augment construct. The modular augment classification developed by the senior authors facilitates application of the various augment sizes and positions to maximize host bone contact with the hemispherical component and provide the required mechanical stability.

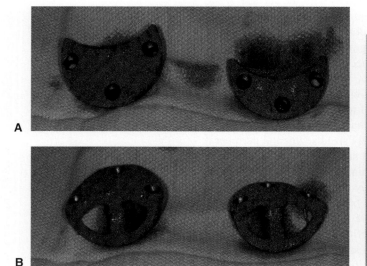

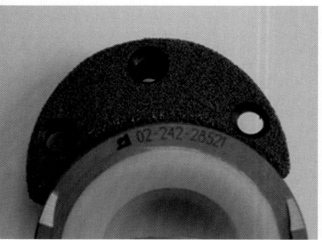

Figure 8. A and **B:** Modular porous tantalum augments of various sizes with fenestrations for supplemental bone graft. **C:** Modular augment with intimate fit on acetabular component of identical radius.

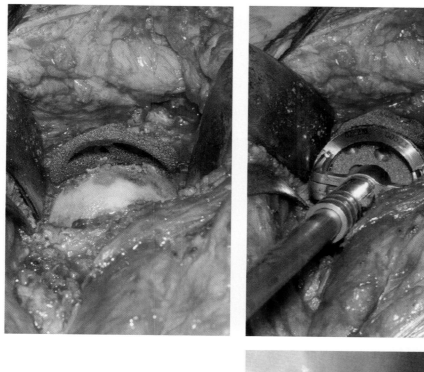

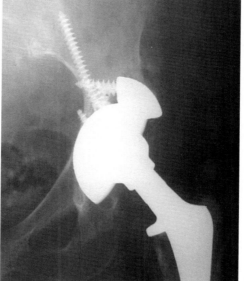

Figure 9. **A:** Superolateral augment in a "flying buttress" or type I configuration with rigid fixation to ilium with screws. **B:** Intraoperative interference fit of hemispherical porous tantalum revision shell into acetabulum supplemented with superolateral augment and the subsequent **(C)** postoperative radiograph of the construct.

A type I modular augment construct is placed superolaterally to fill mild to moderate peripheral rim defects, corresponding to Paprosky type IIB defects (superior and lateral cup migration, with intact anterior and posterior columns and adequate peripheral rim). This augment construct is analogous to the "flying buttress" graft (see Fig. 9).

A type II modular augment construct fills a large superolateral elliptical acetabular defect, analogous to a modular oblong cup. This type II acetabular augment construct is appropriate for reconstruction of Paprosky type IIIA defects (severe superior and lateral deficiency without the necessary 50% host bone contact for mechanical stability).

A type III modular augment construct describes the use of various augments as structural "footings" to provide mechanical stability to a hemispherical component in severe superior and/or medial defects that correspond to large Paprosky type IIA or IIIB acetabular defects (severe superior and medial defects with inadequate host bone for mechanical stability).

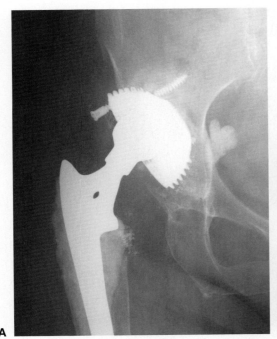
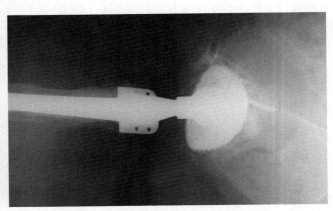

A   **B**

Figure 10. (A) AP and **(B)** lateral radiograph of a loose acetabular component with super-olateral migration of the implant.

Technique

Patient positioning, surgical exposure, component removal, and meticulous acetabular exposure are carried out as detailed in the previous section. In the setting of severe acetabular defects, it is critical to thoroughly remove all periacetabular fibrous tissue and accurately define the extent and location of acetabular defects and remaining host bone suitable for mechanical support of the acetabular implant. The surgeon must then ascertain and classify the defect as detailed in the previous section and formulate an intraoperative plan of acetabular reconstruction. Figure 10 demonstrates a failed acetabular component with severe superior and lateral migration.

Once the acetabulum is exposed and the defect is delineated (see Fig. 11A), reamers of the appropriate size are used to prepare both the hemispherical acetabulum (Fig. 11B) and the associated defect. Large elliptical segmental defects are reamed with hemispherical reamers of diameters corresponding to the proposed augment diameter in order to create an intimate fit of the augment into the defect (Fig. 11C). It is recommended that the surgeon utilize the trial augments to fill the acetabular defects in an attempt to reconstruct a hemispherical cavity to accept a cementless acetabular component. This is accomplished with the use of trial augments and trial sockets, as shown in Figure 12A.

Once the acetabulum and defect have been adequately shaped with the reamers and the appropriate size acetabular component and augment have been selected on the basis of the trials, the porous metal augment and shell can be inserted and secured. The augment can be rigidly attached with acetabular screws to the intact host bone in the defect prior to insertion of the acetabular component or vice versa, whichever facilitates proper interference fit of the implants with optimal mechanical stability (Fig. 12B). Once the first implant is securely attached to bone, bone cement is carefully placed along the surface interface between augment and acetabular shell to prevent motion and subsequent metal debris. If the augment is secured first, the surgeon should fill the fenestrations with morselized allograft or available autograft prior to cementation of the augment to the acetabular shell. The surgeon then inserts the second component and secures the implant rigidly to host bone and adjacent porous metal implant, placing acetabular screws safely and expeditiously prior to cement curing. This facilitates mechanical interference fit and rigid continuity of the entire

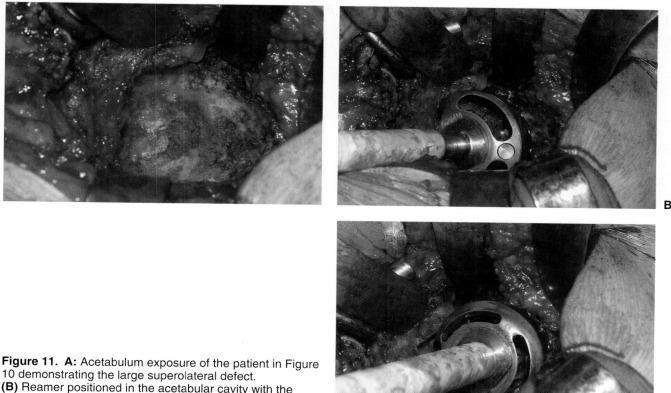

Figure 11. A: Acetabulum exposure of the patient in Figure 10 demonstrating the large superolateral defect.
(B) Reamer positioned in the acetabular cavity with the defect noted superiorly and **(C)** reamer positioned in the superior defect in preparation for the augment.

construct as the cement hardens and interdigitates at the porous interface (see Fig. 13). Furthermore, cementation of the liner over the screw heads creates a "locking screw" construct, with the screws acting as fixed-angle devices that are less likely to back out or angulate. Bone wax is then used to fill in the acetabular screw heads and unused acetabular screw holes to facilitate component removal, should that be necessary in any subsequent revision surgery. An appropriate acetabular liner is then cemented into the porous metal acetabular shell, and the femoral head is reduced (see Fig. 14). Through the correct placement and sizing of the modular porous metal acetabular augments, mechanical stability of the

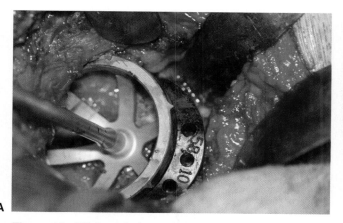

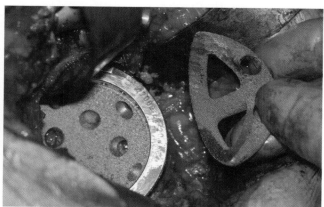

Figure 12. (A) Acetabular and augment trials for the modular porous metal acetabular system, followed by **(B)** insertion of the actual implants of the corresponding sizes.

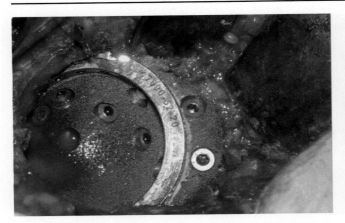

Figure 13. Final construct demonstrating revision shell and superior augment, both with screw augmentation and cement in the associated interface between the two implants.

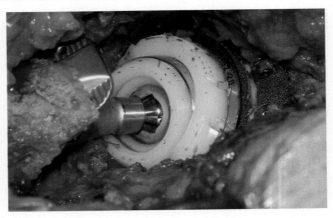

Figure 14. The polyethylene liner is cemented into the revision acetabular component. A large bipolar femoral head is inserted onto retained femoral stem taper and reduced into the liner of accommodating size.

hemispherical component can be obtained with near-normal restoration of the hip center (see Fig. 15), facilitating abductor tension and proper hip biomechanics.

Treatment of large superior and medial acetabular defects (see Fig. 16) follows the same principles as described above for the superolateral defects, with accurate identification of viable host bone for structural support of paramount importance. These defects frequently have a large superomedial defect and may or may not have an intact peripheral rim (see Fig. 17). It is essential that all fibrous debris be removed from within the defect and care be taken to adequately visualize the deepest extent of the bony deficiency to ensure adequate host bone contact with the modular acetabular augments. Careful inspection for pelvic discontinuity should be performed by manual palpation if there is migration of the failed acetabular component medial to Kohler's line or any radiographic evidence of pelvic discontinuity. Once the defect has been accurately debrided and viable host bone has been delineated, this particular acetabular defect is appropriate for a type III modular augment

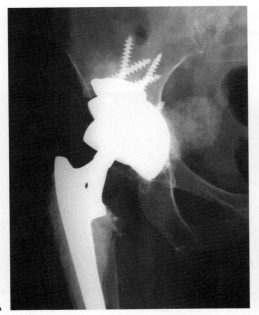

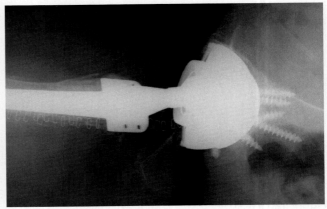

A

B

Figure 15. **(A)** AP and **(B)** lateral postoperative radiographs of acetabular reconstruction depicted in Figures 10 to 14.

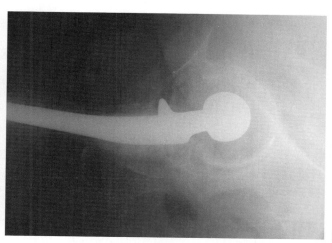

A   B

Figure 16. **(A)** AP and **(B)** lateral radiographs of loose acetabular component with severe superior and medial migration.

construct that utilizes the augments as structural "footings" within the defect to recreate a hemispherical socket that will accommodate a cementless acetabular shell. The modular porous metal augments are seated into the defect with an interference fit (see Fig. 18A), and the augment fenestrations and any associated defects are filled with particulate allograft (Fig. 18B). This is facilitated by using a reamer on reverse (Fig. 18C), creating a smooth, conforming hemispherical socket (Fig. 18D) to facilitate interference fit and mechanical stability of the hemispherical component.

Loose debris are removed from the augment porous metal surface, and cement is carefully placed along that interface with a syringe (see Fig. 19A) to facilitate mechanical interlock and structural continuity of the porous metal shell and augments. Once the hemispherical cup is securely seated into place (Fig. 19B), acetabular screw augmentation is safely performed as described previously in this chapter. The surgeon should be comfortable with and willing to obtain ischial screw fixation, as its contribution to the mechanical stability of the acetabular construct in these challenging acetabular revisions cannot be

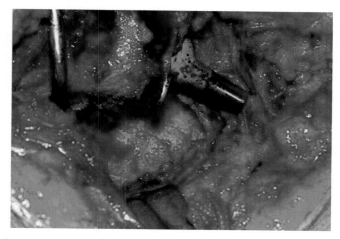

Figure 17. Intraoperative acetabular exposure of the patient in Figure 16 through an anterolateral approach with posterior retraction of the retained well-fixed stem.

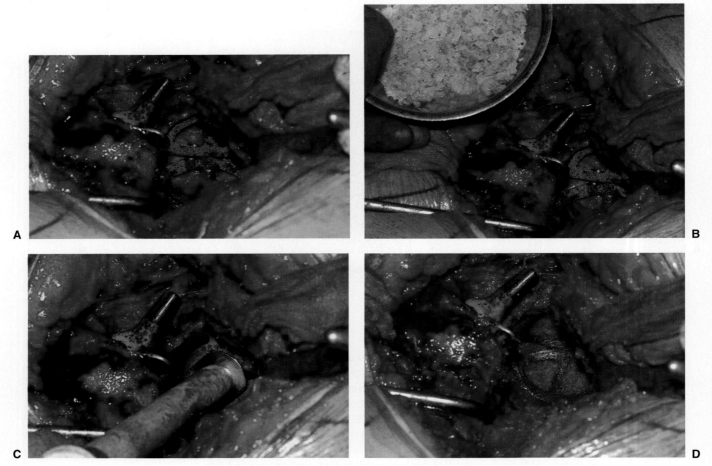

Figure 18. A: Porous tantalum augments placed into the superomedial acetabular defect as structural "footings." **B:** Cancellous allograft is then placed into the augment fenestrations and acetabular cavity and **(C)** impacted with a hemispherical reamer in reverse, which facilitates preparation of a **(D)** well-contoured, structurally supportive, hemispherical cavity to accept the acetabular implant.

overstated. Screw heads and unfilled screw holes are filled with bone wax (Figs. 19C,D), and the acetabular liner is cemented into place, with the outer surface of the liner roughened with a high-speed burr prior to insertion (see Fig. 20). After the cement has cured, the hip is carefully reduced and assessed for stability, range of motion, and impingement. Again, by properly utilizing the modular acetabular augment system and classification, the surgeon can achieve excellent mechanical stability of a cementless hemispherical acetabular component and restore the hip center to near-normal position (see Fig. 21) in these challenging acetabular deficiencies.

POSTOPERATIVE MANAGEMENT

Postoperatively, the patients are admitted to the orthopaedic floor with an abduction pillow, and pain control is obtained via regional nerve blocks and indwelling catheters, with an emphasis on diminished intraoperative and postoperative narcotic use. Typically, hip revision patients at our institution receive a spinal epidural or general anesthesia and a psoas catheter that remains in place for 2 postoperative days. The senior authors have anecdotally observed a dramatic decrease in narcotic usage, increased speed of recovery, and decrease in perioperative medical complications with the induction of regional pain management in revision hip arthroplasty. The abduction pillow remains in place overnight, and the patients

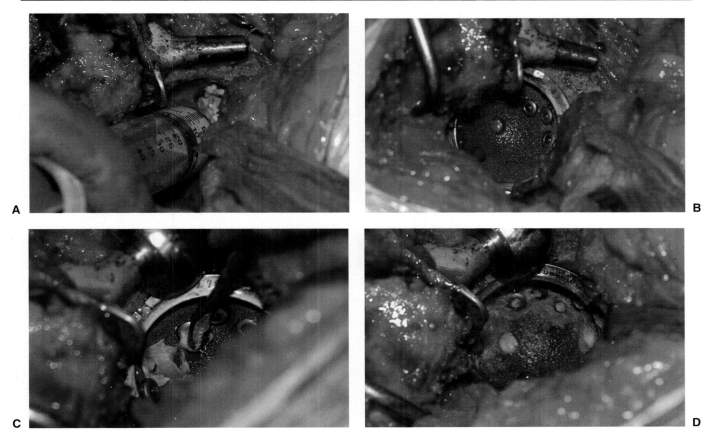

Figure 19. (A) Cement is carefully placed along the porous metal surface of the augment, and the **(B)** porous tantalum revision shell is impacted into place. Screws are placed while the cement is curing, and the **(C and D)** screw heads and vacant holes are filled with bone wax to facilitate removal should that be necessary.

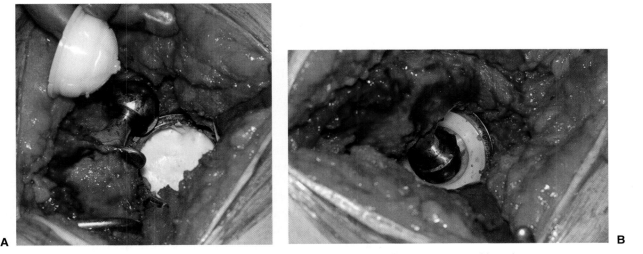

Figure 20. (A) Polyethylene line with a roughened outer surface is cemented into the porous tantalum revision acetabular component and **(B)** the femoral head is reduced into the polyethylene liner once the cement is cured.

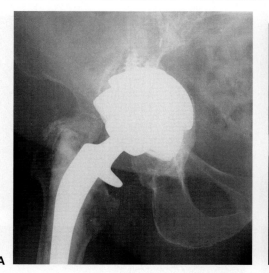
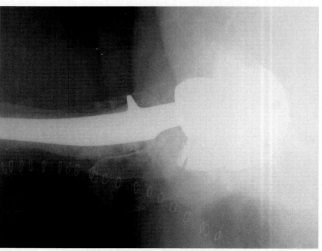

Figure 21. (A) AP and **(B)** lateral postoperative radiographs of the acetabular revision shown in Figures 16 to 20 with restoration of near-normal hip center of rotation.

are up to a chair either the night of surgery or the next morning. While in the hospital, the patients are evaluated and treated by the physical therapy department at our institution and are encouraged to ambulate with assistance and partial weight bearing on the first postoperative day.

REHABILITATION

The patients are allowed to place partial weight on the affected lower extremity, typically not to exceed 40 lbs, for the first 6 to 8 weeks. The patient is required to use either a walker or crutches for assistance and may wean him- or herself to a cane once allowed to bear full weight on the extremity. This may vary with the intraoperative assessment of bone quality and overall stability and fixation of the acetabular construct. Partial weight bearing is maintained to allow osseointegration into the porous metal, as well as protect the hip musculature as it heals from the trauma of revision hip surgery. Upon dismissal from the hospital, the patients do not undergo formal physical therapy, but rather limit their activity to activities of daily living and frequent ambulation for the first 6 to 8 weeks postoperatively, at which time they may begin gentle strengthening exercises targeting hip abductors.

RESULTS

Long-term results of revision acetabular reconstruction with cementless, hemispherical, porous coated, titanium components have recently emerged in the literature (5–7). These reports, with a minimum 10-year follow-up, document combined radiographic and clinical aseptic loosening rates of 3% to 11% with 10-year survivorship rates of 96% to 98% using the same endpoints (5–7). These studies demonstrate that long-term success can be achieved in revision acetabular reconstruction with cementless hemispherical components.

The senior authors' experience at the Mayo Clinic includes 60 revision acetabular reconstructions with a first-generation cementless hemispherical socket (8). At a minimum of 5 years' follow-up, a 12% failure rate was observed in those hips requiring less than 25% coverage from allograft and a 78% radiographic or clinical failure rate in 27 hips requiring greater than 50% allograft coverage at the time of socket revision. In a review of all uncemented acetabular components, including 2,443 revisions performed at the Mayo Clinic over a 15-year period, a steady and increasing rate of acetabular failure requiring rerevision beyond the first decade was observed (8), prompting the authors to seek improvements in acetabular fixation and durability.

The authors currently use a hemispherical porous tantalum shell for the majority of acetabular revisions, and early results are extremely encouraging. In 113 revision acetabular reconstructions treated with a porous tantalum revision shell and multiple screws, there have been no revisions for aseptic loosening, and no radiographic loosening has been observed at a minimum 2-year follow-up (9). Furthermore, at least 20% of these acetabular reconstructions contained bone defects classified as Paprosky type IIIA or IIIB. In addition, the authors currently avoid the use of structural bulk allograft in severe acetabular defects and have obtained excellent early clinical results with the newly developed modular porous metal augment acetabular reconstruction system. In 16 hips implanted with uncemented acetabular components with the use of modular acetabular augments for structural support, there was no evidence of component migration or loosening at a minimum 2-year follow-up (3). Furthermore, 11 of 16 reconstructions in this series were classified as Paprosky type IIIA or IIIB (3). The authors are very encouraged by these excellent early clinical and radiographic results; however, these results must be considered preliminary, as long-term follow-up is currently unavailable. In addition, the biologic and mechanical benefits of porous metal acetabular reconstruction systems offer the treating surgeon an excellent alternative in the challenging setting of complex acetabular revision.

COMPLICATIONS

Because of the complex nature of revision total hip arthroplasty, complications are more frequent than in primary hip surgery. Hip instability with dislocation is one of the most frequent complications encountered, especially in isolated acetabular revision with retention of the femoral component. Intraoperative assessment is critical to ensure proper implant position and that appropriate range of motion is obtainable without evidence of impingement. In addition, abductor muscle integrity and tension should be carefully evaluated and addressed intraoperatively. The authors currently utilize various sizes of large-diameter femoral heads when feasible to increase the impingement-free range of motion and enhance stability. In addition, the judicious use of elevated and offset liners is helpful to enhance stability in this setting. Finally, if an isolated acetabular revision is performed with retention of a monobloc femoral component or implant with a neck taper incompatible with a large-diameter femoral head, a bipolar head that accepts an inner 22-mm head with an outer diameter of 40 mm may be used in a polyethylene liner of a matching diameter to effectively optimize stability (Fig.14).

Nerve injury can occur in revision hip surgery and most commonly involves the sciatic nerve. Careful placement of acetabular retractors is essential, and acetabular screw placement, especially in the posterior column and ischium, should be performed with attention to the pertinent anatomy and safe technique. Because of the frequent elevation of the hip center with acetabular component migration, lengthening of the affected extremity is common as the hip center is returned to its near-normal location via the acetabular revision. In this situation, made more complicated by the frequent scar tissue formation from multiple prior surgeries, the tension on the soft tissue is carefully evaluated as the hip is reduced, and if significant lengthening occurs, the surgeon may consider positioning the knee in a flexion with the hip extended during the immediate postoperative period to remove any undue tension on the sciatic nerve from positioning. Fortunately, the majority of neuropraxias that occur are incomplete and fully recover with time.

Aseptic loosening of cementless hemispherical components utilized in revision acetabular surgery appears to be more frequent than in primary hip arthroplasty. However, the long-term rates of aseptic loosening with porous coated titanium implants are acceptable (3% to 11%) and demonstrate that these implants may be used quite successfully in the challenging setting of revision acetabular reconstruction. Long-term results are needed with porous tantalum acetabular shells to ascertain whether the favorable biological and mechanical characteristics of this material represent an improvement on the long-term success achieved with traditional titanium implants.

Finally, periprosthetic sepsis remains a devastating complication in revision total hip arthroplasty, and prevention is the mainstay of treatment. Careful preoperative evaluation, meticulous attention to soft tissue handling, sterile technique, and timely administration of appropriate perioperative antibiotics are critical to prevention of periprosthetic infection. Furthermore, intraoperative pathology and cultures are followed for 7 days, and oral antibiotics are administered until the final cultures are negative.

RECOMMENDED READING

1. Mitchell PA, Masri BA, Barbuz DS, et al. Removal of well-fixed, cementless, acetabular components in revision hip arthroplasty. *J Bone Joint Surg Br* 85(7):949–952, 2003.
2. O'Rourke MR, Paprosky WG, Rosenberg AG. Use of structural allografts in acetabular revision surgery. *Clin Orthop Relat Res* 420:113–121, 2004.
3. Nehme A, Lewallen DG, Hanssen AD. Modular porous metal augments for treatment of severe acetabular bone loss during revision hip arthroplasty. *Clin Orthop Relat Res* 429:201–208, 2004.
4. Paprosky WG, Perona PG, Lawrence JM. Acetabular defect classification and surgical reconstruction in revision arthroplasty. A 6-year follow-up evaluation. *J Arthroplasty* 9(1):33–44, 1994.
5. Della Valle CJ, Berger RA, Rosenberg AG, Galante JO. Cementless acetabular reconstruction in revision total hip arthroplasty. *Clin Orthop Relat Res* 420:96–100, 2004.
6. Hallstrom BR, Golladay GJ, Vittetoe DA, Harris WH. Cementless acetabular revision with the Harris-Galante porous prosthesis. Results after a minimum of ten years of follow-up. *J Bone Joint Surg Am* 86(5):1007–1011, 2004.
7. Templeton JE, Callaghan JJ, Goetz DD, et al. Revision of a cemented acetabular component to a cementless acetabular component. A ten to fourteen-year follow-up study. *J Bone Joint Surg Am* 83(11):1706–1711, 2001.
8. Lewallen DG. Acetabular revision: technique and results. In: Morrey BF, ed. *Joint Replacement Arthroplasty*. 3rd ed. Philadelphia: Churchill Livingstone, 2003: 824–843.
9. Mardones R, Talac R, Hanssen AD, Lewallen DG. Porous tantalum revision shell in revision total hip arthroplasty. Presented at: American Academy of Orthopaedic Surgeons 2005 Annual Meeting; February 25, 2005; Washington, DC.

30

Acetabular Revision with Structural Allograft

Michael R. O'Rourke, Scott Sporer,
and Wayne G. Paprosky

The most challenging aspect of acetabular revision surgery relates to the management of bone loss that compromises implant fixation and stability. Revision of cemented acetabular components is most commonly related to aseptic loosening with migration of the component correlating with the degree of bone loss. With cementless fixation, the severity of bone loss can be pronounced prior to migration because of osteolysis and stress shielding.

There are several reconstructive options available for revision acetabular surgery including both nonbiologic fixation and biologic fixation. Nonbiologic fixation options include cemented polyethylene cups, superior structural allografts with cemented polyethylene cups, impaction grafting, and total acetabular allografts (1–4). Reconstruction cages are an adjuvant to nonbiologic fixation in many of these circumstances. Biologic fixation options include hemispherical cementless cups at the anatomic hip center, high hip center (>2 cm superior to the native hip center), jumbo cup (66 to 80 mm), oblong cups, cementless hemispherical cup supported by structural allograft ("figure-seven" graft), and modular cementless implant systems (2,5,6). Hemispherical cementless components are the gold standard for the majority of acetabular revisions and have improved outcomes over cemented components when adequate host bone is available. Reliable and durable fixation of cementless acetabular components requires an environment with adequate biologic potential (intimate contact of viable living bone with the implant) and mechanical stability (motion <40 to 50 μm) to allow for bone ingrowth (7). Bone loss can compromise both of these prerequisites for successful use of these implants.

The purpose of this chapter is to review the indications for structural allograft use in revision acetabular surgery. The goals of structural allografts are to restore bone stock and provide initial implant stability. The technique for a "figure-seven" distal femoral allograft with use of a cementless hemispherical component and a total acetabular transplant will be described.

INDICATIONS AND CONTRAINDICATIONS

The indications for acetabular revision include symptomatic aseptic loosening, failure of fixation, sepsis, wear, osteolysis, and instability. Revision may be indicated for the asymptomatic patient in cases of progressive osteolysis, severe wear, or bone loss that is at risk of compromising future reconstructive options. Indications for structural allografts include providing support to a cementless acetabular implant that has the potential for durable fixation if ingrowth occurs and management of massive bone loss where cementless fixation alone is unlikely to be successful. Cementless fixation with a hemispherical cup alone is a risk of failure when the surface area of bone contact is less than approximately 50% to 60%, more than a third of the rim is absent, the trial implant has partial or absent inherent stability (defined below), in the presence of a pelvic discontinuity, or with an absent posterior column.

Contraindications for revision of the acetabular component include severe bone loss precluding allograft fixation or implant fixation, uncontrolled sepsis, or medical comorbidities that preclude the risk of surgery.

PLANNING AND DECISION MAKING

We use a classification system initially described in 1991 based on the severity of bone loss and the ability to obtain cementless fixation for a given bone loss pattern (8). The key to the classification is the ability of the remaining host bone to provide initial stability to a hemispherical, cementless acetabular component until ingrowth occurs (see Table 1). Intraoperative decisions are based on the stability of the trial components. The amount of rim remaining contributes greatly to the stability of the trial and implant.

Table 1. *Description of the Classification System for Acetabular Bone Loss Used to Make Intraoperative Decisions Based on the Location of the Hip Center and the Degree of Inherent Stability Achieved with Trial Components*

Type	Location of hip center	Rim	Columns	Host bone stock	Trial stability	Reconstruction options
I	Anatomic	Fully intact	Intact	>80%	Full inherent stability	Hemispherical cementless cup
II						
IIA	<2 cm superior	Fully intact	Intact	>60%	Full inherent stability	Hemispherical cementless cup (cancellous allograft)
IIB	<2 cm superior	Up to one-third rim defect	Intact	>60%	Full inherent stability	Hemispherical cementless cup (nonsupportive bone graft)
IIC (*protrusio*)	<2 cm superior with medial migration	Fully intact	Intact	>60%	Full inherent stability	Hemispherical cementless cup (medial cancellous allograft)
III						
IIIA	>2 cm superior	Up to one-half rim defect	Usually intact	40–50%	Partial inherent stability	1. Hemispherical cementless cup with structural allograft (number 7 graft) 2. Nonhemispherical cementless modular implant 3. Cage with graft
IIIB	>2 cm superior and medial	Greater than one-half rim defect	Disruption of one or both columns (high risk for discontinuity)	<40%	No inherent stability	1. Large structural allograft, cage, and cemented cup (acetabular transplant) 2. Modular revision cementless implant 3. Custom implants

Inherent Stability

Although some have reported success with line-to-line reaming cementless cups, we believe that in the presence of bone loss, the ability to achieve inherent stability of the implant is necessary to predict durable fixation. Trial components are critical to predict remaining bone stock. Trial cups can have full inherent stability, partial inherent stability, or no inherent stability. With full inherent stability, the surgeon is able to push on the rim of the trial without displacing the trial. A trial reduction can be performed without displacing the trial component. With partial inherent stability, the position of the trial is maintained while the trial inserter is removed; however, loading the rim of the trial implants causes displacement (see Fig. 1). Cup position will not be maintained if a trial reduction is attempted. Finally, no inherent stability is defined as the inability to maintain the trial position without secondary support.

Radiographic Correlation

Preoperative radiographic findings on the anteroposterior radiograph of the pelvis generally can be used to predict the type of defect present, allowing the surgeon to plan for the acetabular reconstruction accordingly. The four criteria on the preoperative radiograph that

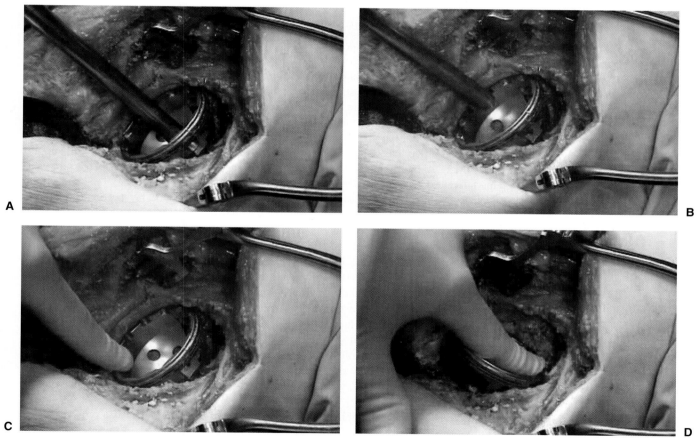

Figure 1. Illustration of partial inherent stability of a trial acetabular component. Partial inherent stability defines a type IIIA bone loss pattern. **A:** Insertion of the trial acetabular implant at the anatomic hip center location with a 45% to 50% rim defect superolaterally. **B:** The trial inserter is removed, and the trial implant remains in the desired location without displacement. **C:** Loading the supported aspect of the trial implant does not cause displacement. **D:** Loading of the unsupported portion of the implant causes displacement of the trial implant.

Table 2. *Radiographic Classification to Predict the Intraoperative Bone Loss Pattern*

Type	Superior migration of hip center (Relative to the SOL)*	Kohler's line (Location of the most medial aspect of the implant)	Ischial osteolysis (Inferior extension relative to the SOL)	Teardrop (Partial when lateral limb missing but medial limb present)
I	Anatomic location (1 cm above SOL)	Lateral	None	Intact
II				
IIA	<3 cm	On or lateral	<7 mm	Intact or partial
IIB	<3 cm	Lateral	<7 mm	Intact
IIC *(protrusio)*	<3 cm	Medial	<7 mm	Partial or absent
III				
IIIA	>3 cm	Lateral	7–15 mm	Partial
IIIB	>3 cm	Medial	>15 mm	Absent

*SOL, superior obturator line.

are important to assess include (a) superior migration of the hip center (acetabular dome), (b) ischial osteolysis (inferior posterior column), (c) teardrop osteolysis (inferior and medial acetabulum), and (d) position of the implant relative to Kohler's line (anterior column) (see Table 2).

Algorithmic Approach

The algorithmic approach to revision of the acetabulum is shown in Figure 2. The initial decision point relates to the superior migration of the hip center prior to revision. If the hip center has not migrated more than 2 cm superiorly, a determination is made as to whether full inherent stability can be achieved with a trial component. If this can be achieved, the defect is a type I or type II. Hemispherical cementless fixation is utilized. If there is migration medial to Kohler's line, the defect would be a type IIC, and rim fixation will support the hemispherical implant in the anatomic location. The authors routinely place screws as an adjuvant to cementless fixation in revision shells.

When the hip center has migrated more than 2 cm superiorly or the surgeon is unable to achieve full inherent stability of the trial, the defect is a type III defect. If a trial component has partial inherent stability, there is generally enough contact with host bone to support ingrowth (type IIIA defect). Type IIIA defects usually have an oblong shape; however, occasionally they are spherical. If spherically remodeled, a large cup may be appropriate with multiple screw fixation. With oblong remodeling of the host acetabulum the options include a number 7 distal femoral graft with a cementless hemispherical cup, a modular nonhemispherical cementless implant, or a high hip center hemispherical cup. When restoration of an anatomic hip center is desired, the former two options are appropriate. With the number 7 structural graft, the goal is to provide support to a hemispherical implant that has partial inherent stability until adequate supportive ingrowth can occur into the cup. One of the advantages of a distal femoral allograft is the restoration of bone for future reconstructions if necessary, which makes it a particularly attractive option in the younger revision patient.

If there is no inherent stability of the hemispherical trial, the defect is a type IIIB. Preoperatively, the radiographic finding of superior migration of the hip center more than 3 cm above the superior obturator line, migration medial to Kohler's line, and moderate to severe ischial and teardrop osteolysis suggests a type IIIB defect and should alert the surgeon to the possibility of a pelvic discontinuity. Judet views of the pelvis can assist in the preoperative determination; however, we have not found them routinely necessary. The intraoperative detection of a pelvic discontinuity is determined by complete removal of the pseudomembrane and identification of remaining bone stock. In the presence of a

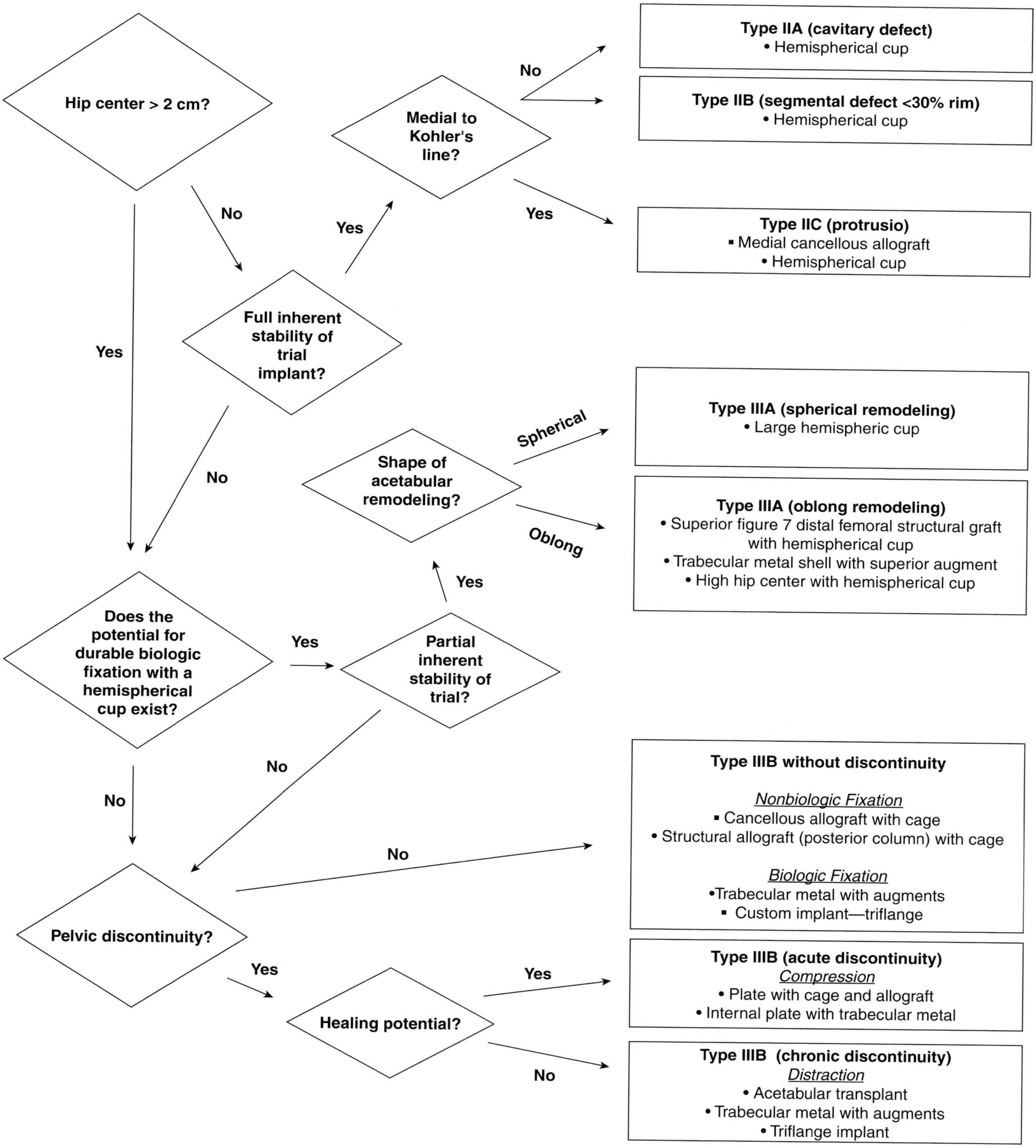

Figure 2. Flowchart illustrating the algorithmic approach to acetabular bone loss decision making.

discontinuity, there is absence of bridging bone and/or a fracture present involving the anterior column, posterior column, and medial wall. In addition, discontinuous motion can be elicited between the superior and inferior aspects of the hemipelvis. When a pelvic discontinuity has been ruled out, the options include nonbiologic fixation with impaction allograft supported with a cage, structural allograft (acetabular allograft or distal femoral allograft) supported with a cage, biologic fixation with a modular cementless system, or a custom implant. In the presence of a pelvic discontinuity, the surgeon must determine whether it appears to be an acute dissociation with a potential for healing or whether it is a chronic dissociation without healing potential. Our determination of healing potential is based on the ability to achieve reduction of the discontinuity gap with compression of the inferior and superior aspects of the hemipelvis. If a reasonable surface area of bone contact is achieved, the judgment is made that a healing potential exists, and compression plating across the dissociation is performed. If a gap persists despite compression, the judgment is made that a healing potential does not exist, and we achieve our reconstruction stability with distraction of discontinuity in combination with secondary support (i.e., posterior column plate and/or cage).

Total acetabular transplants remain a viable reconstructive option in the physiologically younger patient with a type IIIB acetabular defect, and bone stock restoration may be advantageous for future reconstruction.

TECHNIQUES

General Principles

Preoperative planning based on the aforementioned classification system is critical to have the appropriate grafting materials, tools for implant removal, and components at the time of surgery. If significant medial migration is present, consideration of imaging (angiography or computed tomography scanning with intravascular contrast infusion) and possible intrapelvic mobilization of vascular structures is recommended.

Careful patient positioning is required, giving particular attention to the orientation of the pelvis and torso relative to the floor, as internal landmarks often are distorted in the setting of revision surgery. Extensile exposures often are necessary with the incision extending toward the posterosuperior iliac spine. The plane between the iliotibial band and the underlying vastus lateralis and the abductors (often scarred to the iliotibial band) is redeveloped. After identifying the borders of the gluteus medius and gluteus minimus, the plane between the gluteus minimus and the capsule is identified, and the abductors are mobilized anteriorly. We do not routinely expose the sciatic nerve unless dissection through heterotopic ossification is necessary. A posterior capsule flap is developed and maintained for repair following the reconstruction. Intraoperative infection is evaluated with cell count and frozen sections. As a general guideline, a white cell count less than 3,000 predicts the absence of an infection, and one greater than 10,000 predicts the presence of an infection. If the white cell count is between 3,000 and 10,000, we base our decision on the preoperative C-reactive protein level and frozen sections. The posterior flap is retracted, and an anterior capsulectomy is performed. The superior ilium and posterior column are dissected in the subperiosteal plane to obtain the necessary exposure. An extended trochanteric osteotomy might be indicated depending on the visualization and the anticipated reconstruction of the femur. After the removal of existing components, a systematic debridement of granulation tissue and interface membrane is done to assess the entire remaining acetabular bone stock and rule out the possibility of a pelvic discontinuity.

Structural Allograft Selection and Principles

An appropriate graft must be selected to match the mechanical demands of the proposed reconstruction to optimize outcomes. We do not use femoral head allografts when the graft serves a structurally supportive role. Fresh-frozen distal femoral or proximal tibial allografts are used to orient the trabecular patterns of the graft parallel to the direction of load to optimize stress transfer. The grafts are contoured to maximize contact surface area between the host bone and the allograft to optimize union rates. Unnecessary stress risers must be avoided. Temporary fixation with K-wires helps to prevent unwanted shifting of the allograft during fixation. It is important to have separate fixation between the allograft and host bone in addition to implant fixation. Fixation of the allograft generally is accomplished with 6.5-mm screws oriented parallel with one another in the direction of loading without interfering with component placement or fixation.

TYPE IIIA DEFECT: DISTAL FEMORAL STRUCTURAL ALLOGRAFT WITH CEMENTLESS ACETABULUM

The location of the desired hip center is identified, and acetabular reamers are used to size and shape the acetabulum for a hemispherical cementless implant (see Fig. 3). After it is determined that adequate host bone is available to contact the implant, a trial component is placed to determine areas of contact, inherent stability, and location of segmental loss.

The preparation of the allografts starts by trimming the epicondyles so the medial to lateral dimension of the allograft matches the diameter of the acetabular cavity (see Fig. 4). A female reamer is then used that is about 1 to 2 mm larger than the acetabular cavity to ream the distal aspect of the allograft in slight flexion to avoid notching the anterior cortex of the graft and so that the reamed condyles will be directed into the acetabular cavity (see Fig. 5). The metaphyseal portion of the allograft is then cut in the coronal plane to create the shape of the number 7 graft with the anterior aspect of the metadiaphyseal bone left in continuity with the distal condyles (see Fig. 6). The superior aspect of the allograft (anterior cortex) is generally around 5 to 6 cm in length.

The angle between the condyles and the anterior cortex on the posterior aspect of the allograft is contoured with a burr to optimize the contact between the allograft and the host ilium (see Fig. 7). The more of a ledge present between the lateral margin of the ilium and the depth of the acetabular cavity at the site of the defect, the more acute the angle should be (as opposed to obtuse). This "tongue-in-groove" effect will enhance stability at the graft-host junction.

The superior limb of the allograft is contoured to the lateral ilium and secured with Steinmann pins provisionally (see Fig. 8). Use four parallel 6.5-mm cancellous screws with washers. Tap the allograft to avoid fractures. Orientation of the screws is oblique

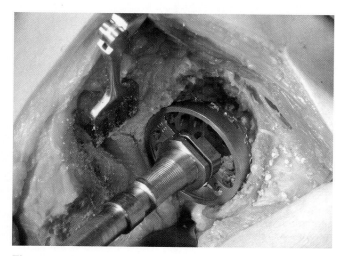

Figure 3. Size the acetabulum at the desired location, and assess the defect location and involvement.

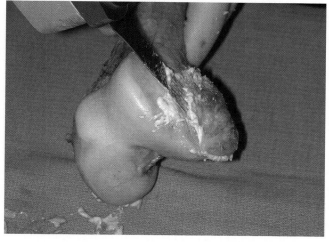

Figure 4. Trim the allograft in the medial/lateral dimension on the basis of the acetabular size by removing the epicondyles with a saw.

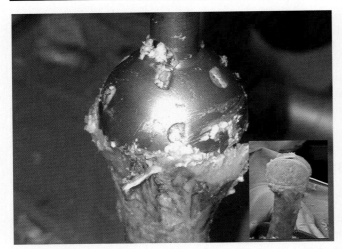

Figure 5. Prepare the distal femur with a female reamer one size larger than the size of the acetabulum. Avoid notching the anterior cortex of the femur by reaming in slight flexion. The inset picture shows the allograft after reaming.

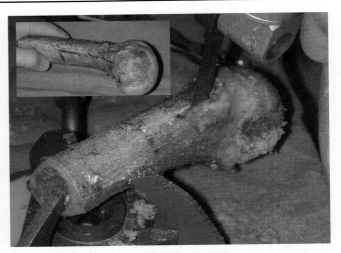

Figure 6. Cut the graft in the coronal plane, leaving approximately 5 cm of the anterior cortex of the femur attached to the distal condyles. The inset picture shows the allograft with the mark for the resection in the coronal plane.

into the ilium in the direction of loading to provide compression of the graft against the remaining ilium. The acetabular cavity then can be reamed to contour the portion of the graft that will contact the component. Smaller reamers initially are used and sequentially increased in size to obtain the dimensions of the desired acetabular cavity (see Fig. 9). Care must be taken to prevent additional host bone removal or inadequate reaming of the allograft, causing failure of contact between the remaining host bone and the component (see Fig. 10). Remaining voids are filled with particulate allograft, and a cementless cup is impacted into the newly sculpted acetabular cavity and fixed with multiple screws for adjunctive fixation (see Fig. 11).

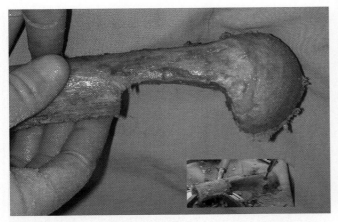

Figure 7. Contour the posterior junction between the condyles and the anterior cortex with a burr to minimize a stress riser. The angle between the condyles and the anterior cortex is dependent on the remaining host bone shelf. If there is a shelf of bone remaining, a more acute angle is contoured in the graft to obtain a tongue-in-groove effect, improving stability between the graft and host bone.

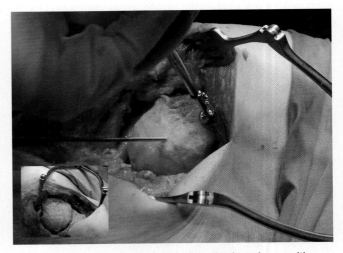

Figure 8. Temporarily fix the graft to the host bone with a Steinmann pin. Drill and tap the graft for placement of 6.5-mm partially threaded screws with washers. At least three screws with washers are placed. The inset shows the allograft in the defect location, and the remaining host rim is visible.

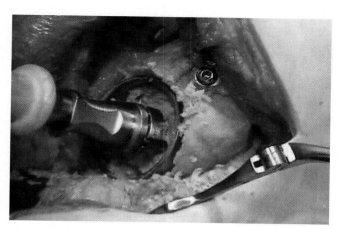

Figure 9. Contour the allograft with a smaller acetabular reamer to create a hemispherical cavity. It is important to ream to, but not into, the remaining host bone so the maximal contact between the implant and the host bone is achieved.

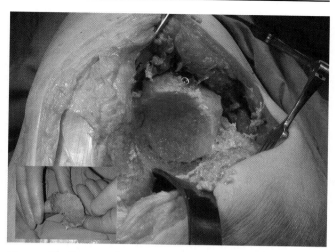

Figure 10. Prepared acetabular cavity with host bone and distal femoral allograft creating a hemispherical cavity. The inset is a removed allograft after final preparation showing the restoration of the rim defect.

TYPE IIIB DEFECT: TOTAL ACETABULAR TRANSPLANT WITH CAGE

Use acetabular reamers to size the acetabular cavity and identify the location of remaining bone to support the allograft (see Figs. 12 and 13). Identify the ledge of bone on the superior ilium that will abut against the allograft. Ream the acetabulum of the allograft on a back table—avoid weakening the graft by excessive reaming. A cage is sized to the allograft prior to placement. The allograft hemipelvis is cut in a curvilinear fashion from the greater sciatic notch to the anterior superior iliac spine to maintain a portion of the ilium attached to the acetabulum (see Fig. 14). The pubic and ischial portions of the allograft are cut distal to the confluence of the acetabulum with enough length to accommodate the inferior defects. Avoid leaving excessive inferior bone on the allograft that prevents optimal

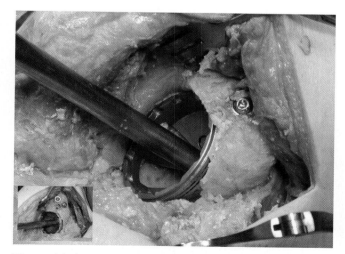

Figure 11. Insert the hemispherical component (trial shown) with press-fit stability and adequate contact with host bone for durable long-term biologic fixation. Multiple screws are placed through the component.

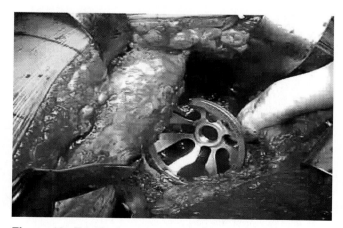

Figure 12. Trial in the desired location (anatomic hip center) illustrating extensive bone loss involving more than 60% to 70% of the rim with a large posterior/superior defect and medial wall defect. The trial lacks inherent stability, and the remaining host bone stock is inadequate to achieve durable fixation with a standard hemispherical cup.

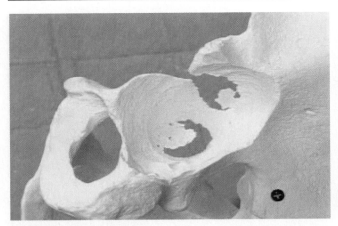

Figure 13. This is a saw bone model with a type IIIB defect similar to the defect illustrated in Figure 12. Notice that greater than 60% to 70% of the rim is absent associated with a large segmental dome bone deficiency.

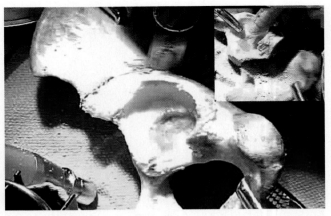

Figure 14. The acetabulum is cut from an allograft pelvis with sufficient ilium to compensate for the bone deficiency and achieve fixation into the remaining host bone. The inset shows the ischial and pubic bone cuts close to the acetabulum, which is necessary to achieve adequate metallization of the hip center.

medialization of the inferior aspect of the graft. Failure to recognize this can result in vertical cup placement and lateralization of the hip center. A groove is made in the superior ilium of the allograft to correspond to the ledge of bone along the superior aspect of the native acetabulum. This tongue-in-groove junction provides a stable buttress between the host and the allograft. A burr is used to "debulk" the inner table of the ilium on the allograft and maintain shelf distally that will fill the defect of the host acetabulum (see Fig. 15). Allograft should be placed with press fit. The graft can be secured with Steinmann pins provisionally. Four 6.5-mm partially threaded screws and washers are then directed obliquely into the ilium from both the intra-articular and lateral ilium aspects of the graft (see Fig. 16). A pelvic reconstruction plate is then contoured to the posterior column with ideally three screws in the native ilium and ischium (see Fig. 17). A cage is recommended to protect all transplants (see Fig. 18). If possible, the inferior flange of a cage is inserted into a slot in the ischium for fixation (Fig. 18). Cement a metal shell or a polyethylene liner into

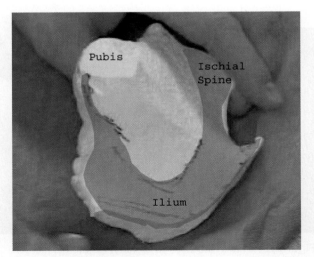

Figure 15. Medial aspect of the allograft showing the areas that need contouring shaded in gray. The inner table of the allograft ilium outlined in this image is burred away, and the outer table is maintained. To improve the stability between the host and the allograft, a "tongue-in-groove" is created when possible.

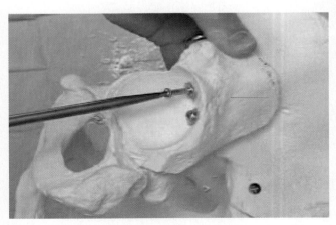

Figure 16. The allograft is secured to the ilium with 6.5-mm partially threaded screws.

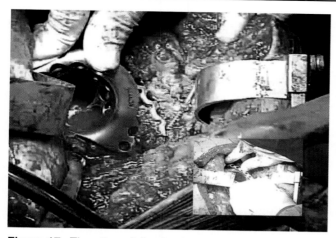

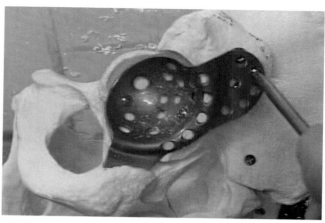

Figure 17. The allograft fixation is achieved with a contoured posterior column pelvic reconstruction plate. In addition, a pelvic reconstruction cage is recommended with a total acetabular transplant. The inferior flange of the cage is slotted into the ischium for fixation.

Figure 18. Saw bone illustrating the placement of the reconstruction cage.

the cage/allograft composite avoiding the tendency to place the component in a vertical and retroverted position (see Fig. 19).

POSTOPERATIVE REHABILITATION

Toe-touch weight bearing is used for 6 to 12 weeks following structural allografting, and there should be a gradual return to full weight bearing over 4 to 6 months. All patients are treated with a hip brace for 6 weeks.

CONCLUSIONS

The prevalence, younger age, and greater life expectancy of the arthroplasty population promise a continued need for solutions for difficult acetabular revisions in the face of bone loss. The algorithmic approach we have outlined is an approach that allows the surgeon to predict findings in the operating room, make plans for treating the expected bone loss patterns, and make appropriate judgments regarding reconstructive technique to achieve the best possible durable treatment. Our preference is to achieve cementless fixation when possible and alternative solutions when initial stability is not achievable.

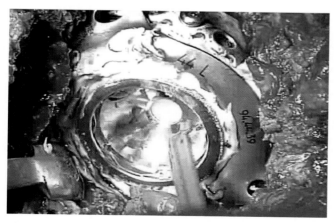

Figure 19. A polyethylene liner or an acetabular shell is cemented into the cage/allograft.

RECOMMENDED READING

1. Gross AE. Revision arthroplasty of the acetabulum with restoration of bone stock. *Clin Orthop Relat Res* 369:198–207, 1999.
2. Paprosky WG, Magnus RE. Principles of bone grafting in revision total hip arthroplasty. Acetabular technique. *Clin Orthop Relat Res* 298:147–155, 1994.
3. Schreurs BW, Busch VJ, Welten ML, et al. Acetabular reconstruction with impaction bone-grafting and a cemented cup in patients younger than fifty years old. *J Bone Joint Surg Am* 86(11):2385–2392, 2004.
4. Shinar AA, Harris WH. Bulk structural autogenous grafts and allografts for reconstruction of the acetabulum in total hip arthroplasty. Sixteen-year-average follow-up. *J Bone Joint Surg Am* 79(2):159–168, 1997.
5. Schutzer SF, Harris WH. High placement of porous-coated acetabular components in complex total hip arthroplasty. *J Arthroplasty* 9:359–367, 1994.
6. Whaley AL, Berry DJ, Harmsen WS. Extra-large uncemented hemispherical acetabular components for revision total hip arthroplasty. *J Bone Joint Surg Am* 83(9):1352–1357, 2001.
7. Pilliar RM, Lee JM, Maniatopoulos C. Observations on the effect of movement on bone ingrowth into porous-surfaced implants. *Clin Orthop Relat Res* 208:108–113, 1986.
8. Paprosky WG, Lawrence JM, Cameron HU. Classification and treatment of the failed acetabulum: a systematic approach. *Contemp Orthop* 22(2):121–130, 1991.

31

Cages

Daniel J. Berry

INDICATIONS/CONTRAINDICATIONS

The role of acetabular antiprotrusio cages for acetabular reconstruction has declined in the last 5 years in North America as the spectrum of difficult acetabular revision problems that can be managed with uncemented porous coated acetabular components has increased (1). Acetabular antiprotrusio cages are used when uncemented components can be predicted to have a high likelihood of failure: circumstances in which adequate mechanical stability cannot be gained with uncemented components or circumstances in which so little biologically active remaining host bone is available that the likelihood of biologic fixation with an uncemented component is remote (2). Uncemented porous coated components have numerous advantages over cages: Uncemented cups are technically easier to implant, are associated with a lower risk of early complications, and have the potential for long-term biologic fixation. Thus, whenever there is sufficient remaining host bone to gain early mechanical and long-term biologic fixation of an uncemented porous implant, an uncemented porous coated component is preferred, and an antiprotrusio cage is not indicated.

The most common indication for antiprotrusio cages is massive acetabular bone loss in revision total hip arthroplasty. In this setting, cages provide a large surface area that spans bone defects, prevents early migration, and helps gain stable early mechanical fixation on the pelvis. Antiprotrusio cages may be indicated in revision total hip arthroplasty when the quality or the activity of remaining host bone is so poor that uncemented fixation will predictably fail. Finally, antiprotrusio cages also infrequently may be indicated in cases of massive bone loss associated with primary hip pathology such as severe posttraumatic defects, previous pelvic radiation, or reconstructions for malignancies.

Currently, antiprotrusio cages are used in less than 5% of acetabular revisions, even in most referral centers where severe acetabular defects are encountered commonly. Recently, antiprotrusio cages have been used in combination with uncemented sockets to enhance initial cup stability.

PREOPERATIVE PLANNING

Determine from the history if there is anything to suggest infection of the hip joint. Document the implants in place, and review previous operative records so that appropriate tools and instruments are available for failed implant removal. Understand the problems that led to failure of the previous reconstruction: This may prevent repeating methodologies that have already failed in a specific patient. Examine the patient carefully to document neurovascular status of the limb and function of the abductor musculature. Templates are available for many modern antiprotrusio cages. Use the templates to determine the anticipated cage size, the anticipated location of the hip center of rotation after reconstruction, and the anticipated need for structural bone grafts.

Radiography

Plain radiographs should include an anteroposterior pelvis film and anteroposterior and lateral radiographs of the entire prosthetic hip joint and the surrounding pelvic and femoral bone that will be instrumented during the planned reconstruction. Oblique pelvic Judet films may be helpful to determine if pelvic discontinuity is present. Computerized tomography with metal artifact reduction can be used to further define bone defects effectively but is not needed routinely. Computerized tomography can help determine whether large structural bone grafts will be needed for the reconstruction and may be useful if these grafts must be ordered in advance by the surgeon. Multiple different bone loss classification schemes are available, but Paprosky's classification method provides a practical approach to understanding the severity of acetabular bone loss in acetabular revision based on plain radiographs. Antiprotrusio cage reconstruction is considered in selected Paprosky type IIIB defects and occasional type IIIA defects. Almost all type I and II defects can be treated with uncemented hemispherical implants.

Routine laboratory testing prior to surgery should include an erythrocyte sedimentation rate and C-reactive protein. Aspirate the hip if the sedimentation rate or C-reactive protein is abnormal or if other features of the patient's history, physical examination, or radiographs suggest infection (early failure of previous implants, radiographic findings typical of infection, a history of wound drainage or wound problems, or constitutional symptoms).

SURGERY

Most surgeons in North America prefer to operate with the patient in a lateral decubitus position, but this surgery also can be performed with the patient in the supine position. Drape the thigh and pelvis area to allow access to the ilium.

Administer intravenous antibiotics prior to wound incision except in exceptional cases in which infection is considered highly likely and confirmatory intraoperative cultures are required.

Operative Approaches

Placement of an antiprotrusio cage requires wide exposure of the ilium and some exposure of the proximal ischium. Cages can be placed through routine anterolateral or posterolateral approaches, but injury to the superior gluteal nerve (which provides innervation to the abductor musculature) is possible when a large cage is placed through an anterolateral or posterolateral approach. In most situations, when an antiprotrusio cage is planned preoperatively and adequate greater trochanteric bone stock is present, the author prefers a transtrochanteric approach. Many transtrochanteric approaches have been described, but a conventional transtrochanteric approach, in which the greater trochanter and abductors are reflected proximally (simultaneously providing good exposure of the joint and protection of the superior gluteal nerve and vessels), has advantages when an antiprotrusio cage is being placed. To perform a conventional transtrochanteric approach, make a straight lateral incision. When possible, use at least a portion of a previous incision. Dissect through the subcutaneous tissue to the fascia. Divide the iliotibial band in the direction of its fibers, and divide the interval between the tensor fascia lata and the gluteus maximus or split the anterior aspect of the gluteus maximus. Reflect the origin of the vastus lateralis from the vastus tubercle. Use an oscillating saw to make a flat or chevron-shaped greater trochanteric osteotomy (see Fig. 1). The osteotomy is made from distal to proximal, and the osteotomy fragment should be about 1 to 1.5 cm thick in most cases. Reflect the greater trochanteric fragment and the abductors proximally. Excise the anterior and superior hip pseudocapsule, and dislocate the hip anteriorly. If the femoral component will be removed, remove it now to gain better access to the joint. If the femoral component will not be exchanged, mobilize the femur to allow access to the acetabulum. Mobilization involves dissection of scar and pseudocapsule from the anterior, medial, and posterior aspects of the proximal femur above the level of the lesser trochanter.

Identify the sciatic nerve, when possible, by palpation or direct visualization. Understanding the exact relationship of the sciatic nerve to the posterior wall of the acetabulum and the ischium may reduce nerve injury risk.

Gain circumferential exposure of the acetabulum by dissecting muscle and hip pseudocapsule from the superior, anterior, inferior, and posterior rim of the acetabulum.

Remove the failed acetabular component, cement, and membrane from the acetabulum. Be careful not to unnecessarily damage or remove bone during this process.

Carefully assess the acetabular bone deficiency with respect to the pattern and magnitude of bone loss. Consider whether a hemispherical porous coated component can be employed. If an uncemented porous coated component can be used, this method is preferred.

If an antiprotrusio cage is chosen, expose about 3 cm of the ilium above the remaining rim of the acetabulum. This is the location in which the flange of the antiprotrusio cage will be placed. Avoid damage to the superior gluteal vessels and nerves. Carefully expose about 1 to 2 cm of the proximal lateral ischium to the level of the proximal hamstring tendon origins. Avoid damage to the sciatic nerve during this part of the exposure by keeping the dissection directly against bone and by understanding the location of the sciatic nerve in the operated patient. Keeping the hip extended and the knee flexed during this exposure relaxes the nerve and may reduce risk of nerve injury. When possible, use trial cage implants to judge the proper

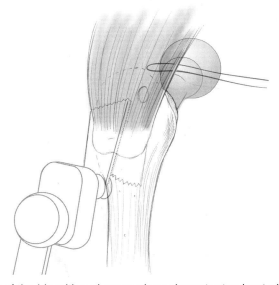

Figure 1. Exposure of the hip with a chevron-shaped greater trochanteric osteotomy. The second saw blade placed is used to mark the path of the first limb of the osteotomy. (After Berry DJ, Müller ME. Chevron osteotomy and single wire reattachment of the greater trochanter. *Clin Orthop Relat Res* 294:155–161, 1993.)

antiprotrusio cage size and to judge the approximate contour and shape of the antiprotrusio cage required to fit the patient's bone. Most pelves in which antiprotrusio cages are necessary are deformed; hence, custom contouring of the antiprotrusio cage usually is necessary.

Make a slot in the ischium for the inferior flange of the antiprotrusio cage. Under exceptional circumstances, the antiprotrusio cage can be placed on the outside of the ischium and fixed with screws. However, in most cases, placement of the inferior flange inside the ischium is preferred for three reasons: (a) It orients the cage more horizontally, (b) the risk of injury to the sciatic nerve may be reduced, and (c) flange fixation inside the ischium (like a blade plate) often is more stable than flange fixation to the outside of the ischium with screws. Place the ischial slot laterally where the root of the ischium meets the peripheral rim of the acetabulum. Avoid medial placement, which leads to flange perforation into the obturator ring. Make the slot with a narrow high-speed burr. Deepen the slot with a curved osteotome that is oriented so that the osteotome curves laterally into the remaining ischium, instead of medially into the pelvis (see Fig. 2). Orient the slot in appropriate anteversion.

Bring the real antiprotrusio cage onto the operative field, and contour the cage to fit the patient's bony pelvis. In most cases, the superior flange needs to be gently bent toward the ilium, and the inferior flange needs to be bent away from the pelvis. Contouring the proximal flange toward the pelvis provides better contact of the flange with the ileum; contouring the inferior flange away from the pelvis allows the inferior flange to slide into the ischium (and not through the ischium and into the obturator ring), as the cup portion of the cage is brought over the rim of the ilium during cage insertion (see Fig. 3).

Use surgical sponges to protect the cage when contouring it with metal-bending instruments. Avoid scratching or damaging the cage, because titanium is notch sensitive. Cages are made out of relatively thin titanium and are at risk for fracture. Avoid bending a cage different directions multiple times because this reduces its strength.

Bone Grafting

Cages frequently are employed in conjunction with cancellous bone graft, which is packed into medial cavitary and segmental bone deficiencies. Cages also are used to pro-

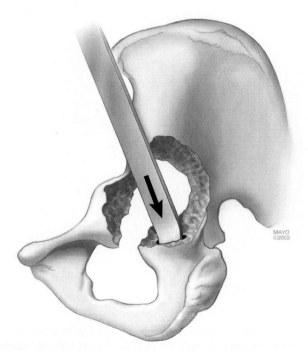

Figure 2. An osteotome is used to make a slot for the inferior flange of the cage in the ischium.

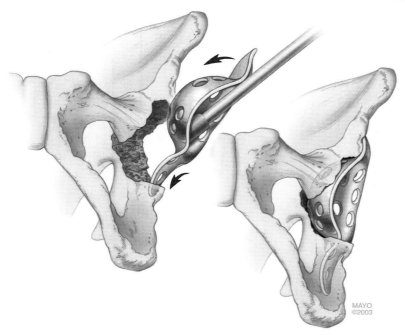

Figure 3. Insertion of a cage into the acetabulum. The cage is inserted from superior and impacted into the ischium.

tect large structural bone grafts. Structural bone grafts include posterior column allografts, large superior allografts, or whole acetabular allografts. If a structural allograft is necessary, bring the allograft onto the field, and contour it to fit the pelvic defect. Fix the allograft to the pelvis with screws. Avoid using too many screws because they take up space needed for cage fixation with screws. Pack remaining cavitary defects in the acetabulum with particulate cancellous bone graft before inserting the cage.

Cage Insertion

Insert the cage into the pelvis from superior to inferior, driving the inferior flange of the cage into the slot in the ischium. As the cup portion of the cage goes over the superior rim of the acetabulum, it will fall into the defect of the acetabulum, and the superior flange can be brought medially to rest against the ilium (Fig. 3). Make sure to insert the cage in appropriate anteversion. Once the cage is seated in the pelvis in appropriate orientation and position, fix the cage to the pelvis with multiple fully threaded 6.5-mm cancellous bone screws. Place the first screws through the dome of the cage and into the ilium; this pulls the cage against the ilium so that the cage rests firmly superiorly against sound host bone or structural allograft. Insert as many screws as possible into the ilium. Put your finger on the pelvis to judge the proper angle of screw placement into the ilium. Screws can be oriented into the posterior column as well as into the lateral ilium and often are 50 to 60 mm in length (see Fig. 4). Be careful to avoid damage to pelvic contents during drilling and screw placement. After inserting a maximum number of dome screws, place transverse screws through the superior flange of the cage into the ilium. These screws typically are short and may interlock with the previously placed dome screws (Fig. 4).

After placement of all the screws, the cage should be very mechanically stable. If it is not extremely stable, the reconstruction will fail because cage reconstruction provides only mechanical implant fixation and biologic fixation cannot be anticipated.

Pack remaining cavitary defects behind the cage with cancellous bone graft. Place trial liners or cemented acetabular components into the cage, and judge the position of the liner or cemented cup necessary to provide optimum hip stability. Use an all-polyethylene ce-

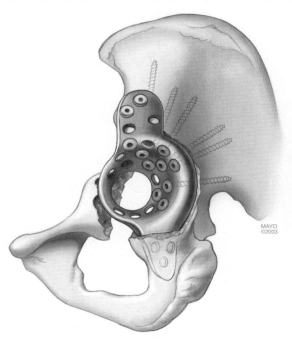

Figure 4. Multiple screws are placed through the dome holes in the cage into the ileum.

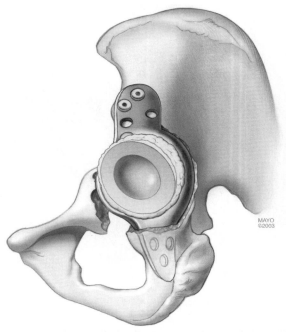

Figure 5. The polyethylene cup is cemented into the cage.

mented acetabular component or a modular acetabular component polyethylene liner that has been contoured on its back surface with a 4-mm burr in a spider-web pattern to improve cement fixation. Occasionally, a porous coated shell can be cemented into the cage, after which a modular liner can be snapped into the metal uncemented shell, which imparts the advantage of many more liner options. An x-ray may be obtained to document cage and screw position prior to cementing the liner into the cage.

Mix methylmethacrylate to a doughy state, then interdigitate the cement into the cage and into the underlying bone graft. Most surgeons prefer to use bone cement that is impregnated with an antibiotic for these large reconstructions. Cement the liner (or metal shell) into the cage in appropriate orientation. The liner can be oriented slightly differently from the cage when necessary. If the liner or metal shell is a little uncovered superiorly, create a buttress of cement (see Fig. 5) between the cage and liner superiorly. Hold the implant in place until all cement has hardened. Complete the femoral reconstruction. Reduce the hip, and confirm satisfactory hip stability. Reattach the greater trochanter to its bed. If soft tissue tension needs to be improved, the trochanter can be advanced. Close the wound over drains.

SPECIAL CIRCUMSTANCES

Use of a Cage in Pelvic Discontinuity

When pelvic discontinuity is present and a cage will be used, special methods are required. Some fixation of pelvic discontinuity is provided by the cage and flanges (3), but many surgeons prefer to gain additional plate fixation of the discontinuity when possible. A plate and a cage together in the pelvis put a great deal of hardware along the posterior wall and column and, therefore, the sequence of reconstruction is important (see Fig. 6).

Gain good exposure of the posterior column. Identify the sciatic nerve. If necessary, a limited dissection of the nerve can be carried out as it courses along the posterior column. The nerve can be scarred to the bone near the discontinuity site, and sometimes it is best identified distally in fat deep to the gluteus maximum tendon insertion. Perform the

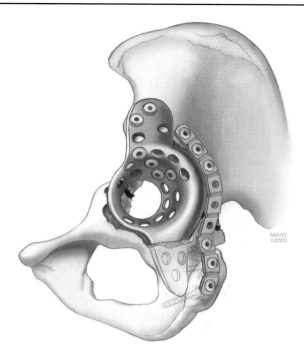

Figure 6. Pelvic discontinuity treated with an antiprotrusio cage and posterior column plate.

dissection with the knee flexed, taking utmost care to avoid damaging the nerve. Define the pelvic discontinuity line, and place autogenous graft (if available) along the nonunion. Perform any necessary structural or cancellous grafting before inserting the cage. After the cage has been inserted, place a posterior column 3.5-mm pelvic reconstruction plate from the ischium to the ilium. Implant the plate after the cage is in place because the plate and screws would inhibit placement of the inferior cage flange if the plate were placed first. Insert at least three screws distal to the discontinuity (in the ischium) and at least three screws proximal to the discontinuity (in the ilium). Compress the pelvic discontinuity line with the plate when possible.

Placement of a Cage with an Uncemented Cup

Recently, uncemented cups have been placed in combination with antiprotrusio cages. This form of reconstruction provides the potential for biologic cup fixation (by virtue of the porous coated hemispherical socket) but can protect a porous coated hemispherical cup from early migration or mechanical failure during the osteointegration process (by virtue of the added fixation provided by the cage).

Use the same exposure as outlined previously for placement of an antiprotrusio cage. Ream the acetabulum to a hemisphere, and implant an uncemented cup. We have performed this technique with a tantalum revision cup that allows elective placement of screws through the cage, through the cup, and into the host bone. Impact the tantalum revision cup into place, and secure it with screws. If a cage is necessary to provide further stability, use trial templates to judge the proper cage size that will fit inside the cup, onto the ilium, and into the ischium. Make the ischial slot, and then implant the cage over the cup. Then place screws through the dome of the cage, through the tantalum shell, and into the ilium. Use a high-speed cutting burr to make holes through the tantalum shell that match those of the cage to facilitate multiple screw placement into the bone of the pelvis. Use further screws to fix the superior cage flange to the ilium. Confirm the position of components with an intraoperative radiograph. When the liner is cemented into the cage, interdigitate the cement through the cage into the underlying tantalum shell, making the liner–cage–uncemented cup become a single unit. Use the same closure as for a conventional antiprotrusio cage.

PITFALLS AND HOW TO AVOID THEM

Injury to the superior gluteal nerve or vessels is possible when conventional exposures rather than a greater trochanteric osteotomy are used. In most cases a greater trochanteric osteotomy is the preferred exposure method to protect these structures.

Injury to the sciatic nerve can occur, particularly if the inferior cage flange is placed on the outside of the ischium. The sciatic nerve also is at high risk during plating of pelvic discontinuity. When necessary, the sciatic nerve can be partially dissected away from the posterior column to ensure that its location is known and that the nerve is protected. The nerve can be identified most easily distally beneath the gluteus maximus, where it usually is surrounded by fatty tissue; the nerve then can be traced proximally to ascertain its course.

Implant the cage in appropriate orientation to provide good hip stability. The polyethyelene cup can be aligned partially independently of the cage—but not completely. If the cage is markedly malpositioned, it can impinge against anterior or inferior soft tissues and cause pain. Be sure the cage is inserted in satisfactory anteversion. A severely deficient posterior column needs to be reconstructed with structural bone graft prior to cage insertion. Making the ischial slot in an anteverted orientation helps ensure satisfactory cage anteversion.

Mechanical cage failure is possible because of loosening or fracture. Avoid excessive bending of the cage during contouring to reduce the risk of fracture. Most importantly, provide sufficient structural mechanical support for the cage to reduce the risk of early mechanical failure or fracture. Support the cage directly against the ilium or superior structural graft, and fix it with the maximum number of screws to avoid early migration and failure as the cage is loaded.

These massive reconstructions probably have an elevated risk of infection. Use appropriate perioperative systemic antibiotic coverage, and consider using antibiotic-impregnated cement to cement the liner into the cage to reduce infection risk.

POSTOPERATIVE MANAGEMENT

Keep most patients touch weight bearing for a period of 2 months and partial weight bearing for a period of 2 more months. Full weight bearing usually is allowed 4 months after surgery. Consider using a hip guide brace during the first 2 months after surgery to protect the greater trochanteric osteotomy (if one was used) and to reduce the risk of early dislocation after this large reconstruction.

What to Tell the Patient to Expect

Anticipated recovery in these complex reconstructions is dictated by the quality of the remaining muscle, the severity of bone loss, and the number of previous surgeries.

RESULTS

Antiprotrusio cages have a higher rate of mechanical failure than porous coated uncemented hemispherical acetabular reconstructions in most series, although it is important to understand that cages commonly have been used selectively for severe bone defects (4). In some European series in which cages were used for most straightforward revisions, the failure rate has been lower. Because cages are not biologically fixed to the pelvis, some failures of this mechanical construct can be anticipated with time. Nevertheless, in many cases, cages can function very well as a stable mechanical construct for long durations.

Selected series of antiprotrusio cages are presented in Table 1.

Table 1. *Failure Rates of Antiprotrusio Cages*

Author	Year	Number of hips	Follow-up in years (Mean)	Results	Comments
Berry and Muller (9)	1992	42	2 to 11 (5)	12% mechanical failure rate	—
Böhm and Banzhaf (10)	1999	26	0.3 to 13 (4.5)	83% worst case survival at 11 years	—
Gill et al. (11)	1998	63	5 to 18 (8.5)	3/63 rerevised because of aseptic loosening 3/63 definite/probable loosening radiographically	—
Perka and Ludwig (5)	2001	63	Mean 5.5	3/63 rerevised for aseptic loosening or deformity 2/63 probable radiographic loosening	Highest failure rate in posterior column deficiencies
Peters et al. (6)	1995	28	Mean 2.8	14% with significant migration (? loose)	Marked acetabular bone reconstitution
Rosson and Schatzker (12)	1992	20	Mean 5.0	No rerevisions Two patients with one broken fixation screw	—
Schatzker and Wong (13)	1999	38	Mean 6.6	Failure rate = 5.4%	—
Udomkiat et al. (14)	2001	18	Mean 5.4	64% survivorship free of mechanical failure at 6 years	Cages selectively used for severe deficiency
van der Linde and Tonino (15)	2001	16	6 to 16 (10)	1 infection No revisions for aseptic loosening	—
Wachtl et al. (16)	2000	38	8 to 21 (12)	1 radiographically loose	—
Winter et al. (17)	2001	38	4.2 to 9.4 (7.3)	No failures	—

Several important findings have emerged from the published series. Perka and Ludwig found that antiprotrusio cages have a higher rate of failure when used in the presence of severe posterior column deficiency; this suggests that structural posterior column grafts should be used to reconstruct large defects if an antiprotrusio cage is used (5). Peters et al. have identified incorporation over time of cancellous bone graft placed medial to antiprotrusio cages, demonstrating the potential for pelvic bone restoration (6). Gross et al. have demonstrated that antiprotrusio cages can effectively protect large allograft prosthetic composite reconstructions of the acetabulum (7,8).

RECOMMENDED READING

1. Berry DJ. Antiprotrusio cages for acetabular revision. *Clin Orthop Relat Res* 420:106–112, 2004.
2. Berry DJ. Acetabular anti-protrusio rings and cages in revision total hip arthroplasty. *Semin Arthroplasty* 6:68–75, 1995.
3. Berry DJ, Lewallen DG, Hanssen AD, Cabanela ME. Pelvic discontinuity in revision total hip arthroplasty. *J Bone Joint Surg Am* 81:1692–1702, 1999.
4. Saleh KJ, Jaroszynski G, Woodgate I, et al. Revision total hip arthroplasty with the use of structural acetabular allograft and reconstruction ring: a case series with a 10-year average followup. *J Arthroplasty* 15:951–958, 2000.
5. Perka C, Ludwig R. Reconstruction of segmental defects during revision procedures of the acetabulum with the Burch-Schneider anti-protrusio cage. *J Arthroplasty* 16:568–574, 2001.
6. Peters CL, Curtain M, Samuelson KM. Acetabular revision with the Burch-Schneider antiprotrusio cage and cancellous allograft bone. *J Arthroplasty* 10:307–312, 1995.
7. Garbuz D, Morsi E, Gross AE. Revision of the acetabular component of a total hip arthroplasty with a massive structural allograft: study with a minimum 5 year followup. *J Bone Joint Surg Am* 78:693–697, 1996.
8. Gross AE, Wong P, Saleh KJ. Don't throw away the ring: indications and use. *J Arthroplasty* 17(4 Suppl 1):162–166, 2002.

9. Berry DJ, Muller ME. Revision arthroplasty using an anti-protrusio cage for massive acetabular bone deficiency. *J Bone Joint Surg Br* 74:711–715, 1992.
10. Böhm P, Banzhaf S. Acetabular revision with allograft bone: 103 revisions with 3 reconstruction alternatives, followed for 0.3–13 years. *Acta Orthop Scand* 70:240–249, 1999.
11. Gill TJ, Sledge JB, Muller ME. The Burch-Schneider anti-protrusio cage in revision total hip arthroplasty: indications, principles, and long-term results. *J Bone Joint Surg Br* 80:946–953, 1998.
12. Rosson J, Schatzker J. The use of reinforcement rings to reconstruct deficient acetabula. *J Bone Joint Surg Br* 74:716–720, 1992.
13. Schatzker J, Wong MK. Acetabular revision: the role of rings and cages. *Clin Orthop Relat Res* 369:187–197, 1999.
14. Udomkiat P, Dorr LD, Won YY, et al. Technical factors for success with metal ring acetabular reconstruction. *J Arthroplasty* 16:961–969, 2001.
15. van der Linde M, Tonino A. Acetabular revision with impacted grafting and a reinforcement ring: 42 patients followed for a mean of 10 years. *Acta Orthop Scand* 72:221–227, 2001.
16. Wachtl SW, Jung M, Jakob RP, Gautier E. The Burch-Schneider antiprotrusio cage in acetabular revision surgery: a mean followup of 12 years. *J Arthroplasty* 15:959–963, 2000.
17. Winter E, Piert M, Volkmann R, et al. Allogeneic cancellous bone graft and a Burch-Schneider ring for acetabular reconstruction in revision hip arthroplasty. *J Bone Joint Surg Am* 83:862–867, 2001.

32

Acetabular Revision: Managing Osteolysis

R. Stephen J. Burnett and John C. Clohisy

INDICATIONS/CONTRAINDICATIONS

Implant particle-induced osteolysis is the major problem that limits the survivorship of total hip arthroplasties and remains the most common indication for revision hip surgery (1). This bone resorptive disorder can result in acetabular failure from aseptic implant loosening or major bone loss around a well-fixed component. With cemented acetabular components, periprosthetic bone resorption usually occurs in a linear pattern, resulting in destruction of the cement–bone interface and eventual implant loosening (2). In contrast, cementless acetabular implants frequently remain osseointegrated with pods of bone ingrowth, yet implant failure ensues secondary to particulate debris access to periprosthetic bone and progressive periacetabular osteolysis (2). This type of aggressive acetabular osteolysis can be clinically silent in early stages, yet it may result in massive bone loss (3) and eventual catastrophic failure of the implant. Thus, there are a variety of acetabular component failure mechanisms, with varying degrees of acetabular osteolysis, that require distinct surgical solutions to optimize treatment results. *The purpose of this chapter is to present our treatment rationale and surgical techniques for the effective management of acetabular implant failure with associated pelvic osteolysis.*

Initial clinical and radiographic evaluation is critical for the appropriate selection of patients for surgical intervention and for initiation of the decision-making process regarding the type of revision surgery needed. Indications for surgery include hip symptoms that are associated with a loose acetabular component or implant failure signs that indicate pending or future failure. Specific treatment options are dependent on the fixation status of the prosthesis, associated bone loss, and implant characteristics. Rubash et al. (4) classify acetabular failures associated with cementless sockets into three distinct types (Table 1). *Type I* cases have a stable functional acetabular shell and can be considered for liner exchange or liner cementation. *Type II* cases are well-fixed components but require revision because of a damaged or nonfunctional acetabular component, and *type III* cases are unstable and require revision. These general categories provide guidelines for a preliminary treatment plan.

Table 1. *Cementless Acetabular Component Classification System*

Type	Description
I	Stable, functional
	Ingrown shell
	Worn polyethylene
	Focal lesion
	Replaceable polyethylene liner
II	Stable, damaged
	Nonfunctional shell due to excessive wear
	Broken locking mechanism
	Nonmodular component
III	Unstable
	Loose component collapsed into lesion

After Rubash HE, Sinha RK, Paprosky W, et al. A new classification system for the management of acetabular osteolysis after total hip arthroplasty. *Instr Course Lect* 48:37–42, 1999 and Maloney WJ, Paprosky W, Engh CA, Rubash H. Surgical treatment of pelvic osteolysis. *Clin Orthop Relat Res* (393):78–84, 2001.

In our practice, pending acetabular failures or progressive osteolysis, in the presence or absence of symptoms, are managed surgically to prevent progression of the osteolytic disease and catastrophic failure. Indicators of pending failure include major polyethylene wear, catastrophic liner failure, or progressive periacetabular osteolysis. These failure types are frequently present in the setting of a well-fixed cementless component, and the surgeon must decide whether to preserve the acetabular shell, to graft around the implant and exchange the articulating surfaces (femoral head and acetabular liner), or to perform a complete socket revision. In general, we recommend retention of well-fixed components if the implant is in good position, the lesion can be adequately accessed for grafting, and the liner can be exchanged or a new liner cemented into place.

Complete component revision is preferred if the acetabular component is loose, the implant is malpositioned, the shell is significantly damaged, the lesion is not accessible for grafting, or it is a massive osteolytic lesion that requires a large grafting procedure (5). Components with suboptimal fixation surfaces should also be considered for complete revision. For example, ongrowth fixation surfaces are at risk for subsequent loosening or socket breakout when associated with major osteolytic lesions. These should be revised, especially in young, active patients. If component revision is being contemplated, the acetabular bone stock is carefully assessed to determine the ease of implant removal and the anticipated remaining bone stock and type of reconstruction needed after shell removal. Loose acetabular components require complete revision with contemporary techniques of bone grafting or bone stock augmentation, depending on the extent and location of acetabular osteolysis and bone loss (6).

General contraindications for surgery include minor osteolytic lesions that can be followed clinically, severe medical comorbidities that place the patient at an unacceptably high risk for major perioperative complications, and concurrent implant infection. Periprosthetic osteolysis can be associated with deep implant infection, and in this clinical scenario, we recommend surgical resection, appropriate antibiotic therapy, and a second-stage reimplantation procedure.

PREOPERATIVE PLANNING

Detailed preoperative planning is essential to the development of an optimal surgical treatment strategy and ensures that the appropriate equipment, implants, and bone graft materials are obtained for the surgical procedure. All surgical options should be considered, and the appropriate materials for each option must be available at the time of surgery. Preoperative planning should first consider patient-specific factors that may affect the type of procedure, the results and risks of the procedure, and the perioperative management of the patient. The medical condition of the patient is assessed preoperatively, and preemptive plans to manage medical comorbidities are made. The patient's hip surgery history is obtained, because this may affect the surgical procedure and the prognosis of the reconstruction. Previous operative notes or hospital records also provide critical information regarding the type of hip implants (manufacturer and component size) and the integrity of the surrounding muscle and bone. The ingrowth surface and track record of the implant should be known. For example, ongrowth cups such those with a hydroxyapatite macrotextured surface may be easier to remove and in most instances should be removed routinely regardless of apparent implant stability because of the poor performance record of this type of implant. Titanium plasma-sprayed components may also be simpler to remove, and recognition will aid in anticipating ease of extraction. Any history consistent or suggestive of hip infection needs to be fully investigated with preoperative labs [erythrocyte sedimentation rate (ESR) and C-reactive protein (CRP)] and a hip aspiration. Physical examination findings of incision type and position, leg length discrepancy, limp, and abductor strength must also be appreciated and considered in the surgical plan. It is important that patients with poor abductor function and a history of previous direct lateral approaches are at risk for abductor incompetence, and a constrained acetabular implant and/or large femoral heads should be available for potential instability problems.

Radiographic evaluation and detailed templating of the case preoperatively are fundamental to a well-orchestrated, comprehensive procedure that addresses the complexities of each case. We obtain standing anteroposterior pelvis, cross-table lateral, frog lateral, and anteroposterior hip views for all patients undergoing revision hip surgery. If the integrity of the anterior and posterior columns is in question, iliac and obturator oblique views can be used to better assess these regions of the pelvis. The iliac oblique projection is extremely helpful in assessing the integrity of the posterior column and the extent of posterior column lytic lesions that are not well visualized with the other radiographic views (Fig. 1). The cross-table lateral radiograph provides further information regarding posterior bone stock and acetabular component version (Fig. 2). Furthermore, computed tomography scanning techniques with artifact reduction have been refined and can accurately define the size and location of periprosthetic osteolytic lesions (7,8). The integrity of the periacetabular bone and the continuity of the posterior column can be assessed in more detail than with plain radiographs. Overall, these imaging studies should determine

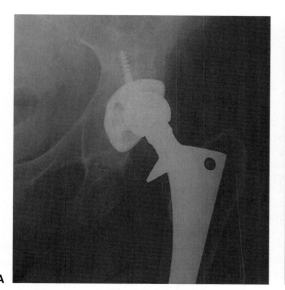
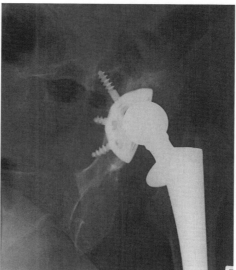

A   B

Figure 1. Anteroposterior **(A)** and iliac oblique views **(B)** of a cementless total hip replacement in a 62-year-old female with mild hip pain. The anteroposterior view demonstrates major polyethylene wear, and the iliac oblique view reveals a major osteolytic lesion of the posterior column.

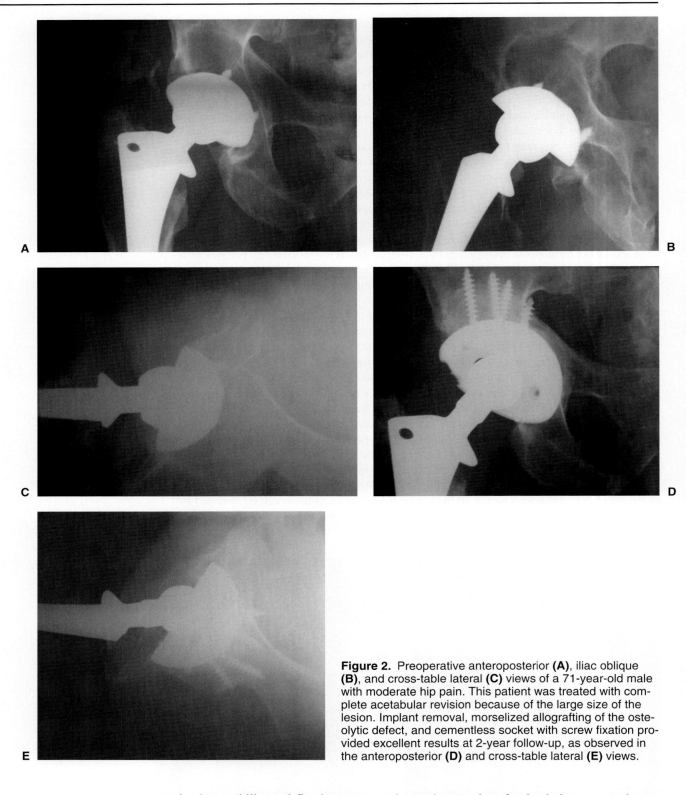

Figure 2. Preoperative anteroposterior **(A)**, iliac oblique **(B)**, and cross-table lateral **(C)** views of a 71-year-old male with moderate hip pain. This patient was treated with complete acetabular revision because of the large size of the lesion. Implant removal, morselized allografting of the osteolytic defect, and cementless socket with screw fixation provided excellent results at 2-year follow-up, as observed in the anteroposterior **(D)** and cross-table lateral **(E)** views.

implant stability and fixation status, estimate the severity of polyethylene wear, characterize periprosthetic bone loss and bone quality, and provide information regarding the type of implant being revised. Acetabular bone deficiency is classified according to the system of Paprosky et al. (6). Radiographic leg length measurements should be correlated with the physical examination findings to decide upon the need for leg length alteration during the procedure.

If preoperative radiographs indicate the acetabular component is well fixed, a preliminary decision regarding retention or revision of the acetabular shell is made (4). In *type I* cases, the liner locking mechanism is intact and functional, and the acetabular component is to be retained. The appropriate liner types and sizes for the implant must be obtained preoperatively. If the liner locking mechanism is not functional or has a poor design, consideration should be given to cementing an acetabular liner into the well-fixed shell. Appropriate liner options (large diameter, offset, constrained) should be available to provide flexibility and address potential intraoperative problems.

In *type II* cases, a well-fixed, cementless acetabular component needs to be revised, and specific plans for implant removal are made preoperatively. Most importantly, the surgeon must assess whether there is adequate bone stock for safe implant removal. The cross-table lateral and iliac oblique views are very informative with respect to bone stock of the posterior column and can be used to determine the risk of implant removal. Specific instruments for acetabular shell removal have been developed (Fig. 3) and can greatly facilitate preservation of bone and continuity of the pelvis during explantation of cementless shells. After implant removal, the revision component is usually 4 to 8 mm larger in the outer diameter. Reconstructive options and preoperative templating are the same as those outlined below for loose acetabular components.

If radiographic analysis indicates that the acetabular component is loose and the acetabulum does not have a major structural defect or pelvic discontinuity, standard acetabular revision techniques are used. In our hands, the vast majority of acetabular revisions are performed with a cementless component fixed with screws. The component size should be templated to optimize fit of the implant into the acetabular bed without removal of excessive host bone. Associated contained osteolytic defects are treated with morselized allografting or a bone graft substitute. The resultant hip center is dependent upon the location of acetabular host bone, and if the hip center is raised to optimize shell contact, an offset liner is considered. On the other hand, major structural defects that compromise rim support of the implant are treated with cementless acetabular components with bulk allografts or modular implant augments. Cage reconstructions are rarely used but may be necessary in cases with a massive contained acetabular defect that is too large for a contemporary acetabular component or in the setting of a pelvic discontinuity with massive periacetabular osteolysis (Fig. 4).

Although the focus of this chapter is revision of the acetabular component, it is understood that thorough templating and preoperative planning are also needed to outline a

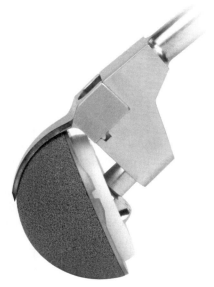

Figure 3. Zimmer Explant Cup-Out Extractor System (Zimmer, Warsaw, IN). Reproduced with permission.

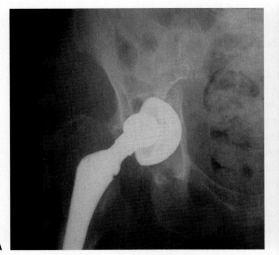
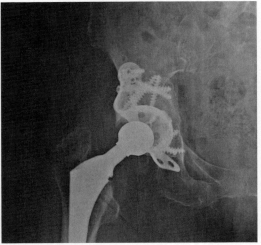

A   B

Figure 4. Preoperative **(A)** and postoperative **(B)** anteroposterior views of the hip in a low-demand 76-year-old female with severe hip pain. The patient had massive periacetabular osteolysis, associated pelvic discontinuity, and poor bone quality. Morselized allografting, reconstruction cage, and cemented socket yielded an excellent result at 3-year follow-up.

definitive plan (and alternative plans) for the femoral side. Specifically, the status of the femoral stem and the potential need for revision are determined. The surgical approach, anticipated implant removal equipment, implant needs, and bone graft options for the femoral side are selected during preoperative planning. If a femoral head exchange is being performed, the appropriate head sizes (including large-diameter heads) should be available for the procedure.

SURGICAL TECHNIQUE

Revision hip surgery can be performed through posterior, lateral, and anterolateral surgical approaches. In complex cases, the extended trochanteric osteotomy, trochanteric slide, or a standard trochanteric osteotomy will facilitate acetabular and femoral exposure. We prefer the posterolateral approach for the majority of cases because of its extensile nature and preservation of the abductor insertion. The extended trochanteric osteotomy is specifically used for cases requiring wide access to the femoral canal and femoral stem. The patient is positioned laterally, and care is taken to protect all bony prominences and peripheral nerves. Prophylactic antibiotics are given before incision unless there is concern about deep implant infection. If this is the case, prophylactic antibiotics are held back until deep cultures are taken. Clinical leg length measurement and/or a leg length caliber are used to assess relative limb length before incision. Previous surgical incisions are incorporated into the revision approach whenever possible. For the posterior approach, the incision is based on the middle greater trochanter, extended distally along the middle femoral shaft, and curved proximally and posteriorly toward the posterior iliac spine. The fascia lata is first incised distally, and the plane between the fascia lata and the underlying vastus lateralis is developed. The dissection is carried proximally in this plane, and care is taken to preserve the abductor insertion as the dissection is carried proximal over the greater trochanter. The sciatic nerve is identified by palpation and protected throughout the procedure. Access to the joint is provided by raising a full-thickness soft-tissue flap of the pseudocapsule and external rotators off the greater trochanter. This soft-tissue sleeve is extended proximally along the posterior margin of the gluteus medius and distally toward the posterior margin of the vastus lateralis. The flap is reflected posteriorly for acetabular exposure and preserved for later repair to enhance stability. The hip is dislocated, the femoral head is removed, and the proximal femur is partially skeletonized for anterior mobilization. If the femoral component is to be revised, it should be removed before acetabular exposure because this will enhance visualization of the acetabulum. If the femoral stem is retained, the femoral neck or a nonmodular femoral head will be an obstacle to exposure and may obstruct access to the acetabulum. In this situation, an anterior capsulotomy is performed, and a subperiosteal "pocket" is created by elevation of the soft tissue off of the anterior column with a Cobb elevator. The femur is retracted anteriorly, and the proximal portion of the implant is positioned in the anterior pocket. Acetabular exposure is then accomplished by excision of scar tissue and the pseudocapsule. Adequate exposure requires complete visualization of the bony acetabular rim and the interface between the modular polyethylene liner and the acetabular shell. Removal of osteophytes or heterotopic bone around the acetabular rim may be necessary to visualize this interface. Curettes, small osteotomies, rongeurs, and a high-speed burr will help the surgeon in the final exposure of the acetabular rim. The extent of the acetabular exposure is dependent on the type of acetabular reconstruction anticipated. Exposure may be confined to the true acetabulum or may involve extensive exposure of the posterior column and supra-acetabular region if a more complex reconstruction is anticipated. Once the acetabular component is exposed, the acetabular liner is removed. A company representative will often provide information regarding liner removal, polyethylene extractor tools, and trial components to assess the reduction once the existing polyethylene has been removed. If a specific extractor is available, then the component may be removed without difficulty. In some designs, tines on the locking mechanism may be retracted and the liner gently pried out of the cup with an osteotome. If removing the component with standard extraction tools is problematic, then an alternative method must be used. The key principle at this point is to remove the polyethylene liner without damaging the acetabular component. For example, polyethylene with locking rings or cold-flow interference-fit liners may be difficult to extract. A 3.2-mm drill in the apex of the polyethylene may be used to create a hole to insert a 6.5-mm cancellous screw. The screw is inserted, and upon contact with the metal shell, the liner is forced out of the locking mechanism. This technique will fail if the screw is inserted into a screw hole. The locking mechanism is often damaged with this technique, and a new ring replacement must be anticipated preoperatively. If these techniques fail, the surgeon may be required to section the polyethylene with a high-speed pencil-tip burr into quadrants and remove the pieces separately. Careful attention to locking mechanism damage must be observed during this technique, and creation of undersurface metal defects must be carefully avoided. Damage to the existing locking mechanism may be incurred during these alternative removal techniques, and new locking mechanisms must be available for insertion. Secondary damage to the cup or the need to revise the acetabular component must be anticipated, and implants must be available for this at the time of revision.

Assessment of cup stability intraoperatively can be performed by several methods but is completely dependent on adequate exposure of the implant–bone interface. Grasping the edge of the cup with a Kocher clamp and attempting to move it for the purpose of detecting motion at the bone–implant interface is an effective test for shell osseointegration. Alternatively, pressure on the rim of the component with a Cobb elevator may demonstrate movement of the cup. It must be emphasized that wide exposure and careful examination of cup stability are critical to making a sound intraoperative decision regarding whether to retain or revise the implant. Once the fixation status has been determined, the definitive treatment plan is made by considering the size and location of the osteolytic defect, the stability of the implant, and the capability for exchanging the liner (4,5,9).

For implants that are well fixed, the decision to retain or revise the acetabular shell is dependent upon several variables. In general, we retain acetabular components that are well positioned, have an intact liner locking mechanism or can accommodate a cemented liner, and have an accessible osteolytic lesion (*type I* cases). After liner removal, the edges of the acetabular implant are clearly demarcated, any osteolytic pathways that lead to retroacetabular disease are identified, and the membrane of the osteolytic channels and cavities are debrided (Fig. 5). Screws in the acetabular shell are removed, and screw holes can be utilized to access lesions behind the acetabular component. Rarely, a cortical window is needed to access the osteolytic lesion. On occasion, the superior or posterosuperior aspect of a well-fixed shell may have an osteolytic membrane that extends to the cortical margin of the supra-acetabular region. If the cup is well fixed, this area may be windowed and provide access to

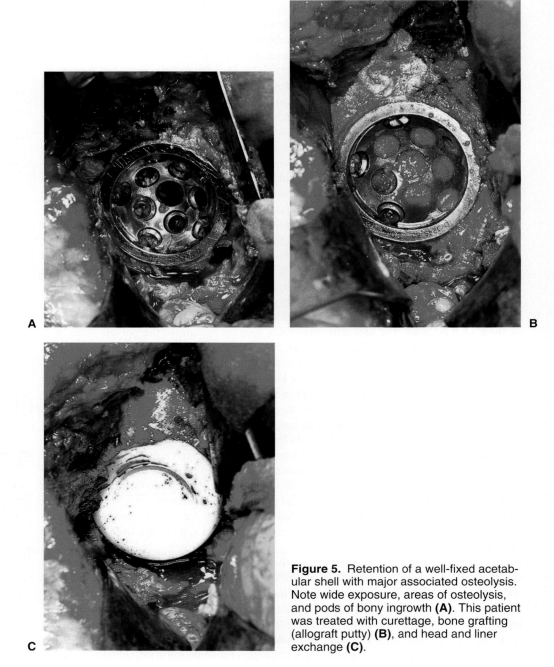

Figure 5. Retention of a well-fixed acetabular shell with major associated osteolysis. Note wide exposure, areas of osteolysis, and pods of bony ingrowth **(A)**. This patient was treated with curettage, bone grafting (allograft putty) **(B)**, and head and liner exchange **(C)**.

an area of osteolysis and allow direct visualization for curettage and bone grafting (Fig. 6). If a cortical window is required, it is imperative not to compromise the structural support of the acetabulum. The lytic granuloma and membrane are removed with appropriate curettes, a pituitary rongeur, and small suction tip. After meticulous debridement, the cavity is packed aggressively with morselized allograft or a bone graft substitute. The goal is to effectively fill the void with the bone graft material. To date, the optimal graft type(s) has not been found, and we currently use morselized allograft in the majority of cases.

New technical developments and the ability to access osteolytic lesions have improved with the availability of specialized instruments for treating contained osteolytic cavities. Ideally, such a system of instruments should allow safe debridement and curettage of a lesion, visualization of lesional filling with either bone graft (or bone substitute), and a means of pressurizing or filling contained defects.

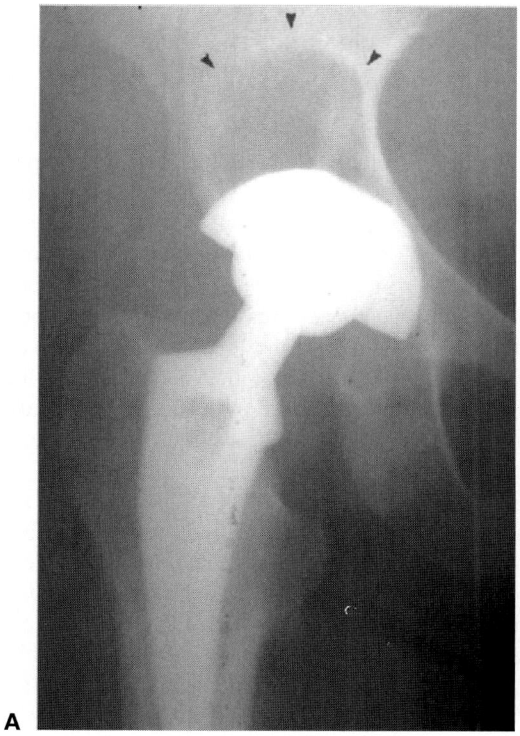

A

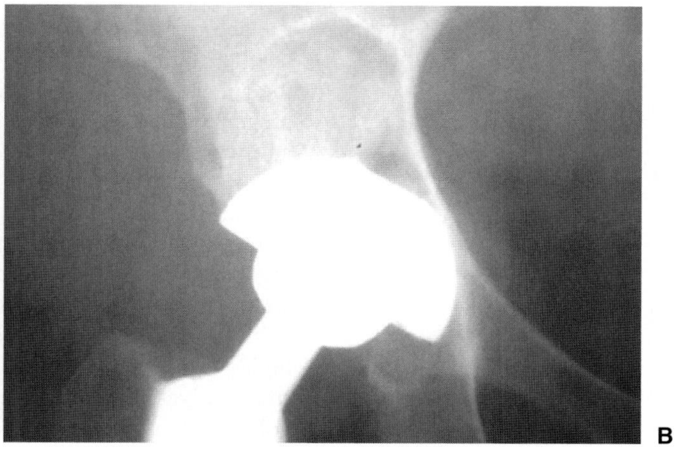

B

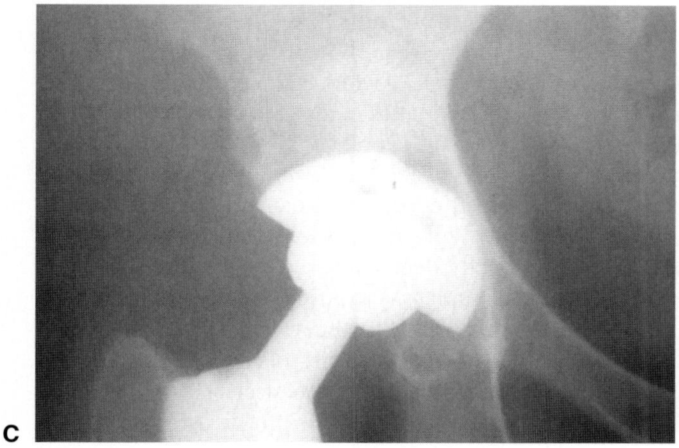

C

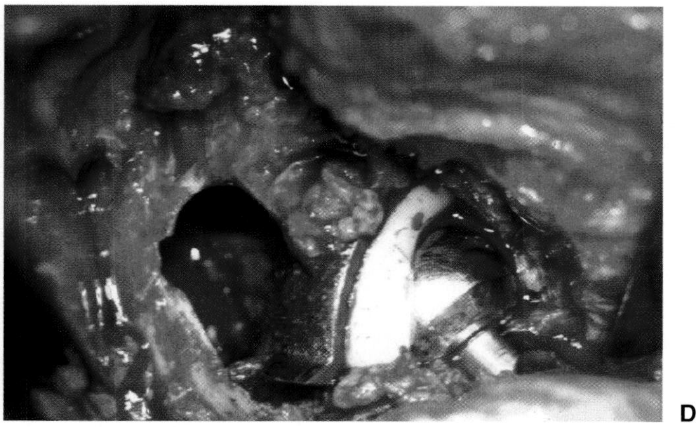

D

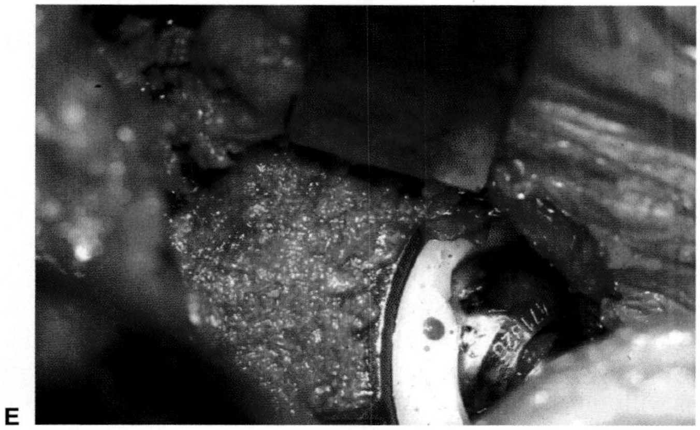

E

Figure 6. Access to an acetabular osteolytic lesion and grafting through direct cortical communication. Anteroposterior radiographs: **(A)** preoperative, **(B)** postoperative, **(C)** 1 year postoperative. **(D)** Intraoperative cortical window. **(E)** Filling of defect with bone graft.

Once the grafting is completed, liner and head trials are conducted for optimal leg length and hip stability. If the liner locking mechanism is intact, the liner is impacted into position. With some acetabular components, the liner locking ring will need to be replaced or locking tines may have to be bent to better stabilize the new liner. If the locking mechanism is ruined or is not compatible with the desired liner, then cementation of the liner is considered. With this technique, the inner surface of the acetabular shell is prepared by washing and drying. The backside of the liner is roughened with a high-speed burr to improve the cement–polyethylene bond. A liner that is at least 2 mm smaller in diameter than the inner diameter of the shell is used. Cement is placed within the acetabular component, and a layer is also spread over the backside of the polyethylene liner. The liner is placed in the acetabular shell and held in position with constant pressure until the cement has polymerized. It is critical to ensure that the liner is well seated within the acetabulum and flush with the acetabular rim. If the liner is cemented in a prominent position, there is risk for impingement and early loosening or dislodgement. A common technical mistake is to place an excessive amount of cement within the acetabular shell, which can prevent full seating of the polyethylene liner.

Once the acetabular liner is implanted, the femoral head is placed and the hip is reduced. Large-diameter femoral heads are preferred in the majority of cases because of the known high incidence of postoperative dislocation after head and liner exchange (10,11). The added stability and greater impingement-free range of motion may make the use of longer-skirted head sizes unnecessary. It should be emphasized that with the development of highly cross-linked polyethylenes, the temptation to use a larger head for stability and sacrifice polyethylene thickness is experimental. The authors still recommend a minimum polyethylene thickness of 6.5 mm because thin liners may be more susceptible to fracture and accelerated polyethylene wear. The hip is reduced, and a final leg length and stability check is performed. With the posterior approach, we carefully check for anterior impingement of the greater trochanter and femoral neck, which can be debrided to increase the impingement-free range of motion in flexion and internal rotation. The posterior soft tissue flap is closed with nonabsorbable suture through drill holes in the greater trochanter and to the posterior margins of the gluteus medius and vastus lateralis.

Well-fixed acetabular components that require revision pose a more significant surgical challenge (*type II* cases). Implants that are malpositioned, have a damaged shell, or are not amenable to liner exchange need to be extracted and revised to a new acetabular component. Actual implant removal can be technically demanding and carries the risk of iatrogenic bone loss around the acetabulum. The implant is exposed, and the implant–bone interface is debrided as described above. Sharp, curved acetabular gouges can effectively dislodge the acetabular component but do have an associated risk of removal of an excessive amount of acetabular bone, despite meticulous technique. Newer osteotome instruments that rotate around the center of the cup axis and sharp, low-profile osteotomes with incremental sizes have shown promise in achieving effective cup extraction with limited bone destruction (Fig. 3). The bone–implant interface is disrupted around the circumference of the acetabulum, and sequentially longer, curved blades remove the osseointegrated bone toward the apex of the acetabular component. The implant is not forced out of the bony bed until it is grossly loose and easily extracted. Once the component is removed, the remaining acetabular bone stock and bone deficiencies are assessed. The most common osseous defect after implant removal is in the medial wall, which is commonly deficient, especially if the extracted implant was osseointegrated medially. It should be noted that even with careful technique, major acetabular deficiencies can be created at the time of implant removal, and all reconstructive options should be available to the surgeon when a well-fixed acetabular component is being removed. In most cases, there remains adequate host bone to accommodate a cementless acetabular component fixed with screws. The acetabular bed is reamed with hemispherical reamers until peripheral "purchase" is obtained. Underlying defects are grafted with morselized allograft or an appropriate bone graft substitute. The graft is compressed by reverse reaming, and the acetabular component is impacted into position with a press-fit technique. Shell fixation is supplemented with acetabular screws (Fig. 7). If a significant structural defect is present that requires grafting, acetabular augmentation can be accomplished with a structural allograft or a prosthetic

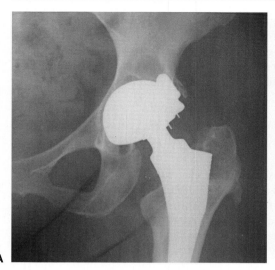
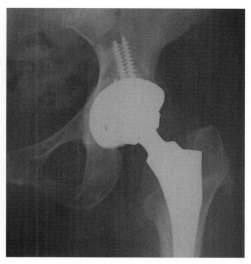

A   B

Figure 7. Anteroposterior preoperative **(A)** and postoperative **(B)** radiographs of a 38-year-old female with hip pain and acetabular lysis. The patient had a large posterior column lesion and had a complete revision because of her young age and large inaccessible osteolytic lesion. Note the minimal periacetabular bone loss after implant removal and revision.

build. The defect is prepared by reaming, and an appropriately sized structural graft or trabecular metal augment is fixed to the pelvis with screws. Cementless acetabular fixation can then be used. If a trabecular metal augment is used, the interface between augment and acetabular shell is stabilized with cementation.

When acetabular osteolysis is associated with a loose acetabular component, bone defect classification and conventional acetabular revision techniques are applied (*type III* cases) (6). The defect size may be underestimated on plain radiographs, and CT scanning may demonstrate the extent of the lesion more clearly. If the cup proceeds to migrate medially, the eventual outer acetabular diameter may decrease or become less than that of the component, making removal of this type of cup a challenging task. This will require removal of obstructing bone around the rim of the acetabulum before the removal of the cup. A cup that migrates into an osteolytic lesion will usually remain loose; however, on rare occasions, the cup may become partially ingrown in its new location, and removal can be more difficult than anticipated. Similarly, the loose, unstable acetabular component will create a defect that is significantly larger than that anticipated from preoperative radiographs, and the surgeon must recognize this and have fixation options available. As outlined above, cementless acetabular revision is the mainstay treatment for these cases. Large, porous cups with screws are preferred when available host bone coverage is at least 50%. Occasionally, prosthetic augments or a bulk allograft may be required to provide adequate structural support. Rarely, a massive structural allograft (distal femur or acetabulum) and reconstruction cage may be required (Fig. 4).

POSTOPERATIVE MANAGEMENT AND REHABILITATION

The details of postoperative management for revision hip patients are dependent upon the surgical approach and type of reconstruction performed. Patients treated with implant retention, grafting, and head/liner exchange are able to recover quickly from surgery. Nevertheless, these patients are at a relatively high risk for dislocation (10,11), and hip abduction bracing is used to protect the hip during the early healing phase. These patients are weight bearing as tolerated and are braced for 6 weeks. Active hip strengthening exercises are started when the brace is discontinued, and for the posterior approach hip precautions are continued for 3 months. Patients with structural grafts or major morselized grafting are treated with limited weight bearing, which is increased progressively to full weight bearing over the first 3 months. If a massive allograft and cage reconstruction are performed, protected weight bearing may be extended for up to 6 months. Trochanteric osteotomies are protected with touch-down weight bearing for 6 weeks and 50% weight bearing for an additional 6 weeks. Active hip abductor strengthening is started at 3 months in these cases. Overall, abduction bracing for 6 weeks is recommended in the majority of hip revision patients.

RESULTS

Clinical results of acetabular revision surgery have markedly improved over the past 2 decades, primarily because of cementless acetabular fixation. For cases with adequate host bone to support a cementless socket fixed with screws, intermediate- to long-term follow-up results have been very encouraging. Results of more recent techniques with retention of the acetabular shell and exchange of the femoral head and liner have been reported at early follow-up (10–13). For example, Maloney et al. described the early results of head and liner exchange in 35 hips followed for an average of 3.3 years. None of these hips failed, and stable fixation was maintained in all cases. Clearly, longer-term follow-up will be important to an objective assessment of the efficacy of this surgical strategy.

COMPLICATIONS

Complications associated with hip revision surgery have been well documented in the literature and include thromboembolic events, dislocation, intraoperative fracture, infection, neurovascular problems, and medical problems. In managing periacetabular osteolysis, specific complications of note include hip dislocation, cemented liner dissociation, and acetabular fracture or bone deficiency associated with implant removal. Rates of dislocation after head and liner exchange can approach 25% (10); thus, stability at surgery must be carefully assessed and addressed intraoperatively. Meticulous closure of the posterior pseudocapsule and postoperative bracing are routinely used for the posterior approach. Alternatively, some authors recommend the anterolateral approach to decrease the dislocation rate (13). Liner dissociation after cementing into a well-fixed shell can be avoided by full seating of the implant to prevent rim impingement. Acetabular fracture or a structural defect resulting from removal of a well-fixed implant can be very problematic and significantly complicate revision surgery. These problems are best avoided with the use of effective explant tools and a careful surgical technique. The above complications underscore the importance of preoperative planning, obtaining the necessary surgical equipment before the procedure, and having appropriate implant options at the time of surgery.

RECOMMENDED READING

1. Clohisy JC, Calvert G, Tull F, et al. Reasons for revision hip surgery: a retrospective review. *Clin Orthop Relat Res* Dec(429):188–192, 2004.
2. Zicat B, Engh CA, Gokcen E. Patterns of osteolysis around total hip components inserted with and without cement. *J Bone Joint Surg Am* 77(3):432–439, 1995.
3. Maloney WJ, Peters P, Engh CA, Chandler H. Severe osteolysis of the pelvic in association with acetabular replacement without cement. *J Bone Joint Surg Am* 75(11):1627–1635, 1993.
4. Rubash HE, Sinha RK, Paprosky W, et al. A new classification system for the management of acetabular osteolysis after total hip arthroplasty. *Instr Course Lect* 48:37–42, 1999.
5. Mehin R, Yuan X, Haydon C, et al. Retroacetabular osteolysis: when to operate? *Clin Orthop Relat Res* (428):247–255, 2004.
6. Paprosky WG, Perona PG, Lawrence JM. Acetabular defect classification and surgical reconstruction in revision arthroplasty. A 6-year follow-up evaluation. *J Arthroplasty* 9(1):33–44, 1994.
7. Leung S, Naudie D, Kitamura N, et al. Computed tomography in the assessment of periacetabular osteolysis. *J Bone Joint Surg Am* 87(3):592–597, 2005.
8. Puri L, Wixson RL, Stern SH, et al. Use of helical computed tomography for the assessment of acetabular osteolysis after total hip arthroplasty. *J Bone Joint Surg Am* 84-A(4):609–614, 2002.
9. Maloney WJ, Paprosky W, Engh CA, Rubash H. Surgical treatment of pelvic osteolysis. *Clin Orthop Relat Res* (393):78–84, 2001.

10. Boucher HR, Lynch C, Young AM, et al. Dislocation after polyethylene liner exchange in total hip arthroplasty. *J Arthroplasty* 18(5):654–657, 2003.
11. Griffin WL, Fehring TK, Mason JB, et al. Early morbidity of modular exchange for polyethylene wear and osteolysis. *J Arthroplasty* 19(7 Suppl 2):61–66, 2004.
12. Maloney WJ, Herzwurm P, Paprosky W, et al. Treatment of pelvic osteolysis associated with a stable acetabular component inserted without cement as part of a total hip replacement. *J Bone Joint Surg Am* 79(11):1628–1634, 1997.
13. O'Brien JJ, Burnett RS, McCalden RW, et al. Isolated liner exchange in revision total hip arthroplasty: clinical results using the direct lateral surgical approach. *J Arthroplasty* 19(4):414–423, 2004.

Special Techniques

PART VII

Special Techniques

33

PROSTALAC for Infection

Finnbar Condon, Bassam A. Masri, Donald S. Garbuz, and Clive P. Duncan

INDICATIONS AND CONTRAINDICATIONS

Two-stage exchange arthroplasty remains the standard of care in North America for the management of the chronically infected total hip arthroplasty. In cases where the patient is severely immunocompromised, has dementia, has multiple resistant organisms, or is frail, medically unfit, or elderly and cannot tolerate two major surgical procedures, alternative treatment options are considered. These include suppressive antibiotics, excision arthroplasty, or one-stage exchange arthroplasty.

Two-stage exchange arthroplasty is a technique designed to ensure, as much as possible, resolution of the infection prior to implanting a definitive revision total hip arthroplasty. To that end, the implants in the infected hip are removed, along with all other foreign material at the first stage. The patient is then treated with a 6-week course of intravenous antibiotics (the interval period), and definitive implants are subsequently implanted after the surgeon has deemed the hip to be infection-free (second stage). The interval period, which is a minimum of 6 weeks in duration, and has been reported to be as long as 1 year, can be difficult for the patient and the health care team. A short limb with poor muscular control results from the excision arthroplasty performed at the first stage. Furthermore, scarring and shortening make the second-stage procedure difficult. Beginning in 1986, we have addressed these concerns by use of the concept of an articulating spacer. Placed at the time of arthroplasty resection, this spacer holds the limb out to length, improves rehabilitation between stages, and simplifies the second stage by reducing soft tissue contractures. Our temporary articulated spacer has been referred to as the Prosthesis of Antibiotic-Loaded Acrylic Cement (PROSTALAC, DePuy, Warsaw, IN) and is currently approved by the U.S. Food and Drug Administration and by Health Canada (see Fig. 1). Apart from the functional and surgical advantages already stated, this system uses the high doses of organism-specific antibiotic powder in the cement, thus potentially improving the infection control rates. Furthermore, with the presence of a facsimile of a hip replacement during the interval period, we can delay the second stage by an additional 6 weeks for a total of 3 months to ensure resolution of the infection and its lack of recurrence after the systemic antibiotics are stopped.

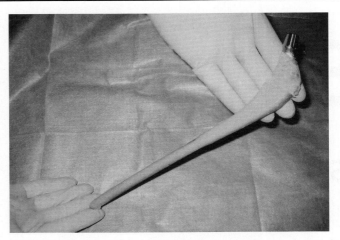

Figure 1. The PROSTALAC hip antibiotic-loaded articulated temporary spacer.

Despite the advantages of the PROSTALAC system, not every patient with a proven or suspected chronic infection at the site of a hip replacement is a suitable candidate. Frail elderly patients in whom a cemented revision total hip arthroplasty is feasible may be best served with a one-stage exchange arthroplasty. Similarly, patients with a limited life expectancy or who are institutionalized because of uncorrectable disability and who are unlikely to benefit from revision total hip arthroplasty may be best served with suppressive antibiotics or excision arthroplasty.

The purpose of this chapter is to outline the surgical technique of two-stage exchange arthroplasty using the PROSTALAC system.

PREOPERATIVE PLANNING

The algorithms used to diagnose infection following joint arthroplasty and the evidence supporting these rationales have been outlined in earlier publications from this and other centers. The preoperative plan should include the following steps:

1. Determine the infecting organism and identify the appropriate antibiotics to be used within the cement intraoperatively and systemically postoperatively. In dealing with the case where infection has been confirmed, it is desirable that the organisms responsible for the infection be identified before surgery by aspiration of the joint. The antibiotic to be used within the cement can be customized according to the sensitivity profile of the organism. In the vast majority of patients, a mixture of tobramycin and vancomycin is the preferred antibiotic combination. It has been shown by many groups that tobramycin elutes well from bone cement, allowing very high concentrations within the joint, without substantial systemic absorption. These high local levels are sufficient for most organisms that cause infection within total hip replacements. Furthermore, with *Staphylococci* being the most common organisms, vancomycin is a suitable antibiotic. While the elution of vancomycin is not as good as that of tobramycin, our group has shown that the addition of tobramycin enhances the elution of vancomycin, a process that we have termed "passive opportunism." The typical doses that we use are 2.4 to 3.6 g of tobramycin and 1 to 1.5 g of vancomycin per package of bone cement. It has also been shown that antibiotics elute better from Palacos cement (Biomet Orthopaedics, Ried B. Kerzers, Switzerland) than from Simplex cement (Stryker, Kalamazoo, MI). For this reason, we recommend the use of Palacos cement with the PROSTALAC system. In cases where neither tobramycin nor vancomycin are deemed suitable, other antibiotics may be added provided that they are available in sterile powder form, are thermostable, have been shown to elute from bone cement, and do not have a high risk of inducing

allergic reactions. Postoperatively, a suitable bactericidal antibiotic should be used for a minimum of 6 weeks. We prefer to obtain the assistance of an infectious diseases consultant for the postoperative antibiotic therapy. In the situation where we are unable to identify the organism preoperatively, we use the above-mentioned combination of vancomycin and tobramycin, as these have been shown to be effective against most of the common organisms implicated in hip arthroplasty infection.

2. Determine a safe strategy for implant and foreign body removal. In preparation for the procedure, we obtain the following radiographs:

   AP pelvis, to include the full length of the stem, all cement, and restrictors
   Lateral radiograph of the hip, also including the full stem and all cement
   AP and lateral radiographs of rest of femur (selective)
   Judet views of pelvis (selective)

These radiographs allow us to map the location of all foreign material, plan on its removal, and assess the presence and severity of any bone stock deficiency. The full range of exposures used in aseptic revision hip surgery is applicable also in revision procedures for the management of infection, and these have been outlined in earlier chapters. We prefer an extensile approach, not infrequently employing an extended trochanteric osteotomy (ETO), which allows safe removal of all implants and cement without further compromise of the bone stock. It has to be stressed, however, that these extensile exposures should respect the blood supply to the femur and the proximal femur should not be devascularized, as development of an infected sequestrum may contribute to the risk of infection recurrence. The chosen exposure is designed to allow removal of all cement and foreign material at the time of the first stage. In our experience, the implants are more often than not well fixed and are not loose. The techniques for removing well-fixed implants have been described elsewhere and are beyond the scope of this chapter. If a substantial amount of intrapelvic cement is present within the pelvis, consideration has to be given to the use of a retroperitoneal approach if the safe removal of the cement cannot be achieved from within the hip joint. In such cases, a preoperative arteriogram and consultation with a vascular surgeon may be prudent.

3. Plan for the insertion of the definitive PROSTALAC components. We template the femur and acetabulum preoperatively to assess the degree of bone loss and choose the most likely PROSTALAC implants that will best fit the diaphysis and fill the metaphysis of the femur. On the acetabular side, we aim to insert the PROSTALAC component at the normal level of the hip joint center of rotation. If there is a substantial degree of bone loss, particularly superiorly with proximal migration of the existing acetabular component, we plan to fill the bone defect with antibiotic-loaded bone cement. In general, we do not require more than one package of antibiotic-loaded cement for fixation of the PROSTALAC acetabular component. However, in cases of substantial bone loss (Paprosky type III defects), an additional package of antibiotic-loaded cement may be required to fill the defect and allow restoration of the anatomic or near-anatomic center of rotation of the hip joint.

On the femoral side, the length of an osteotomy, if required to remove an implant or cement, is determined preoperatively by the amount of foreign material to be removed. However, this does not preclude the surgeon from taking into consideration the length of the implant to be used at the second stage and planning the osteotomy in such a way that the osteotomy ends at least 4 to 5 cm above the end of the porous coating of an extensively porous coated stem of an appropriate length. If a longer osteotomy is mandatory for the safe removal of cement or implant, then the surgeon should use the longer osteotomy. The length of the PROSTALAC stem is determined by the need for an osteotomy and its length. If no osteotomy is required and there is no substantial bone loss in the proximal femur, a standard length PROSTALAC stem may be used. Longer stems may be used for hips with bony defects or in those requiring an ETO. Any areas of weak bone or osteotomies should be bypassed by at least two to three cortical diameters. The final step in the plan is to ensure that a PROSTALAC stem will actually fit. Most hips will accommodate a PROSTALAC stem. The minimum canal diameter for a long PROSTALAC stem is 13 mm. Patients with a femoral canal that cannot be reamed up to 13 mm are not suitable for the PROSTALAC system, and an alternate technique should be used.

PROSTALAC SYSTEM OVERVIEW

The PROSTALAC system consists of a core femoral implant, available in four stem lengths, and is coated with antibiotic-loaded acrylic cement using a size-specific mold to make the final composite, custom-made antibiotic-loaded implant. These four lengths are 120, 150, 200, and 240 mm.

The 120-mm stem relies on proximal fit and fill for fixation. For this reason, it is available in five composite sizes, each with its own broach (see Fig. 2), designated as sizes 1 through 5 to ensure maximum versatility. These stems have neutral version and are available in two offsets, standard and high (see Fig. 3). The required offset is determined by preoperative planning and intraoperative trialing. The offset is determined by the core implant used. Only one core implant is required for all five sizes, and the various sizes are obtained by using a size-specific mold (see Fig. 4).

The longer stems are made by using a bowed core stem, which is available in right and left configurations, and a single mold is used to manufacture the appropriate length stem by using a "bullet" inside the mold to convert a longer stem into a shorter stem (see Fig. 5). Each longer stem uses a separate core to allow making a 150-, 200-, or 240-mm stem. Since these longer stems rely on three-point fixation within the diaphysis, only one size is available. In cases where the stem is not stable, a bolus of antibiotic-loaded cement is used to manufacture a collar that would support the stem at its junction with the host bone. This is particularly applicable in cases of significant bony deficiency (see Fig. 6). In most cases, unless extra buildup is required, a single 40-g mix of antibiotic-loaded cement is sufficient for even the longest PROSTALAC stem. The standard DePuy cemented stem centralizers (Cementralizer, DePuy, Warsaw, IN) may be attached to the tip of the PROSTALAC stem to centralize it within the mold. Size one through five 120-mm stems use 11- through 15-

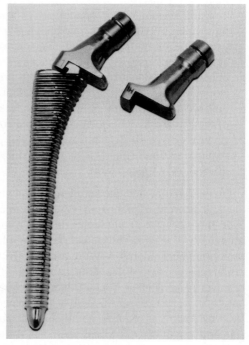

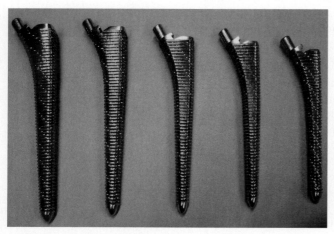

Figure 2. The five broaches available for the five sizes of the 120-mm stem.

Figure 3. The two offset options on the 120-mm stem, standard and extended.

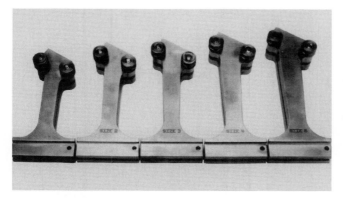

Figure 4. The five molds available for the 120-mm composite.

mm centralizers, and the longer stems use a 13-mm centralizer. These centralizers ensure an even cement mantle around the PROSTALAC component, avoid a stress riser at the tip of the PROSTALAC metal stem, and prevent the occurrence of a fracture of the cement tip at the time of either stem insertion or stem extraction. This step is optional.

The femoral head used with the PROSTALAC system is a standard 32-mm Articuleze head with a 12/14 taper (DePuy, Warsaw, IN) and is available in multiple neck lengths ranging from +1 to +17 mm in length. Since the cup is a snap-fit constrained design, exact replication of leg lengths and soft tissue balancing is not essential, and it is seldom necessary to use the long femoral necks. It is important that the dedicated PROSTALAC trial heads be used instead of the standard Articuleze trial heads. The dedicated PROSTALAC trial heads are 30 mm in diameter instead of 32 mm. This allows dislocation from the constrained socket after a trial reduction.

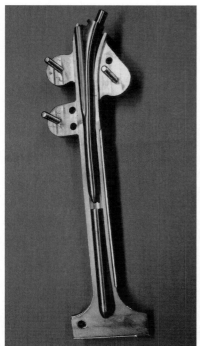
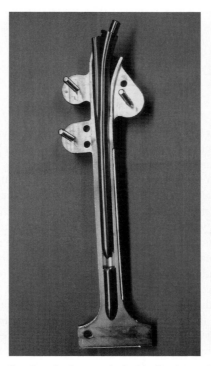
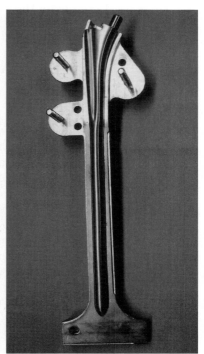

A,B   **C**

Figure 5. A: The 150-mm trial composite stem is demonstrated in the long-stem mold with the appropriate "bullet" filling the distal void. **B:** The 200-mm trial composite stem is demonstrated in the long-stem mold with the appropriate "bullet" filling the distal void. **C:** The 240-mm trial composite stem is demonstrated in the long-stem mold; in this case, no "bullet" is required.

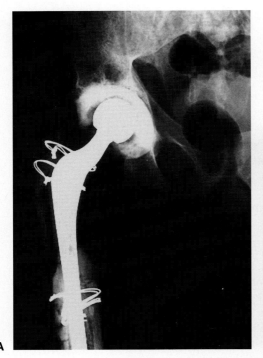
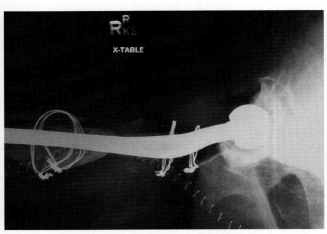

Figure 6. A: Anteroposterior radiograph in a man with a deficient proximal femur; the PROSTALAC composite is supported by a "collar" of cement. **B:** Lateral radiograph of the same patient.

The acetabular component comprises a one-piece ultrahigh-molecular-weight polyethylene (UHMWPE) snap-fit acetabular component (inner diameter 32 mm, outer diameter 44 mm). This component is designed to capture the femoral head and to prevent postoperative dislocation.

SURGICAL TECHNIQUE

Approach

The patient is positioned in the lateral decubitus position with anterior and posterior supports. An extensile approach should be utilized, as already discussed in the section on preoperative planning. Technical details of the various approaches have been outlined in another chapter and elsewhere in the literature and will not be repeated; however, the important nuances, as they apply to the management of infection, will be emphasized.

Upon entering the hip joint, multiple cultures are obtained and are sent for definitive histopathology to confirm the presence of infection and also for culture and sensitivity. The surgeon should target the most inflamed tissue. We obtain at least three specimens but occasionally obtain more if further inflammation or purulence is encountered elsewhere in the procedure. Administration of antibiotics should be withheld until after the specimens are obtained for culture.

We favor the posterolateral approach as our initial exposure because it can be extended into virtually any extensile exposure. While the anterolateral approach has been extended into an ETO by some authors, this will by necessity either strip the lateral femoral fragment of its blood supply or cut into the substance of the vastus lateralis, potentially reducing the blood supply to the lateral femoral fragment. Because of the presence of infection, we prefer to maintain as much blood supply to that fragment as possible; hence our choice of the posterolateral approach. In performing the ETO, we only reflect the vastus lateralis off the femur for about 1 cm anterior to the lateral intermuscular septum. An osteotomy from posterior to anterior is then created incorporating about one third of the cortical width of the femur. Great care is taken not to damage the junction between the greater trochanter and the lateral femoral cortex. Furthermore, we round off the distal end of the osteotomy to minimize the stress riser effect.

In general, it may be preferable to work on the acetabulum before performing the extended trochanteric osteotomy, unless the osteotomy is required for acetabular exposure.

Implant Removal

The implants are removed with specialized instruments according to general principles of avoiding further bone loss or fracture. Many techniques beyond the scope of this chapter have been described to remove well-fixed implants, and these principles are the same whether the revision is for septic or aseptic reasons. When managing infection, however, it is imperative to remove all foreign material.

Acetabular Debridement and Preparation

Once the acetabular component and cement are removed, we use a combination of curettes, rongeurs, and Cobb elevators to remove all the osteolytic membrane, soft tissue debris, and foreign material from the socket. Gentle reaming is then performed to further debride the socket. The point of reaming is not to remove bone and create a hemispherical surface for implant fixation. Instead, the reamers are used as mechanical debriders and can be thought of as motorized curettes. At this point, we evaluate the host bone for its quality and quantity, information that helps us in planning the second stage. It is important for the surgeon to note the extent of bone loss and to determine the strategy required for implant fixation at the second stage. This should be recorded in the operative note to facilitate the planning of the second stage. If the surgeon encounters pelvic dissociation, the posterior column should be plated using 3.5-mm pelvic reconstruction plates.

Femoral Debridement and Broaching

The femoral canal is debrided using rongeurs, curettes, burrs, and/or reverse hooks until we are satisfied that the canal is completely clear of all debris circumferentially. The canal is then gently reamed using flexible reamers over a guide wire to further debride the medullary canal. When using the 120-mm stem, the surgeon then sequentially broaches up to the broach size that gives reasonable stability and reconstitution of leg lengths. If preoperative planning suggests that a longer stem is necessary, the canal is reamed up to 13 mm in diameter using flexible reamers, and trial stems are then inserted. On occasion, there will be a mismatch between the bow of the stem and the bow of the femur, making it difficult to insert the PROSTALAC stem. In such cases, the canal is reamed in 0.5-mm increments with further attempts at inserting the PROSTALAC stem. Prior to doing that, however, it is important to ensure complete removal of cement from within the medullary canal, as this is a common reason for difficulties with PROSTALAC stem insertion. An intraoperative radiograph may be extremely helpful, particularly when an ETO is not performed.

Once the femoral preparation is completed, all trial implants are removed, and the entire field is further debrided to remove any potentially contaminated, dead, or devitalized tissue and is then irrigated with up to 9 L of sterile normal saline. While one team is performing this final debridement and irrigation, a most critical part of the procedure, a second team prepares the PROSTALAC stem using the specialized molds. The operation can continue while the cement is setting on the back table.

Femoral Implant Molding Process

The appropriate femoral mold is chosen on the basis of the required stem size and length. For a 120-mm stem, the final broach that was used will define the final size of the composite required to fill the canal. The components of the mold are similar, whichever size is being used, except that with the longer stem options, the larger mold is used and the

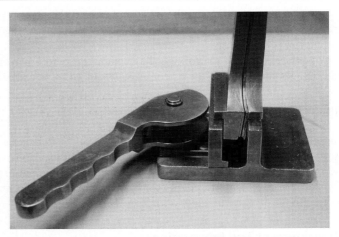

Figure 7. Base and jaw of long stem open, demonstrating how compression is achieved.

tip is filled with a metal "bullet" of differing size depending on whether a 150- or 200-mm stem is needed. No "bullet" is needed with the 240-mm stem.

The mold consists of a base with a removable jaw and a compression handle that attaches to the base and closes the jaws on the mold (see Fig. 7). The stem itself fits into a two- or three-part mold, depending on whether it is a short stem or longer stem. All metal portions of the mold that will be in contact with any cement should be liberally coated with sterile mineral oil to facilitate release of the finished product.

The 120-mm molds are completely assembled, cement is mixed, and while it is at a doughy stage, it is inserted into the mold and gently pressurized to ensure complete filling of all voids (see Fig. 8A). The appropriate offset stem is then used, and the appropriate centralizer is attached. The stem is then inserted centrally within the upright mold into the correct amount of anteversion as determined by the fit of the broach within the femur (Fig. 8B). Once the cement is completely set, the two pieces of the mold are pried open using a periosteal elevator,

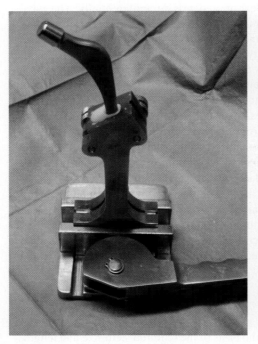

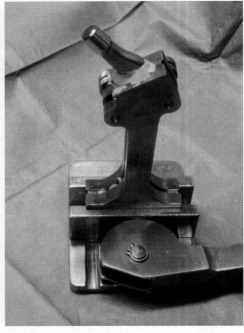

A   **B**

Figure 8. A: A 120-mm core implant being advanced into antibiotic-loaded cement within closed mold. **B:** Final seated position of core implant in mold, while cement is polymerizing. *(continues)*

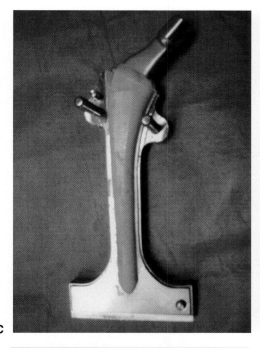

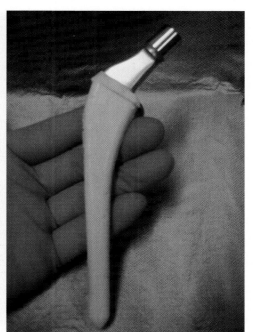

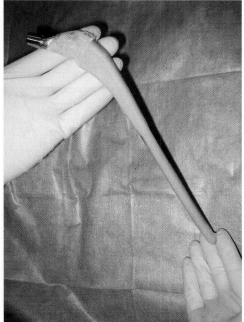

Figure 8. *(continued)* **C:** Opened mold, revealing satisfactory cement mantle on composite stem. **D:** Final 120-mm PROSTALAC composite stem after removal from mold and trimming. **E:** Final 240-mm PROSTALAC composite stem after removal from mold.

and the stem is removed (Figs. 8C, D). If the stem is difficult to remove, a gentle tap on the neck of the prosthesis with a 1-lb mallet will remove the stem from the mold.

The longer stems are manufactured in a similar manner (Fig. 8E). An alternate method is to insert the cement and the stem into the lubricated open mold. The mold is then closed on top of the stem and cement.

Acetabular Component Insertion

The antibiotic-loaded cement is placed in the acetabulum at a relatively advanced stage of polymerization, usually about 5 to 6 min, depending on exact consistency, so as to avoid deep intrusion into bone. The cement is not fully pressurized but achieves stability by

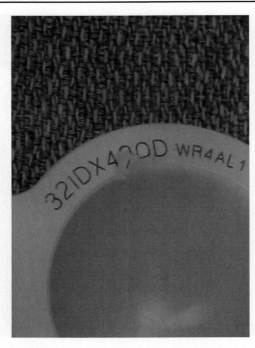

Figure 9. Close-up of snap-fit constrained acetabular cup, with "nibble" removed.

interference fit and interdigitation with surface irregularities of the acetabular walls. Deep intrusion makes removal problematic at the second stage, with the potential for further bone stock loss. Any substantial bone defects are filled with cement. Because of the constrained nature of the socket, a small amount of polyethylene is removed from the inferior rim of the cup to allow air and fluid to escape at the time of definitive reduction and to allow appropriate capture of the femoral head (see Fig. 9).

The cup is pressed into the bed of cement in the desired position of 40 degrees of lateral opening and 20 degrees of anteversion. The position is maintained with the acetabular inserter in a standard fashion until full polymerization has occurred. The inserter must have a diameter of less than 32 mm.

Femoral Head Insertion and Reduction

Once the acetabular component is inserted, a final trial reduction is performed. Once satisfactory reconstruction is achieved, the definitive PROSTALAC stem is inserted, and a final trial reduction with the PROSTALAC 30-mm head is made. The final Articuleze 32-mm head is then inserted in place of the trial, and the hip is reduced. The reduction maneuver is a bit different from a standard hip reduction. Once the head is on the mouth of the socket, the hip is abducted further to allow the rim of the femoral head to pass the rim of the socket. At this stage, axial pressure on the greater trochanter allows final seating of the femoral head. The surgeon will then both feel and hear a satisfying clunk, ensuring a stable and complete reduction. We aim to keep the leg about 5 to 10 mm short at this stage to allow final fine-tuning of leg lengths at the second stage. The snap-fit constrained articulated design assists us in achieving this.

Wound Closure

The ETO, when used, is closed in the usual manner, and wound closure is achieved in routine fashion, ensuring a watertight closure of the deep tissue. Wound drainage fluids should not be reinfused during or after the insertion of the PROSTALAC system, as they contain high levels of antibiotics, which the patient may also be receiving intravenously, and toxicity can result. A cell saver should not be used for the same reasons, as well as because of the presence of infection. We generally do not use suction drains so as to avoid removal of the antibiotic-rich fluid. In exceptional circumstances, if the use of a drain is deemed unavoidable by the surgeon, we connect the drain to a bile bag without suction, which serves as an overflow reservoir. We also instruct the recovery room and ward staff not to empty the bag. This ensures that the high levels of antibiotics are not sucked out, discarded, and replaced with lower levels. This occurs because of the rapid logarithmic decline of antibiotic elution from bone cement as a function of time. The bile bag and drain are then discarded on the first postoperative day. The use of a drain with this system should be the exception rather than the rule.

POSTOPERATIVE MANAGEMENT

In the standard case, mobilization is commenced on the first postoperative day and toe touch weight bearing only is allowed over the succeeding days. If a good press fit is achieved, up to 50% weight bearing may be allowed. It is essential, however, that the patient understand the temporary nature of the PROSTALAC system and the need for protected weight bearing while awaiting the second stage.

A peripherally inserted central line (PICC line) is placed before the surgery or soon after, and the patient is seen by the infectious diseases team and by a home intravenous therapy coordinator. Appropriate arrangements are made for 6 weeks of home intravenous therapy, and the patient is discharged between 4 and 7 days after surgery, as the wound swelling is settling. At the completion of the 6-week course of antibiotic therapy, erythrocyte sedimentation rate (ESR) and C-reactive protein (CRP) are obtained, and the patient is seen in follow-up. Four weeks later, the ESR and CRP are repeated, and if the ESR and CRP are trending downward or have returned to normal, the hip is deemed infection-free, and reimplantation is planned for 2 weeks subsequently. We used to perform routine aspirations prior to reimplantation; however, the yield from these aspirations is so low that we now prefer to only perform aspirations in suspicious cases.

REHABILITATION

The emphasis between stages is on safe patient mobility, general physical well-being, and good analgesic coverage and homeostatic and nutritional balance. Formal rehabilitation is usually left until after the second procedure. If these measures are adopted, the patients present back for the second stage, prepared and fit for another major surgery.

RESULTS

In 1997, we reported on 48 patients with an average follow-up of 43 months and a minimum follow-up of 2 years. Infection recurred in 3 patients (6.25%). In that series, two of the three recurrent infections had a different organism from the original infecting organism. Thirty-seven patients (77%) had a Harris hip score over 80 at the time of final review, an average improvement of 30 points on their preoperative score.

COMPLICATIONS

The general complications possible following primary and revision hip surgery have been extensively dealt with elsewhere and are, in general, no different when revision is for aseptic reasons.

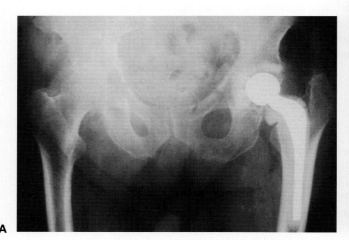
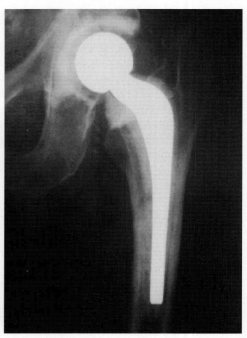

A   B

Figure 10. A: Anteroposterior radiograph of both hips demonstrating a 120-mm PROSTA-LAC 3 months postoperatively in 2000. **B:** The same patient, 3 years later, having decided against a second, definitive reconstruction, because of significant comorbidities. Apart from a little subsidence, little untoward has happened otherwise.

Specific complications associated with the PROSTALAC system include the following.

1. Implant subsidence: This may not be a very significant issue unless it leads to an unstable hip. Revision to a larger-diameter component may be an option.
2. Dislocation: This can be in two forms. The head can dislocate from the snap-fit socket, or the acetabular component with its cement attached can dislocate from the acetabulum.

Open reduction is generally required, though depending on the timing, the second stage can be performed if the ESR and CRP have returned to normal and aspiration is negative for infection. If a recurrent problem, it may not be possible to proceed with the PROSTALAC system, and an alternative management pathway is chosen. This may involve reverting to antibiotic-loaded beads as the interim measure. This option is rarely needed in our hands.

3. Failure to eradicate the infection: This can necessitate a longer period between stages, different antibiotic therapy, or both. A second attempt at management with another PROSTALAC articulated spacer, with the added antibiotics tailored to updated organism sensitivities, is possible; very occasionally, an older, frail patient, unfit for prolonged repeat surgery, may opt to retain the PROSTALAC composite system long-term and reduce weight bearing permanently (see Fig. 10).

RECOMMENDED READING

1. Duncan CP, Beauchamp C. A temporary antibiotic-loaded joint replacement system for management of complex infections involving the hip. *Orthop Clin North Am* 24(4):751–759, 1993.
2. Duncan CP, Masri, BA. The role of antibiotic-loaded cement in the treatment of an infection after a hip replacement. *J Bone Joint Surg Am* 76(11):1742–1751, 1994.
3. Fitzgerald RH Jr. Revising the infected total hip: surgical techniques. In: Steinberg ME, Garino JP, eds. *Revision Total Hip Arthroplasty.* 1st ed. Philadelphia, Pa: Lippincott Williams & Wilkins, 1999: 419–434.
4. Haddad FS, Masri BA, Garbuz DS, Duncan CP. The treatment of the infected hip replacement. *Clin Orthop Relat Res* 369:144–156, 1999.

5. Masri BA, Duncan CP, Beauchamp CP. Long term elution of antibiotics from bone cement. *J Arthroplasty* 13(3):331–338, 1998.
6. McAlinden MG, Masri BA, Duncan CP. Management of the infected total hip arthroplasty: a North American perspective. In: Bourne R, ed. *Controversies in Hip Surgery.* 1st ed. New York: Oxford University Press, 2003: 289–310.
7. Spangehl MJ, Younger ASE, Masri BA, Duncan CP. Diagnosis of infection following total hip arthroplasty. *J Bone Joint Surg Am* 79(10):1578–1588, 1997.
8. Spangehl MJ, Masri BA, O'Connell JX, Duncan CP. Prospective analysis of pre-operative and intraoperative investigations for the diagnosis of infection at the sites of two hundred and two revision total hip arthroplasties. *J Bone Joint Surg Am* 81(5):672–683, 1999.
9. Spangehl MJ, Hanssen AD, Osmon DR. Diagnosis and treatment of the infected hip arthroplasty. In: Morrey B, ed. *Joint Replacement Arthroplasty.* 3rd ed. New York: Churchill Livingstone, 2003: 856–874.
10. Younger ASE, Duncan CP, Masri BA, McGraw RW. The outcome of two-stage arthroplasty using a custom-made interval spacer to treat the infected hip. *J Arthroplasty* 12(6):615–623, 1997.
11. Younger ASE, Duncan CP, Masri BA. Treatment of infection associated with segmental bone loss in the proximal part of the femur in two stages with use of an antibiotic-loaded interval prosthesis. *J Bone Joint Surg Am* 80(1):60–69, 1998.

JOINT EDUCATION LIBRARY

1 FEB 2006

NORTH MANCHESTER
GENERAL HOSPITAL

Index

Page numbers in *italics* indicate figures. Page numbers followed by "t" indicate tables.